At-Risk Children & Youth: Resiliency Explored

At-Risk Children & Youth: Resiliency Explored has been co-published simultaneously as *Child & Youth Services,* Volume 29, Numbers 1/2 2007.

Monographs from *Child & Youth Services*®

For additional information on these and other Haworth Press titles, including descriptions, tables of contents, reviews, and prices, use the QuickSearch catalog at http://www.HaworthPress.com.

1. ***Institutional Abuse of Children and Youth,*** edited by Ranae Hanson (Vol. 4, No. 1/2, 1982). *"Well researched . . . should be required reading for every school administrator, school board member, teacher, and parent." (American Psychological Association Division 37 Newsletter)*

2. ***Youth Participation and Experiential Education,*** edited by Daniel Conrad and Diane Hedin (Vol. 4, No. 3/4, 1982). *A useful introduction and overview of the current and possible future impact of experiential education on adolescents.*

3. ***Legal Reforms Affecting Child and Youth Services,*** edited by Gary B. Melton, PhD (Vol. 5, No. 1/2, 1983). *"A consistently impressive book. The authors bring a wealth of empirical data and creative legal analyses to bear on one of the most important topics in psychology and law." (John Monahan, School of Law, University of Virginia)*

4. ***Social Skills Training for Children and Youth,*** edited by Craig LeCroy, MSW (Vol. 5, No. 3/4, 1983). *"Easy to read and pertinent to occupational therapists." (New Zealand Journal of Occupational Therapy)*

5. ***Adolescent Substance Abuse: A Guide to Prevention and Treatment,*** edited by Richard E. Isralowitz and Mark Singer (Vol. 6, No. 1/2, 1983). *"A valuable tool for those working with adolescent substance misusers." (Journal of Studies on Alcohol)*

6. ***Young Girls: A Portrait of Adolescence Reprint Edition,*** Gisela Konopka, DSW (Vol. 6, No. 3/4, 1985). *"A sensitive affirmation of today's young women and a clear recognition of the complex adjustments they face in contemporary society." (School Counselor)*

7. ***Adolescents, Literature, and Work with Youth,*** edited by J. Pamela Weiner, MPH, and Ruth M. Stein, PhD (Vol. 7, No. 1/2, 1985). *"A variety of thought-provoking ways of looking at adolescent literature." (Harvard Educational Review)*

8. ***Residential Group Care in Community Context: Insights from the Israeli Experience,*** edited by Zvi Eisikovits, PhD, and Jerome Beker, EdD (Vol. 7, No. 3/4, 1986). *A variety of highly effective group care settings in Israel are examined, with suggestions for improving care in the United States.*

9. ***Helping Delinquents Change: A Treatment Manual of Social Learning Approaches,*** Jerome S. Stumphauzer, PhD (Vol. 8, No. 1/2, 1986). *"The best I have seen in the juvenile and criminal justice field in the past 46 years. It is pragmatic and creative in its recommended treatment approaches, on target concerning the many aspects of juvenile handling that have failed, and quite honest in assessing and advocating which practices seem to be working reasonably well." (Corrections Today)*

10. ***Qualitative Research and Evaluation in Group Care,*** edited by Rivka A. Eisikovits, PhD, and Yitzhak Kashti, PhD (Vol. 8, No. 3/4, 1987). *"Well worth reading. . . . should be read by any nurse involved in formally evaluating her care setting." (Nursing Times)*

11. ***The Black Adolescent Parent,*** edited by Stanley F. Battle, PhD, MPH (Vol. 9, No. 1, 1987). *"A sound and insightful perspective on black adolescent sexuality and parenting." (Child Welfare)*

12. ***Developmental Group Care of Children and Youth: Concepts and Practice,*** Henry W. Maier, PhD (Vol. 9, No. 2, 1988). *"An excellent guide for those who plan to devote their professional careers to the group care of children and adolescents." (Journal of Developmental and Behavioral Pediatrics)*

13. ***Assaultive Youth: Responding to Physical Assaultiveness in Residential, Community, and Health Care Settings***, edited by Joel Kupfersmid, PhD, and Roberta Monkman, PhD (Vol. 10,

No. 1, 1988). *"At last here is a book written by professionals who do direct care with assaultive youth and can give practical advice."* (Vicki L. Agee, PhD, Director of Correctional Services, New Life Youth Services, Lantana, Florida)

14. ***Transitioning Exceptional Children and Youth into the Community: Research and Practice,*** edited by Ennio Cipani, PhD (Vol. 10, No. 2, 1989). *"Excellent set of chapters. A very fine contribution to the literature. Excellent text."* (T. F. McLaughlin, PhD, Department of Special Education, Gonzaga University)

15. ***Family Perspectives in Child and Youth Services,*** edited by David H. Olson, PhD (Vol. 11, No. 1, 1989). *"An excellent diagnostic tool to use with families and an excellent training tool for our family therapy students. . . . It also offers an excellent model for parent training."* (Peter Maynard, PhD, Department of Human Development, University of Rhode Island)

16. ***Helping the Youthful Offender: Individual and Group Therapies That Work,*** edited by William B. Lewis, PhD (Vol. 11, No. 2, 1989). *"In a reader-friendly and often humorous style, Lewis explains the multilevel approach that he deems necessary for effective treatment of delinquents within an institutional context."* (Criminal Justice Review)

17. ***Specialist Foster Family Care: A Normalizing Experience,*** edited by Burt Galaway, PhD, MS, and Joe Hudson, PhD, MSW (Vol. 12, No. 1/2, 1989). *"A useful and practical book for policymakers and professionals interested in learning about the benefits of treatment foster care."* (Ira M. Schwartz, MSW, Professor and Director, Center for the Study of Youth Policy, The University of Michigan School of Social Work)

18. ***Perspectives in Professional Child and Youth Care,*** edited by James P. Anglin, MSW, Carey J. Denholm, PhD, Roy V. Ferguson, PhD, and Alan R. Pence, PhD (Vol. 13, No. 1/2, 1990). *"Reinforced by empirical research and clear conceptual thinking, as well as the recognition of the relevance of personal transformation in understanding quality care."* (Virginia Child Protection Newsletter)

19. ***Homeless Children: The Watchers and the Waiters,*** edited by Nancy Boxill, PhD (Vol. 14, No. 1, 1990). *"Fill[s] a gap in the popular and professional literature on homelessness. . . . Policymakers, program developers, and social welfare practitioners will find it particularly useful."* (Science Books & Films)

20. ***Being in Child Care: A Journey into Self,*** edited by Gerry Fewster, PhD (Vol. 14, No. 2, 1990). *"Evocative and provocative. Reading this absolutely compelling work provides a transformational experience in which one finds oneself alternately joyful, angry, puzzled, illuminated, warmed, chilled."* (Karen VanderVen, PhD, Professor, Program in Child Development and Child Care, School of Social Work, University of Pittsburgh)

21. ***People Care in Institutions: A Conceptual Schema and Its Application,*** edited by Yochanan Wozner, DSW (Vol. 15, No. 1, 1990). *"Provides ample information by which the effectiveness of internats and the life of staff and internees can be improved."* (Residential Treatment for Children & Youth)

22. ***Assessing Child Maltreatment Reports: The Problem of False Allegations,*** edited by Michael Robin, MPH, ACSW (Vol. 15, No. 2, 1991). *"A thoughtful contribution to the public debate about how to fix the beleaguered system . . . It should also be required reading in courses in child welfare."* (Science Books & Films)

23. ***Information Systems in Child, Youth, and Family Agencies: Planning, Implementation, and Service Enhancement,*** edited by Anthony J. Grasso, DSW, and Irwin Epstein, PhD (Vol. 16, No. 1, 1993). *"Valuable to anyone interested in the design and the implementation of a Management Information System (MIS) in a social service agency. . ."* (John G. Orme, PhD, Associate Professor, College of Social Work, University of Tennessee)

24. ***Negotiating Positive Identity in a Group Care Community: Reclaiming Uprooted Youth,*** Zvi Levy (Vol. 16, No. 2, 1993). *"This book will interest theoreticians, practitioners, and policymakers in child and youth care, teachers, and rehabilitation counselors. Recommended for academic and health science center library collections."* (Academic Library Book Review)

25. ***Travels in the Trench Between Child Welfare Theory and Practice: A Case Study of Failed Promises and Prospects for Renewal,*** George Thomas, PhD, MSW (Vol. 17, No. 1/2, 1994). *"Thomas musters enough research and common sense to blow any proponent out of the water. . . .*

Here is a person of real integrity, speaking the sort of truth that makes self-serving administrators and governments quail." (Australian New Zealand Journal of Family Therapy)

26. **The Anthropology of Child and Youth Care Work,** edited by Rivka A. Eisikovits, PhD (Vol. 18, No. 1, 1996). *"A fascinating combination of rich ethnographies from the occupational field of residential child and youth care and the challenging social paradigm of cultural perspective." (Mordecai Arieli, PhD, Senior Teacher, Educational Policy and Organization Department, Tel-Aviv University, Israel)*

27. **The Occupational Experience of Residential Child and Youth Care Workers: Caring and Its Discontents,** edited by Mordecai Arieli, PhD (Vol. 18, No. 2, 1997). *"Introduces the social reality of residential child and youth care as viewed by care workers, examining the problem of tension between workers and residents and how workers cope with stress." (Book News, Inc.)*

28. **Boarding Schools at the Crossroads of Change: The Influence of Residential Education Institutions on National and Societal Development,** Yitzhak Kashti (Vol. 19, No. 1, 1998). *"This book is an essential, applicable historical reference for those interested in positively molding the social future of the world's troubled youth." (Juvenile and Family Court Journal)*

29. **Caring on the Streets: A Study of Detached Youthworkers,** Jacquelyn Kay Thompson (Vol. 19, No. 2, 1999). *"An empowering work which discloses youths' voices, body, mind, and ways of being-in-their-worlds. . . . This book has the potential to enrich youthwork in any setting." (Tania Chalhub, PhD, Professor, Pontifical Catholic University, Rio de Janeiro, Brazil)*

30. **Intergenerational Programs: Understanding What We Have Created,** Valerie S. Kuehne, PhD (Vol. 20, No. 1/2, 1999). *"Groundbreaking work in multidisciplinary intergenerational programming. Newman and Brummel provide a grounding in history and human development and offer examples of cross-cultural experience. The contributors apply intergenerational programming to everyday situations, and they reach into the future with social policy, evaluation, and the beginnings of a theoretical framework." (Annabel Pelham, PhD, Professor/Director, Gerontology Programs, San Francisco State University)*

31. **Working with Children on the Streets of Brazil: Politics and Practice,** Walter de Oliveira, PhD (Vol. 21, No. 1/2, 2000). Working with Children on the Streets of Brazil *is both a scholarly work on the phenomenon of homeless children and a rousing call to action that will remind you of the reasons you chose to work in social services.*

32. **Innovative Approaches in Working with Children and Youth: New Lessons from the Kibbutz,** edited by Yuval Dror (Vol. 22, No. 1/2, 2001). *"Excellent. . . . Offers rich descriptions of Israel's varied and sustained efforts to use the educational and social life of the kibbutz to supply emotional and intellectual support for youngsters with a variety of special needs. An excellent supplement to any education course that explores approaches to serving disadvantaged children at risk of failing both academically and in terms of becoming contributing members of society." (Steve Jacobson, PhD, Professor, Department of Educational Leadership and Policy, University of Buffalo, New York)*

33. **Residential Child Care Staff Selection: Choose with Care,** Meredith Kiraly (Vol. 23, No. 1/2, 2001). *"Meredith Kiraly is to be congratulated. . . . A lucid, readable book that presents the fruits of international experience and research relevant to the assessment and selection of child care workers, and which does so in a way that leads to practical strategies for achieving improvements in this important field. This book should be read by anyone responsible for selection into child care roles." (Clive Fletcher, PhD, FBPsS, Emeritus Professor of Occupational Psychology, Goldsmiths' College, University of London; Managing Director, Personnel Assessment Limited)*

34. **Pain, Normality, and the Struggle for Congruence: Reinterpreting Residential Care for Children and Youth,** James P. Anglin (Vol. 24, No. 1/2, 2002). *"Residential care practitioners, planners, and researchers will find much of value in this richly detailed monograph. Dr. Anglin's work adds considerably to our understanding of the residential care milieu as a crucible for change, as well as a scaffolding of support that transects community, child, and family." (James Whitaker, PhD, Professor of Social Work, The University of Washington, Seattle)*

35. **A Child and Youth Care Approach to Working with Families,** edited by Thom Garfat, PhD (Vol. 25, No. 1/2, 2003). *"From ethics to data, from activities to support groups, from frontline to*

being in family homes–it's all here." (Karl W. Gompf, BSc, MA, Consultant in Child and Youth Care, Red River College, Winnipeg, Manitoba, Canada)

36. ***Themes and Stories in Youthwork Practice,*** edited by Mark Krueger (Vol. 26, No. 1, 2004). *"If you ever wanted to know what youth care work is, you should read this book. If you ever wondered what it can be, you should read it again. Useful to the practitioner, student, or teacher interested in discovering the depth of this work, this book offers a refreshing perspective from the traditional control and authority approaches so common in our field. It presents youth work as a living, vibrant, and personal experience of discovery for the youth and the worker. If you don't read it you are missing something important in your own education and development. It defines the possibilities of the field. In an eloquent and lyrical fashion, Krueger and his associates lead us through the experience that is youth work. This book is not for the superficial. It is for those who are truly interested in exploring the depth of this experience that we call youth work."* (Thom Garfat, PhD, Co-editor of CYC-Net International and Relational Child and Youth Care Practice; Editor of A Child and Youth Care Approach to Working with Families)

37. ***Working Relationally with Girls: Complex Lives/Complex Identities,*** edited by Marie L. Hoskins, PhD, and Sibylle Artz, PhD (Vol. 26, No. 2, 2004). *"Bringing together both reports of original research findings and reviews of the existing literature, the authors provide a rich understanding of how young women's gender identity is shaped by the intersection of their relational orientation and environmental forces existing in the lifespace. A major contribution of this book is the explicit attention to the challenge of exploring what is unique and individual among young women while attempting to build theory that incorporates the impact of gender as a powerful social category that profoundly influences individuals' experiences."* (Naomi B. Farber, PhD, MSW, Associate Professor, University of South Carolina School of Social Work)

38. ***Group Care Practice with Children and Young People Revisited,*** edited by Leon C. Fulcher and Frank Ainsworth (Vol. 27, No. 1/2, 2005; Vol. 28, No. 1/2, 2006). *"Will have and richly deserves a resonance and a ready audience on both sides of the Atlantic and beyond."* (Mark Smith, MA, CQSW, MEd, Lecturer in Social Work, School of Social and Political Studies, University of Edinburgh)

39. ***At-Risk Children & Youth: Resiliency Explored,*** Niall McElwee (Vol. 29, No. 1/2, 2007). *A detailed examination of the research into the risk and resiliency of children and youth in Ireland.*

At-Risk Children & Youth: Resiliency Explored

Niall McElwee

At-Risk Children & Youth: Resiliency Explored has been co-published simultaneously as *Child & Youth Services,* Volume 29, Numbers 1/2 2007.

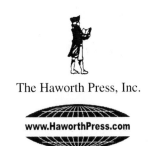

The Haworth Press, Inc.

www.HaworthPress.com

At-Risk Children & Youth: Resiliency Explored has been co-published simultaneously as *Child & Youth Services,* Volume 29, Numbers 1/2 2007.

The development, preparation, and publication of this work has been undertaken with great care. However, the publisher, employees, editors, and agents of The Haworth Press and all imprints of The Haworth Press, Inc., including The Haworth Medical Press® and Pharmaceutical Products Press®, are not responsible for any errors contained herein or for consequences that may ensue from use of materials or information contained in this work. With regard to case studies, identities and circumstances of individuals discussed herein have been changed to protect confidentiality. Any resemblance to actual persons, living or dead, is entirely coincidental.

The Haworth Press is committed to the dissemination of ideas and information according to the highest standards of intellectual freedom and the free exchange of ideas. Statements made and opinions expressed in this publication do not necessarily reflect the views of the Publisher, Directors, management, or staff of The Haworth Press, Inc., or an endorsement by them.

Library of Congress Cataloging-in-Publication Data

McElwee, Niall.
    At-risk children & youth : resiliency explored / Niall McElwee.
        p. cm.
    "Co-published simultaneously as Child & Youth Services, Volume 29, Numbers 1/2 2007."
    Includes bibliographical references and index.
    ISBN 978-0-7890-3381-9 (hard cover : alk. paper) – ISBN 978-0-7890-3382-6 (soft cover : alk. paper)
    1. Problem youth–Services for. 2. Youth with social disabilities. 3. Youth with social disabilities–Counseling of. 4. Juvenile delinquency. 5. Child welfare. I. Child & youth services. II. Title. III. Title: At-risk children and youth.
HV1421.M38 2007
362.74–dc22

2007033145

The HAWORTH PRESS Inc.
Abstracting, Indexing & Outward Linking
PRINT and ELECTRONIC BOOKS & JOURNALS

This section provides you with a list of major indexing & abstracting services and other tools for bibliographic access. That is to say, each service began covering this periodical during the year noted in the right column. Most Websites which are listed below have indicated that they will either post, disseminate, compile, archive, cite or alert their own Website users with research-based content from this work. (This list is as current as the copyright date of this publication.)

- **Academic Search Premier (EBSCO)**
  <http://search.ebscohost.com> 2006

- **CINAHL (Cumulative Index to Nursing & Allied Health Literature) (EBSCO)** <http://www.cinahl.com> 2001

- **CINAHL Plus (EBSCO)** <http://search.ebscohost.com> 2006

- **Educational Research Abstracts (ERA) (Taylor & Francis)** <http://www.tandf.co.uk/era> 2002

- **MasterFILE Premier (EBSCO)** <http://search.ebscohost.com> . . 2006

- **Psychological Abstracts (PsycINFO)** <http://www.apa.org> . . . 1997

- **Social Services Abstracts (ProQuest CSA)** <http://www.csa.com> 2006

- **Social Work Abstracts (NASW)** <http://www.silverplatter.com/catalog/swab.htm> 1982

- **Sociological Abstracts (ProQuest CSA)** <http://www.csa.com> . 1990

- *Academic Source Premier (EBSCO)* <http://search.ebscohost.com> 2007

- *Biological Sciences Database (ProQuest CSA)* <http://www.csa.com> 2006

- *Cambridge Scientific Abstracts (now ProQuest CSA)* <http://www.csa.com> 2006

(continued)

(continued)

(continued)

Bibliographic Access

- *Cabell's Directory of Publishing Opportunities in Educational Psychology and Administration* <http://www.cabells.com/>
- *Cabell's Directory of Publishing Opportunities in Psychology* <http://www.cabells.com>
- *Magazines for Libraries (Katz)*
- *MedBioWorld* <http://www.medbioworld.com>
- *MediaFinder* <http://www.mediafinder.com/>
- *Ulrich's Periodicals Directory: The Global Source for Periodicals Information Since 1932* <http://www.bowkerlink.com>

Special Bibliographic Notes related to special journal issues (separates) and indexing/abstracting:

- indexing/abstracting services in this list will also cover material in any "separate" that is co-published simultaneously with Haworth's special thematic journal issue or DocuSerial. Indexing/abstracting usually covers material at the article/chapter level.
- monographic co-editions are intended for either non-subscribers or libraries which intend to purchase a second copy for their circulating collections.
- monographic co-editions are reported to all jobbers/wholesalers/approval plans. The source journal is listed as the "series" to assist the prevention of duplicate purchasing in the same manner utilized for books-in-series.
- to facilitate user/access services all indexing/abstracting services are encouraged to utilize the co-indexing entry note indicated at the bottom of the first page of each article/chapter/contribution.
- this is intended to assist a library user of any reference tool (whether print, electronic, online, or CD-ROM) to locate the monographic version if the library has purchased this version but not a subscription to the source journal.
- individual articles/chapters in any Haworth publication are also available through the Haworth Document Delivery Service (HDDS).

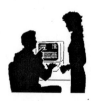

As part of Haworth's continuing commitment to better serve our library patrons, we are proud to be working with the following electronic services:

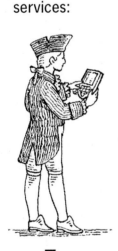

AGGREGATOR SERVICES

EBSCOhost

Ingenta

J-Gate

Minerva

OCLC FirstSearch

Oxmill

SwetsWise

FirstSearch

SwetsWise

LINK RESOLVER SERVICES

1Cate (Openly Informatics)

ChemPort (American Chemical Society)

CrossRef

Gold Rush (Coalliance)

LinkOut (PubMed)

LINKplus (Atypon)

LinkSolver (Ovid)

LinkSource with A-to-Z (EBSCO)

Resource Linker (Ulrich)

SerialsSolutions (ProQuest)

SFX (Ex Libris)

Sirsi Resolver (SirsiDynix)

Tour (TDnet)

Vlink (Extensity, formerly Geac)

WebBridge (Innovative Interfaces)

ChemPort

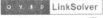

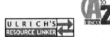

ABOUT THE AUTHOR

Niall McElwee is Director of Relational Research & Consulting based in Galway, Ireland. He is the founding editor of the *Irish Journal of Applied Social Studies* and is the author/co-author of over a dozen books and reports on various child and youth care/human services themes. Dr. McElwee is a regular visitor to Canada where he has recently been appointed Adjunct A/Professor at the University of Victoria, BC. He is married to Susan and has a son called Conor. They live in Athenry, Galway, Ireland.

Dedication

To Susan, my wonderful wife of ten years and my best friend. We have shared many trials and tribulations. We have made it thru together.

To our bonny son, Conor, aged five, who came into the world during the course of this book. His presence in our home reminds me of the really important things in life.

To my mother, Christine, who sparked an interest in children and youth at risk all those years ago. Her memory is strong with us.

To my father, Joe Snr, who has taken a great interest in all my work in child and youth care.

To my Parents-in-Law, Peter and Maura McKenna. It's never too late to get a new family. I scored gold.

At-Risk Children & Youth: Resiliency Explored

CONTENTS

Foreword

My first thought as I begin to write this is that of appreciation. I see it as a compliment and great honour to be allowed to address readers of this volume. In these chapters you will become acquainted with aspects of the work in which I was engaged for almost three decades and from which I obtained enormous satisfaction.

Congratulations to Niall on this work. When he learned of the work of the Youth Encounter Project (St. Augustine's School), he was most anxious to observe at first hand the young people who were at risk and were wrapped, so to speak, in this alternative school. Little was written till then of how these young people responded to interventions; everyone knew of what the at-risk boy or girl, boys especially, thought of the formal school system. Niall's questioning and observations made us much more aware of the nature, extent and depth of the pain of the "at risk" child in our midst. He set about informing himself not so much of the formal life of the school but, more importantly, the informal where he saw pupils relax at centres of recreation around Limerick city or on the campsite by the sea.

The academic, as Niall found, was so important to every individual. The majority of those enrolled in the Y.E.P. had poor school experiences prior to their involvement with us. They were, in many cases, the second generation with such. They saw school in the most negative light as they did authority figures, teachers included. Absenteeism was condoned. Being illiterate was tantamount to being "totally" stupid. Most of us were unaware of this desire within our students, to be the same as others and be able to read and write. A grandmother of some of the students was herself illiterate. I assisted her in her joyous journey to basic

[Haworth co-indexing entry note]: "Foreword." Hanna, John. Co-published simultaneously in *Child & Youth Services* (The Haworth Press, Inc.) Vol. 29, No. 1/2, 2007, pp. xxv-xxvi; and: *At-Risk Children & Youth: Resiliency Explored* (Niall McElwee) The Haworth Press, Inc., 2007, pp. xix-xx. Single or multiple copies of this article are available for a fee from The Haworth Document Delivery Service [1-800-HAWORTH, 9:00 a.m. - 5:00 p.m. (EST). E-mail address: docdelivery@haworthpress.com].

xix

literacy. In a local publication she wrote, "Now I am coming up in the world for I have learned to read and write."

The poor literacy and numeracy skills and the lack of interest of the initial cohort of children made it imperative to establish a centre where each experienced success and a degree of fun. The multi-disciplined staff, envisaged by the Department of Education in 1977, allowed the vital "care" dimension. Good food, a safe environment, despite its strict rules, made school a nice place to be. Daily on the floor it was easy to observe our therapy at work. A visitor for one day only, Fr. Eddie Fitzgerald, writing for his magazine entitled his article "A Happy Place to Learn." That was in 1999. Niall had observed that same spirit earlier when he began his study.

Behind all of the seeming thrills and spills of the school there was the more serious at-risk aspects. Living as we all did in the Limerick of Frank McCourt we were aware of the inevitability and outcomes of those living on the edge, nay dangerously on the edge. We were aware of all of life's ills being posted to the same addresses; we were part of the failure of diverse systems which individuals so badly needed to have some chance and quality of life. But optimism for the future far outweighs for me the recalling of serious and sober milestones on the road of those decades. Good team members at staff level, management, past pupils, volunteers, and the good will of local business would all compel me to continue for further decades! Yes I do jest!

Thank you, Niall, for your support and the direct commendation at the time of your study for the Y.E.P. You made the wider community aware of the at risk and disadvantaged and our society's and community's need to share its resources with them. It is a matter of great satisfaction for both of us, I know, to read that the Task Force on Student Behaviour in Secondary Schools (Department of Education and Science) published 14 March, 2006, recommends that "The Y.E.P. model to be extended in a limited number of urban areas where numbers of potential referrals are substantial enough to warrant this development."

I am confident that this work will impact on all those who have the welfare and happiness of the at-risk cohort at heart.

John Hanna
Principal/Director
Limerick Y.E.P., 1977-2004

Acknowledgements

This book has been in gestation for a decade. Ten years is a long time in anyone's count and there are several people who made sure that this book finally got published. Firstly, I want to thank sincerely the children, youth and families in Limerick, Ireland for their willingness to be involved in this study. Their stories are variously humorous, sad, hopeful and, always, inspiring.

The now retired Director of St. Augustine's Special School in Limerick City, John Hanna has become a great friend to my family. His selfless dedication and commitment to the children, youth and their families is truly inspirational. John walks this earth with undying compassion for disadvantaged youth. To be in his company is to hear an Encyclopaedia of knowledge on Limerick families. I thank him for access to the project over the past decade and for his friendship.

My wife, Susan McKenna, an extraordinary child and youth care practitioner (and that's not just coming from me but from many youth with whom she has worked). Our conversations over the years about "doing" child and youth care have provided me with much to consider in terms of the fit between theory and practice. Susan has displayed endless patience both with her service users and me.

My son, Conor, reminds me on an hourly basis of the importance of relationship. My study is "out of bounds" for him and this is, of course, his favourite room in our house. Our home is all too quiet when he is not there.

Dr. Thom Garfat, for his early comments on this manuscript where his assistance was much appreciated.

This book started its life in a caravan in County Cork, Ireland, during a St. Augustine's summer camp in the mid-1990s and ended in Victoria on Vancouver Island, Canada, a decade later. I would like to express particular gratitude to my editor at the Haworth Press, Dr. Doug Magnuson, for his excellent work, effortless patience and critical eye. Doug indicated an interest in reshaping my Doctorate into a book and stuck with the project with great tenacity. His visits to Ireland are well anticipated.

As in time honoured tradition, any mistakes or limitations in this book are my own.

Irish Association of Social Care Educator's Lifetime Achievement Award Presentation to John Hanna

By Dr. Niall McElwee
President, Irish Association of Social Care Educators
7.10.2004

It is appropriate that this presentation is being made in a year when the Olympics have just been held, for I cannot think of any one individual who brings those lofty ideals of fair play, truth and honour to his life and his work.

This presentation is being made to John Hanna formerly Director of St. Augustine's Special School, Limerick City, Ireland. John is originally from Northern Ireland but has lived in Limerick for three decades. John recently retired from service to the Limerick Youth Encounter Project and I want to mark this tonight.

I first came across John Hanna as a supervisor to students on practica from Waterford Regional Technical College back in 1992. He has since taken students from many colleges across the country and has always provided excellent supervision and a nurturing environment–so many of you will know his name at least. But let me personalise things for a moment.

John Hanna is child and youth care to his core. He is an inspiration to any of us educators and those practitioners and supervisors here who are in the field. He is a constant advocate for change and has been, quite

[Haworth co-indexing entry note]: "Irish Association of Social Care Educator's Lifetime Achievement Award Presentation to John Hanna." McElwee, Niall. Co-published simultaneously in *Child & Youth Services* (The Haworth Press, Inc.) Vol. 29, No. 1/2, 2007, pp. xxix-xxxi; and: *At-Risk Children & Youth: Resiliency Explored* (Niall McElwee) The Haworth Press, Inc., 2007, pp. xxiii-xxv. Single or multiple copies of this article are available for a fee from The Haworth Document Delivery Service [1-800-HAWORTH, 9:00 a.m. - 5:00 p.m. (EST). E-mail address: docdelivery@haworthpress.com].

rightly, a critic of successive governments who have done all too little, too late for children and youth "at risk."

I had the opportunity to work closely with John Hanna in 1995 when I took part in the summer programme at his project as I was commencing research at that time. John was endlessly patient with me and always facilitated my questions about why something was done or, indeed, not done in a particular way. Indeed, much to the humour of the children and youth I was allocated a caravan for my laptop whilst they had only tents. But, they soon made it up to me by threatening to shave off my eyebrows and set me on fire! I survived the experience and have continued to work with him over the years. In fact, I married one of his child and youth care workers!

There are dozens of Limerick families who owe John Hanna a great deal. For some children and youth, John has been, quite literally, the difference between life and death. John has been the difference between personal and professional success and failure, between his graduates staying in Ireland or emigrating, between success or failure in life itself.

John has sat in cold courtrooms, he has attended dreary Department of Education and Science meetings and passionately pleaded for his children. John has sat through thousands of parent/child meetings.

And always, always, always, John has engaged with everyone with good humour, deep and genuine respect and an open tolerance. John has touched more people than he will ever know. John is an inspiration to anyone who would consider a career in child and youth care and this is why we celebrate his career tonight.

His work since 1977 in the Youth Encounter Project (which remains hidden down a Limerick Lane) was not glamorous; his charges were not always thankful for his interventions, his parents were not always there for their own children and the Department of Education and Science was not always supportive. But, John kept going because he believed in what he was doing. He taught me early in my academic career that everyone deserves not one chance–but several chances. We just have to look harder sometimes.

I have been spending quite a time considering what I might say that would be eloquent, but remembering that John remains a teacher at heart and will probably give me some feedback later tonight on my speech I hope to have done him some justice!

Perhaps another one of our IASCE members, Dr. John Ennis, has already written it best in one of his wonderful poems.

"Choreograph the daily griefs, dramas, joys, the little harms
and let them know our love for them is sound:

We that have known the ripple and the wingspan in the arms
The attempts at flight that never leave the ground."

John Hanna, our Association salutes your work as a professional and
you as a person. May your retirement be blessed with all you would
want. May your work be continued. May your legacy in Limerick ring
true.

There is no gold wristwatch for you here tonight. No garish golf set.
These are not you. Instead, we offer you a simple yet elegant print; a Picasso which is of an Owl. It signifies your wisdom as an educator (and
may I say John that I chose this without Susan's help).

REFERENCE

Ennis, J. (1994). Vedic, from *Down in the Deeper Helicon.* Dublin: Dedalus.

Chapter 1

Snowflake Children

SUMMARY. Taking account of the needs and views of children is problematic, particularly in Ireland where children have been "owned" by their parents and social policy has been directed at the family rather than the individual child. The 1980s and 1990s may be said to be the decades where abuse, in its many forms, reared its head and Irish society was forced to sit up and take notice of our distressed children and young people. In particular, we became interested in children and youth at risk. Child and youth care practice, as with other caring occupations, forms a vital element of both the voluntary and statutory social and health care provision systems in Ireland and is in constant evolution. Partly because of this new interest in risk, it came under a public lens of examination that tended to focus almost exclusively on the negative. Broadly at the same time, social scientists in Europe had become interested in what Beck labelled the "risk society" with parallels between both discussions.

My research for this book took place in the context of Ireland emerging from a history of neglect towards vulnerable populations of at-risk children and youth. Moreover, there has been a breakdown in trust in expert systems at a time when "the public's knowledge has become radicalised and they have become experts of sorts" (Giddens, 1991, p. 3). The Irish public is no longer prepared to blindly trust in expert systems or past powerful organisations, such as the Catholic Church, and society has begun to think in whole terms. It is a tragic paradox that many public policy makers have lost confidence in their ability to provide for children and youth at-risk when scientific knowledge has never been more advanced

[Haworth co-indexing entry note]: "Snowflake Children." McElwee, Niall. Co-published simultaneously in *Child & Youth Services* (The Haworth Press, Inc.) Vol. 29, No. 1/2, 2007, pp. 1-27; and: *At-Risk Children & Youth: Resiliency Explored* (Niall McElwee) The Haworth Press, Inc., 2007, pp. 1-27. Single or multiple copies of this article are available for a fee from The Haworth Document Delivery Service [1-800-HAWORTH, 9:00 a.m. - 5:00 p.m. (EST). E-mail address: docdelivery@haworthpress.com].

Available online at http://cys.haworthpress.com
© 2007 by The Haworth Press, Inc. All rights reserved.
doi:10.1300/J024v29n01_01

and we should be more able to protect them. This deeply affects child and youth care. doi:10.1300/J024v29n01_01 *[Article copies available for a fee from The Haworth Document Delivery Service: 1-800-HAWORTH. E-mail address: <docdelivery@haworthpress.com> Website: <http://www.HaworthPress. com> © 2007 by The Haworth Press, Inc. All rights reserved.]*

KEYWORDS. Children and youth at risk, resiliency, child and youth care, Youth Encounter Projects

> In our times, birds fall down hardly noticed in the world.
>
> –John Ennis, *Goldcrest Falling* (2006)

> There is a widespread sense that everything has been tried and has failed and that nobody is very clear about how to advance into an increasingly bleak future. (Langan, 1995, p. xv)

My cell phone rings incessantly but I smile when two numbers come up on it. The first is my wife, Susan's, number because I am guaranteed to hear something positive and affirming and my four-year-old son, Conor, usually wants a chat with his Dad about such important matters as the goldfish tank needs changing, the birds have eaten all the nuts, or Darth Vader is really a "goodie" not a "baddy." Those two voices make my day. The second number belongs to St. Augustine's Youth Encounter Project, and I know it is my friend, John, calling to fill me in on the latest educational developments for youth in Ireland. Ironically, I met both my future wife and John in a child and youth care centre in Limerick in the early 1990s and since then we have worked together, researched together, and lobbied together for over a decade. And this past decade has seen many changes.

In that time, there have been profound shifts in the social typography of our country. Ireland was for centuries one of the highly traditional agrarian, poorer, underdeveloped and small countries of Europe, but this has changed utterly over the past couple of decades. For more than a century and a half, we experienced constant out-migration. When we joined the European Union (EU) in the mid-1980s things started to get better, and we became less insular as a people in every respect. We now have a booming high-tech sector, the return of thousands of our citizens who once could not locate work at home, tens of thousands of migrant workers from the new Europe, and a youthful population recently coined as the "expectocracy" so high are their expectations for life

(McWilliams, 2005). Our unemployment remains low in a European context (some 4.1%), but Limerick is one city that has had to suffer high unemployment rates and poverty over the decades. It is also a city that has received more than its share of negative coverage in the media.

Locating Limerick

Ireland's principal river is the Shannon, which begins in the north-central area, flows south and southwest for about 386 km, and empties into the Atlantic. At the end of the Shannon lies the City of Limerick with a population of some 80,000, made famous by the short poems (Limericks) and, more recently, by one Pulitzer Prize winning book that divided the country: *Angela's Ashes* by Frank McCourt. It is ironic that *Angela's Ashes* is fundamentally about risk and resiliency, for it is in this city that the fieldwork for my own study took place. Limerick has a tough reputation in Ireland and, as with all tough places; there are pockets of those who thrive and do well and those who do not. Why is this? What can be done to assist children and youth to achieve their potential? How can the community respond instead of simply leaving it to the individual?

A Connection with Rivers

St. Augustine's School began as a Youth Encounter Project in 1977. It is a mixed school. It is situated app. 300 meters from the Lock Gates of the new marina in Limerick City. We are a small Post Primary school. We have a huge interest in the Shannon "River of Dreams" project. We are greatly influenced by our proximity to the river and our programmes have a strong outdoor and marine connection. Our picture shows our sailing boat "The Little Mermaid" with some of our students and Pat Lawless, the well known round the world sailor. (http://www.riverofdreams.ie/schools/19587Q/fs_og_main.htm)

SNOWFLAKE CHILDREN

After fifteen years involved in child and youth care, my experience is that most parents take their parenting roles very seriously. A new arrival in the family is a time of great excitement and wonder for all involved. Generally, the new child will be afforded every opportunity to progress and prosper in life and, although sacrifices will have to be made, in the long term it will be worth the considerable effort. These fortunate children are not the ones discussed in this study. Instead, my argument focuses on children of a lost generation. I call them *snowflake children.*

The metaphor of a snowflake seems particularly appropriate for this study, as snow is a commodity we tend to remember for either the pleasure it gives us or the significant disruptions it causes. A snowflake evokes for most Irish people images of purity, uniformity, transience, and isolation. For children, it presents an opportunity to play with homemade sleighs and, generally, a school vacation for a couple of days. Snowmen can be built, rubber tyres can be used to hurtle down slopes at death-defying speeds, and snowballs can be thrown at innocent passer-bys.

Where the metaphor fits well with my study is that a snowflake's shape (called "habit" by meteorologists) is determined by both temperature and the amount of water vapour in the air at any time. As snow crystals descend, they may meet up with one another, forming aggregations. If a snow crystal encounters cooled water droplets on its descent, it can become grouped into snow pellets. A two-foot square of snow ten inches deep contains about a million snowflakes. It is difficult for meteorologists to predict snow falls with any certainty, because the heaviest snow amounts fall in surprisingly narrow bands that are on a smaller scale than observing networks and forecast zones. A second complicating factor is that there are extremely minute temperature differences defining the boundaries between rain and snow.

It is widely held that every snowflake that falls is unique. This is also certainly the case with each new infant that is born, but where the snowflake falls will overwhelmingly determine what will happen to it. If an individual snowflake is fortunate enough to fall in a country field, it will probably remain white and pure until the weather changes and it melts or a wandering farm animal tramples on it changing its texture, shape, and colour. If a child is born into a family that is already experiencing severe problems, stresses, and chaos (what may be termed a negative family climate) the child, like the snowflake, is statistically more likely to be swept away, to have its identity changed, to become blemished, dirtied, and trodden on than a child born into a family unit that is secure in itself. Unfortunately, few people consider a blemished snowflake beautiful. And yet they have their own beauty.

It has long been accepted in child and youth care literature that families with very many problems to contend with face discord (Garfat, 1998; Garfat & McElwee, 2004; Maier, 1979; McElwee, 1996a; McElwee & Monaghan, 2005; Redl & Wineman, 1952). Such families are often termed "multi-agency units" where the quality of life within the family, because of the vast amounts of stress, may be poor and inconsistent. For me, family is key but families cannot merely "dismantle the integrity of past experiences and instead must seek to integrate sets of already interwoven biographies" (Anglin & Glossop, 1987, p. 3). Thom Garfat and I have argued that family is what you consider it to be (Garfat & McElwee, 2004) and, in this case, family is St. Augustine's Special School, Limerick City, Ireland. More of this later.

We all experience positive and negative phenomena in our lives, making each of us special and unique. Various child and youth care authors suggest that the more positive experiences we have as youngsters, the more likely we are to be positive adults (Maier, 1979), and the more negative experiences we have the more likely we are to be resentful and bitter about a system that we perceive has failed us (McElwee, 1996b; McElwee & Monaghan, 2005). Essentially, this book suggests that many Irish children and youth find it extraordinarily difficult to thrive because their personal and familial lives are overly preoccupied with adversity, they consistently receive the (subtle and unsubtle) message that they are unproductive, and there are too few protective factors in place in the community for them which allow them to develop the necessary skills and knowledge to be resilient.

But, of course, it is more complicated than this and many children and youth prosper despite their total environments. This is crucial in attempting to understand the resiliency perspective as it plays itself out in Limerick housing estates, lanes, and apartment blocks.

Indeed, 30% of Irish children have been identified as having a high risk of living in poverty and, by the mid-1990s, Ireland had the highest rates of child poverty of any EU member state (Nolan, 2000). Childhood means different things to different people and this is only too obvious when one travels around the world. In some countries it is normative behaviour for a twelve year old to work in leather shops, in other countries in it is normative behaviour for a child to sit in school for eight hours a day and in other countries, twelve year olds are in armed militia. It is my contention that many of the young parents in this and related studies have never been allowed to experience childhood themselves (in the sense of making sense of the world through normal exploratory play and being free from what we might loosely term adult concerns and responsibilities). They subsequently fail to engage fully in what are understood as effective parenting roles when the time comes for them to parent. It seems to me that if we are to reach children and youth who are at-risk, we must engage on a much deeper level than heretofore with their parent/s and caregivers.

THE BREAKDOWN IN TRUST IN EXPERT SYSTEMS

After the Irish famine in the mid-1840s, the Catholic Church emerged as a powerful and intimidating force, and it exerted tremendous influence in Irish politics and society up until the 1980s. In the early years of what was called the Irish Free State, governments were at pains to prove their loyalty and commitment to the Catholic hierarchy, and it was difficult to raise issues related to maltreatment and abuse where clergy were involved. The 1980s and 1990s, however, witnessed a public discourse around vulnerable, invulnerable and at-risk youth populations which was both vague and confused. It is now acknowledged that there are important connections worth teasing out around the concepts and constructs of children and young people at-risk actively seeking out desired risk and living in a risk society as, indeed, is working in the risk society for child protection and welfare personnel (Beck, 1992; Coates, 2003; Ferguson, 1997; Giddens, 1992; McElwee, 2001; Ungar, 2002).

Over the past fifteen years, I have been struck by the fact that children and young people who are deemed to be at-risk in very many areas of their lives and, crucially, early in their lives, often end up in care of the State later in their lives whether in foster care, residential care, youth diversion projects, the special school system, or prison despite the many and varied interventions made on their behalf. I have wondered why this is the case when the expert lens had already declared that something should be done to avert this occurrence.

RISK AS AN ORGANISING CONCEPT

One continually hears the terms "at-risk," "risk," and "risky" associated with children and youth and their various behaviours but often without much clarity. I suggest that risk, in the context of children and young people and their families, remains surprisingly under-theorised in Irish research, and there are several unresolved definitional issues in employing such terminology in relation to school-going children (Combat Poverty Agency, 1995; McElwee, 2006). Who is at-risk? From what are children at risk? Why are only *some* students perceived to be at risk? What roles do the school and teachers play, in the context of child and youth care provision, in the risk debate more generally?

Risk has now been identified as a key organising concept in discourse on young people, and there has been a movement towards viewing how the social context of risk might be mediated as opposed to the traditional focus on risk behaviours only. The term *at-risk*, as distinct from *risk*, has been taken from the fields of epidemiology and insurance (Baizerman, 1990; Richardson et al., 1989) and has recently been adapted to fit into the education debate but with a significant amount of ambiguity.

An ecological approach to understanding children at-risk includes family background, personal characteristics of the child, the school context, and the social behaviour of children (Boyd, 1993; McElwee, 1996; McElwee, 2006). All of these phenomena interact to create conditions that can place children at-risk of failing to achieve their academic potential, dropping out of school, and/or having limits placed on their ability to function as productive adults in society.

I suggest in this book that pupils are placed at-risk *when they experience a significant mismatch between their circumstances and needs, and the capacity or willingness of society to accept, accommodate, and respond to them in a manner that supports and enables their maximum social, emotional, and intellectual growth and development.*

My overwhelming experience is that it is children and youth living in poverty and on the margins of society who constitute the majority of those who do not benefit fully from formal education. There is an over-representation of individuals from unskilled and manual social class backgrounds among those leaving formal education with few or no qualifications and this is borne out with the participants in this study. In some Irish classrooms, 20% of the children are now from non-national backgrounds, asylum-seeking backgrounds, and are economic immigrants. Whilst this has long been the norm in other countries, it is new to Ireland.

There are literally hundreds of areas of risk that one could spend one's time usefully researching (Ungar, 2004; Werner & Smith, 1992). Reports of children and adolescents in Ireland failing in the formal education system, coming from chaotic families, being placed in residential care, being addicted to alcohol and/or drugs, sleeping rough on our streets, and/or getting involved in prostitution and crime in a wider sense are now commonplace (McElwee & Monaghan, 2005; Wolin & Wolin, 1996). Despite this, there is little research on teasing out risk, at-risk, and resiliency in a specifically educational context or on the connections between the school environment and social work (Gilligan, 1998; 2000) and child and youth care practice (McElwee, 2000; Ricks & Garfat, 1989).

As the central explorations of this study are at-risk and resiliency, it seems appropriate to ask, "Where does this leave risk and resiliency in the anthropologically strange existence of Irish children and youth and, in the context of this study, pupils from the largely forgotten Youth Encounter Project system?" In many ways, the analytical vocabulary to investigate, describe, and understand risk and resiliency with (in) the lives of the children and youth was inadequate, and I had to rethink how one might approach such subject material. Nonetheless, I was and remain aware that researching childhood resilience is powerful as it can "promote hope rather than despair, empowerment rather than alienation, survival rather than victimisation, and pro-action rather than reaction" (Dryden, Johnson & Howard, 1998, p. 30).

MOVING THE YOUTH ENCOUNTER PROJECTS CENTRE STAGE IN THE AT-RISK DEBATE

What is termed the primary education sector in Ireland comprises national schools, special schools, and non-aided private primary schools. There are 3200 national schools of which more than 300 have classes for pupils with special needs, and 106 are Special Schools. These schools cater to some 444,300 pupils. Primary schools, which account for the education of 98 percent of children in the primary sector, are staffed by over 21,800 teachers.

This study engages with concepts and constructs of at-risk as they apply and are used within child and youth care interventions across a number of systems whilst concentrating on special education for marginalised children and youth. The Youth Encounter Projects in the Irish educational setting receive particular attention as they were established specifically to engage with children considered by the Irish Department of Education and Science's Special Education section to be at-risk and have not yet been formally written about. This understanding of at-risk includes those "considered to be at risk because of truancy and related problems of poverty, poor home life, and incipient involvement in crime" (Egan & Hegarty, 1984, p. 1).

The profile of children and youth attending Youth Encounter Projects have been labelled variously as "culturally deprived," "socially disadvantaged," "at-risk," "intellectually deprived" and "minoritized." Such children are rarely considered as potentially productive members of society, and the Directors of these projects have a constant battle to access resources for their pupils. Indeed, it could be argued that the majority of intervention strategies for children at-risk in Ireland interpret at-risk in a narrow sense, such as scholastic achievement within the formal school system (National Forum for Early Childhood Education, 1998, pp. 76-77) as opposed to a more ecological and child-centred understanding, despite the rhetoric of politicians. I attempt here to bridge this gap.

Twilight Children?

The Limerick Leader newspaper runs a column where it repeats head-lines and stories from the past. In 2001, it noted a heading from 1981 that read *Twilight Children out in the Cold?* The report went on to detail, "The highly successful Limerick Youth Encounter Project, which caters for the education of disadvantaged children, is to close on September 30. The project, which has run its four-year course, is to be closed down because the Limerick Youth Service Board can no longer accommodate the staff and children at its headquarters in Lower Glentworth Street. The Department had been searching for premises, but were unable to find one before the September 30 deadline. This, in effect, means that the 25 children, who range in age from 12 to 16, will be out on the streets by the end of the month" (8.9.2001). Thus, the project has battled to sur-vive right from the outset.

The Youth Encounter Project system was long considered by De-partmental officials to be working well but "doing so on a wing and a prayer," and their formal evaluation is finally under way. As with all in-tervention projects with at-risk children and youth, one might expect that the Youth Encounter Projects would have been formally assessed by external sources at some stage, but this was not the case. Indeed, I was informed that a number of civil servants based with the Department of Education and Science in Athlone were given an evaluation brief but only "as a tag on an already overloaded agenda." The recently published report on school discipline has recommended that the Youth Encounter Projects be expanded into some other areas (Task Force on School Dis-cipline, 2006).

Over the past ten years in Ireland, another area of at-risk in special education, intellectual impairment, moved centre stage for the Irish media, the court system, and the public due, in particular, to a high-profile case which resulted in the Irish State being sued by Kathleen Synnott, the mother of a male with autism, for its failure to provide full educa-tional services.

RESEARCH PROBLEMS:
FROM THE GENERAL TO THE SPECIFICS OF THIS STUDY

As noted earlier, the study explores the domains of risk, at-risk, and resilience concepts that have broad interest for social policy formulators in the areas of child protection and welfare and special educational youth initiatives. It focuses on Limerick, Ireland, for its empirical work. We have learned that despite the ever-growing body of research on risk and resilience, there are serious definitional ambiguities of the terms risk factors, protective mechanisms, vulnerability, and resilience. This has resulted in a large and inconsistent set of variables being used to study the trajectories through life of children and youth growing up under adversity or following exposure to trauma (Anthony & Cohler, 1987; Luthar, 2001; McElwee, 2006; Ungar, 2004). To take but one example, the American commentator on resilience, Norman Garmezy (1991) defines resiliency as *"the maintenance of competent functioning despite an interfering emotionality"* (p. 466). It is clear that if educators, youth workers, and human services personnel target the perceived, potential, and existing positive attributes of the child, success will be both greater and long-term.

The study explores five major questions around risk discourse:

1. What is actually meant in the social scientific discourse by risk?
2. From where do the concepts and constructs of risk and resiliency, as applied to child and youth care and "special" education, derive?
3. How does the current climate of risk consciousness affect child and youth care professionals?
4. How does one Youth Encounter Project in Limerick City understand at-risk and "resiliency" and engage with its pupils?
5. How does one particular group of respondents who attended a special educational project make sense of risk, at-risk and resilience?

The Purpose of the Study

As With a number of commentators, I take the view that resilience is as much dependent on structural conditions, relationships and access to social justice as it is with their individual characteristics (see Ungar, 2005). The study attempts to further explore resiliency by uncovering the nature of young people's attitudes towards risk involvement/non-involvement and to explore a range of factors associated with risk at various levels. I explore these research questions by drawing together two distinct bodies of knowledge: the theoretical discourse on risk from the social sciences, and the discourse on child and youth care institutions and practices in the Republic of Ireland as they pertain to children at-risk attending the Youth Encounter Projects. The research questions identified here are important on several theoretical and practical grounds. The study of resilience has been more generally focused on children than on adolescents and, at the same time, there is a consensus amongst social service providers that a disturbingly high percentage of Irish children and adolescents are condemned to live lives of adversity and are ill-equipped to merge into the labour force on completion of their formal schooling (Bates, 1996; Egan & Hegarty, 1984; Lynch, 1999). Nationally, social exclusion of early school leavers has been noted as a major source of concern with the decline of traditional employment opportunities combined with a process of "qualification inflation" (National Economic and Social Forum Report, 1997, p. 3; National Economic and Social Forum Report, 2002).

Secondly, at-risk children and young people now present a formidable challenge to social policy analysts, educators, and researchers because, as this study suggests, childhood and adolescence have become politicised and radicalised and risk is continually understood and discussed in a negative context where the emphasis is on *blame* (Hendrick, 1981; Garfat & McElwee, 2004). At the same time, the study of young people's problems often commands a low budget and even lower status amongst one's peers (Casas, 1995; U.S. Department of Education, 1997; Hill & Tisdall 1997).

Thirdly, this study concurs with the international literature by recognising that the Republic of Ireland is by no means unique having an at-risk population of youth catered for poorly by the State across a number of areas such as child and youth care and special education (see Durrant, 1993; Garfat & McElwee, 2001). The American experience, to take but one example, has also sustained "years of disastrous, persistent ... unintentional biases" (U.S. Department of Education, 1997, pp. iv-v).

Fourthly, the traditional emphasis in the literature towards focussing on individual pathology of at-risk children and young people is set alongside a broader socio-economic and cultural environment. The study's emphasis on the individual perspectives and subjective experiences of the interviewees will hopefully facilitate a more enlightened approach towards child and youth care prevention and intervention strategies. Nonetheless, this study provides unique empirical data on Youth Encounter Projects at St. Augustine's in Limerick where there has been an absence of grounded data since 1984 and on the family and individual profiles of the participants. It also features narratives from interviewees on how they experience life in Limerick.

Finally, this study is the first study of its kind to be conducted in an Irish context. Its theoretical importance hinges predominantly on the explorations of risk, at-risk, and resilience at the outset of the research and the fact that the research participants were permitted to define the parameters of their risk lifestyles. This approach, being inherently objective, facilitates a working epistemology that locates meaningful reality within the immediate settings of young people's daily lives.

LOCATING AN INTEREST
IN AT-RISK CHILDREN AND YOUTH

Child and youth care workers are still relatively free to write from an experiential perspective. In taking the courage to share their own experience in working with young people, they have an opportunity to generate a body of knowledge that promotes understanding, caring, and respect. The "truth" to be discovered is the revelation of what is rather than the attainment of should be or the illusion of what might be. In peeling back the layers of their own experience, child and youth care workers can make a unique contribution to our understanding of how it really is to work with troubled kids. They can tell the untold stories of childhood and adolescence, albeit from the "truth" of their own perspective. Surely the time has come for us to re-examine our discipline that moves from the inside out. The prescriptions for such writing may seem vague, but the first step is definitive and unambiguous–look in the mirror, look beyond, and tell it as it is. (Fewster, 1991, pp. 61-62)

The catalyst for interest in pursuing this study arose from four experiences, the first was reading Nicola Madge's edited book, *Families at Risk* (1983), whilst studying at University; second, my experiences visiting in excess of 350 child and youth care practica for children and young people at-risk throughout Ireland, England, Scotland, Sweden, Romania, Morocco, and Canada beginning in the early 1990s; third, coming across a somewhat obscure Report on the Youth Encounter Projects and Children at-risk completed in 1984 by Gerard Egan and Mary Hegarty in a corner of a store area in St. Augustine's School, and; fourth, reading child and youth care literature advocating a resiliency rather than a risk driven approach to "hidden" populations.

In her influential book, Madge (1983) put forward an alphabetical risk model she terms the "ABC of risk," and I have been drilling this into my students since! Although this model is over twenty years old and Madge does not contend that the model is necessarily complete, she argues the model (both singly and cumulatively) could be used as, or to identify, indicators or predictors of risk by social service providers.

Madge considered risk appropriate to families where it seems likely that difficulties will arise, in other words, where the risk probability could be represented statistically. Madge saw this risk being evident when parents, for a variety of reasons, could not meet the needs of their children and when the children displayed signs of disturbance or a failure to meet normal developmental milestones. The language that Madge uses in describing risk is worth mentioning here as she writes, "... this is because most family life takes place behind closed doors, and partly it is because the enormous variations in both good and less good parenting complicate accurate family assessments" (p. 5).

Madge (1983) further notes that there are two areas where one may direct energy in assessing whether or not a family is experiencing problems: Where it is evident that parents are not able, for whatever reasons, to meet the needs of their children, and if there are obvious signs of disturbance shown by the children themselves.

Coffield et al. (1983) found that there was no single intervening factor acting as a transmitter of deprivation. At the end of their particular study, the research team concluded that there were four main features of families at-risk:

1. The families were overloaded with problems whose very complexity seemed to defeat them.
2. They had no resources, material, emotional, or social.
3. They had become stigmatised.
4. Their family patterns of early marriage, large families and child rearing seemed to militate against them. (p. 26)

I wondered how risk, as discussed by Madge and her colleagues in the UK, translated and mirrored in the Irish context, if at all. Such an ecological understanding of risk was *partly* addressed by the aforementioned 1984 Report. However, I felt that risk in child and youth care and educational discourse was something to which Irish observers have not given enough attention.

As with Coffield et al.'s study (1983) in the UK, I suggest that there has been an over-emphasis on distinguishing between structural and individual divisions that have more to do with academic traditions in psychology and sociology than the lives of families considered to be at-risk. The very multiplicity of disadvantage leaves an indelible mark on all their lives. Both child-centred and middle class child-rearing practices had little currency and are inappropriate in the milieu of poverty and the *cycle of disadvantage* thesis. The Limerick interviewees in this study could be seen as extended family members of the families described by Wilson, and I set out to explore why this might be the case.

The Egan and Hegarty Report

It is surprising that there is such a dearth of academic material devoted to the Youth Encounter Projects, as they have operated for over twenty-five years and the subject areas of risk, at-risk and resiliency are increasingly gaining in popularity. The one significant piece of completed dedicated research thus far on the Limerick City Youth Encounter Project remains the Egan and Hegarty Report published in 1984, just seven years after they were set up and, literally, hundreds of children have passes through its doors.

Referring to the Youth Encounter Projects in general, it observed that *further research should be commissioned to assess the contribution of the Youth Encounter Projects to special education and that past students should be assessed* [italics added] (Egan & Hegarty, 1984). Despite their recommendations, the Youth Encounter Projects have not been formally (re)studied even though it has become obvious that the children and young people from these "special" schools have disproportionately high rates of academic failure compared to the general population and have tended to end up in trouble with their parents, custodians, community and police on a regular basis (Mid-Western Health Board, 1991). They are a highly visible population in terms of their access of social services.

Egan and Hegarty (1984) found that the Youth Encounter Projects fitted into an ecological tradition of compensatory education where "home, school, peer-group, community, and society at large are considered as interlocking environments constituting a single system, and problems of individual behaviour are considered in the light of the environmental factors which might be responsible for them" (p. 185). In terms of child and youth development, then, ecology refers to a supportive social network involving friends, families, neighbours, and both formal and informal carers.

It is my contention that many existing prevention programmes are under-resourced, fragmented, narrow in focus, reactive rather than proactive, and their overall design fails to have any real impact in assisting the children to attend school, study, sit, and pass examinations such as the Junior Certificate and Leaving Certificate. They fail, in the main, to inculcate youth with notions of deferred gratification and to build on resiliency in all its aspects because the youth feel the interventions are not grounded in their experience of the world.

Child and Youth Care Practice Environments

The second influence on my choice of topic was visiting child and youth care centres in a number of countries. This has been a humbling experience as I have witnessed the service user profiles of youth in care. Often, such youth share a number of characteristics with the children and youth attending the Youth Encounter Projects in Ireland. I have visited interviewees in residential child care centres, in centres for young offenders, and in prison. I have visited others in community programmes and others who have established families of their own.

In 1997, I was approached by the Good Shepherd Community of Sisters and asked to research the area of prostitution for them. This ultimately resulted in the publication of a book (McElwee & Lalor, 1997) and from this a committee and a small organisation was established to attempt to befriend people working in prostitution. I was involved in this project for several years and, in my capacity as Chair of the project, attended and spoke at several conferences and seminars in the general area of working with vulnerable populations. Again, I noticed that the international project workers were increasingly focussing on resiliency perspectives, as opposed to risk pathologies, and I attempted to utilise some of their ways of working into my own project.

Literature on Risk and Resiliency

The final significant influence on my choice of topic arose out of my teaching and research for programmes I lectured on at the Waterford Institute of Technology from 1992-2001 and, since 2001, at the Athlone Institute of Technology. I teach modules in professional child and youth care, therapeutic interactional analysis, and relational research and have enjoyed reading up on international approaches to social care and child and youth care provision. I noticed that the Irish models are overly-dependent on a problem-based focus and that the North American literature had evolved more to a resiliency and strength/solutions-based approach in their teaching of this area (Coates, 2003; Garfat, 1998; Ungar, 2004). I was determined to explore why this might be the case and was introduced to the work of key authors in these systems that have greatly influenced my own thinking and academic work (see Garfat & McElwee, 2001; 2004).

THE ERA OF PRODUCTIVE CHAOS:
LINKING THE EMPIRICAL DISCUSSION ON RISK
TO THE THEORETICAL DEBATE

Quite simply, risk means different things to different people with the first decade of sociological discussion on risk being marked as one of "productive chaos" (Machlis & Rosa, 1989). The central feature of our dangers at the beginning of this new millennium is that they are perceived to be rapidly changing and risk has become public, pervasive, compelling and inescapable (Beck, 1992; Coates, 2003; Hacking, 1982; Parton, 1985, 1991). Is the ozone layer really being depleted? Are all the continents becoming warmer? Are ice caps melting? Are hundreds of species going to be wiped out over the forthcoming century because of our failure to predict risk outcomes?

Already, animal and plant species are being wiped out on a daily basis (in fact, human activity has caused the extinction of one million species in the past twenty five years and 10%-40% of all species are threatened with extinction) and the reproductive capabilities of animals are being affected by our released toxins from industrial processes, and Cohen (1997) has suggested that we must redefine what it means to be a citizen of Earth. This is replicated in all areas of our lives such as consumerism, where Russell (1998) calculates some years ago that "we now consume more in one year than we did in the whole period from the birth of Christ to the dawn of the industrial revolution" (p. 43).

A comprehensive theory is required, therefore, which is capable of integrating the technical analysis of risk and the cultural, social and individual response structures that shape the public experience of risk (Kasperson et al., 1988). This is particularly the case with regard to children and youth because, although it sounds corny, they really are our future.

A VIGNETTE ON CHILDREN POWER

Perhaps it is worth telling a little story here to illustrate this point. Globally, humans have transformed 50% of land on earth to deserts, cities, farms or pastures. Ireland lags behind many countries in its appreciation of environmental matters. We have all the rhetoric but at the same time have been fined recently by the European Union for failing to put the rhetoric into practice. One particular private company in the north east of Ireland has become very successful because it quickly realised that the way to educate families about environmental issues was to reach the children. So, representatives called to all the primary schools in the area and invited the children out to their Plant. The children came in groups and were hugely impressed by what they saw. They became the moral police in their homes as their parents were not socialised in an era that was receptive to the idea that one must sustain one's environment. Children throughout the area took great pride in accompanying their parents to the recycle site and showed them how to recycle all the household goods. That one company now has over sixty recycled products. The children are aware that they are living in a global environment. Thus, in this instance, the children can contextualise risk outside of their immediate experiences.

METHODOLOGY

A separate chapter more fully detailing the methodology of this study is included later. In this section, I briefly comment on some aspects of the methodology to illustrate the fact that new pathways for analysis have been created in relation to youth at-risk in the Irish context. The French sociologist, Emile Durkheim (1915), identified the everyday world as a "world of social facts" and suggested, "It is a reality of *sui generis* formed through collective representations that span space and time" (pp. 28-29). This book is based on a detailed study with a cohort of youth in inner city Limerick where access to data (1977-2000) was available concerning their involvement with what is termed a "special" school or Youth Encounter Project. In all, over 227 children attended the school between 1977 and 1995 when this study commenced. Within these figures, a sample of seventeen pupils that took part in a summer programme was chosen. These ex-pupils were followed up and interviewed at length over a two-year period.

The analysis of interview data was conducted utilising an adaptation of frameworks analysis, a system of coding and analysis developed by Ritchie and Spencer (1994) in the UK at the National Centre for Social Research that I have been using for the past number of years. Qualitative methodology was chosen as it was felt that this would lend authenticity to the narratives of the young people. The transcript excerpts used in this study are exemplars of much larger bodies of text identified through frameworks. Material is divided into various thematic chapters intended to portray a comprehensive picture of both adversity and resiliency. The analysis is carried out in the context of key contemporary studies of risk. A distinction is made between recent sociological concepts of politicising of risk, at-risk, trust, blame, and child care practice through a socio-ecological perspective. The role of experts and expert systems in generating risks, the role of these experts and expert systems in solving risk, as well as "fear of risk" and "globalising" of risk are assessed.

FRAMING A DISCUSSION ON RISK: FEAR OF FAILURE

Parton et al. (1997) argue that child protection and welfare discourse in the 1990s was framed in a context of risk and that social policy reform must take cognisance of this fact. It could be argued that what has increasingly informed child and youth care practice in Ireland is fear of failure and a fear of being very publicly blamed by the media for, what is termed in research, issues of competency. This equates with the global sociological discussions on risk. Such fears in child and youth care are based on practice experiences where child protection and welfare and child and youth care personnel have been publicly belittled, scapegoated, and blamed as with the Cleveland, Orkney and Beckford cases in the UK in the 1980s and Trudder House, Madonna House, and the McColgan case in Ireland in the 1990s. In the UK, social workers, health authorities, education, and the courts were criticised in a radical manner that was new for all concerned and had far reaching consequences for the way child protection and welfare was to be approached thereafter. The rule of optimism, so favoured by practitioners in their dealings with families, was actively challenged in early reports, and social workers were asked to use both the law and authority invested in them to much greater degrees and alter their attitudes (Wroe, 1988). In relation to the oft-quoted Jasmine Beckford case, for example, the Government Report concluded that her death was "both a predictable and preventable homicide" (1985, p. 287). The report on Kimberley Carlile noted that UK social work practice was dominated by an historical approach dividing child care from child health, which made little sense in the context of child protection (London Borough of Greenwich, 1987, p. 13).

Removing children from the home environment is taken very seriously by all Irish social workers and child care workers as is placing children in "special" schools such as the Youth Encounter Projects (Bates, 1996; McKenna, 1996). Amazingly, despite all the emerging literature and inquiries focusing on risk, a question that is rarely asked by researchers is, "How do children themselves perceive risk in their lives?" (Ferguson & O'Reilly, 2001; McElwee, 2001).

This is a hugely important question in terms of framing a risk consciousness around special education for at-risk children and young people in this country. There is a great deal of public emphasis on listening and promoting the views of children and yet their voices have been largely absent in the framing of policies and practices until very recently. On a positive note, the National Children's Strategy (Department of Health and Children, 2001, p. 6) outlines one of its goals where "children will have a voice in matters which affect them and their views will be given due weight in accordance with their age and maturity." It remains to be seen how this will translate into practice for the majority of at-risk children and young people, but this study will, at least, assist in raising considerably the profile of youth at-risk as my aspiration is that its publication will interest many in the academic and policy communities.

BREAKING THE CYCLE: CHALLENGING THE RELUCTANCE TO STUDY AT-RISK CHILDREN

The failure of schools to prepare children and young people adequately for the workplace is a common theme in international research as is the cost effectiveness of certain schools. How, then, can schools create zones of resiliency around at-risk children? How can schools establish both protective factors and intervention strategies at the same time whilst getting on with the main task of teaching accredited subjects? How can they attract children and adolescents whilst creating and maintaining an environment where scholarly work can be undertaken?

There is some positive news. The Irish National Anti-Poverty Strategy (1997), *Sharing in Progress,* and the revised National Anti-Poverty Strategy (2002), *Building an Inclusive Society,* represent a major policy initiative by the Irish State to place the needs of the poor and socially excluded at the top of the national agenda in government policy development and action. Three key targets have been set in the revised National Anti-Poverty Strategy (2002): (1) To halve the proportion of pupils with serious literacy difficulties by 2006, (2) To reduce the proportion of the population aged 16-64 with restricted literacy to below 10 to 20 percent by 2007 (restricted literacy being defined as falling below 200-225 on the International Adult Literacy Survey scale or equivalent), and (3) To reduce the number of young people who leave the school system early, so that the percentage of those who complete upper second level or equivalent will reach 85 percent by 2003 and 90 percent by 2006.

One initiative for disadvantaged populations or at-risk children that precedes such enlightened thinking is the Youth Encounter Project, of which there are four: one in Limerick, two in Dublin, and one in Cork. The realities of the children's exposure to and experience of education in its broadest sense has to be actively negotiated and adapted to fit into their own particular worldviews. The Youth Encounter Projects recognise that the potential of the school environment is very strong as a protective mechanism. They are, thus, resiliency led.

THE STUDY:
A SOCIO/ECOLOGICAL, RISK-FOCUSED APPROACH

This study argues that children and parents are compromised to significant degrees by their environment. The ecological frame of reference is increasingly common in the at-risk literature (Bronfenbrenner, 1979; Garbarino, 1982; Garfat & McElwee, 2004; Jack, 1998; McElwee, 1996b; Ungar, 2002) to evaluate interactions between individuals and their social environments to see how functioning is undermined or enhanced (Garbarino & Sherman, 1980). This approach acknowledges that one cannot alter one aspect of family functioning without altering other aspects of family relations. The nature and character of the phenomena under study have a number of contextual factors that cannot be ignored. Education, as a process, occurs both inside and outside the formal school environment and is *affected* as opposed to being *determined* by a number of factors (Hixson & Tinzmann, 1990; U.S. Department of Education, 1997). Social ecological research also illustrates that social networks can act as protective barriers from the negative impacts of marginalisation and poverty, but also that they can be stressful and contribute to harm to children (Cochran, 1993).

In his early work Bronfenbrenner (1979) argued that changes in the exo-system and macro-system have both reciprocal and bi-directional influences on all other ecological systems. Children and young people are continually affected (albeit, to differing degrees) by even the smallest changes in their environments. Because of this, ecological systems theory has much to contribute to understanding why some children end up significantly at-risk whilst others do not. It is in the accumulation of a number of recurring negative stressors, or influences, that the risk profile increases for a child as additional burdens, traumas, and tragedies weigh heavily on any individual.

In relation to Ireland, recognition of these factors has been the trend in literature on resiliency over recent years (Gilligan, 1998; 2000; McElwee, 2004). Parents are now openly encouraged to participate in education and other aspects of their children's lives in relation to youth services more generally (Forkan, 2001; Garfat & McElwee, 2004). Certainly, the work of many professionals involved in this study has been unique in terms of the totality of the human experience seen and recorded in case files, care plans, and team plans for children categorised as at-risk. Of course, some children and adolescents do not perceive themselves as being in the slightest bit of risk or danger and regard work with them as an unwelcome intrusion into their lives (Dunphy, 2006). One's professional training in child policy, protection and welfare, and child care/social care should prepare one for this fact. It often does not. The 1980s and 1990s redefined, redesignated, and reconstructed child protection and welfare. The resultant fragmentation and confusion is surely the challenge facing young at-risk children in general and the children of St. Augustine's Special School in particular.

DELIMITATIONS AND KEY ASSUMPTIONS

When one compares the findings of risk and resiliency-related research carried out in Ireland with that of commentators in the United States (US Department of Education, 1997) and in the UK (Donaldson, 1978; Gilles, Elwood, & Hawtin, 1985; Rutter; 1979), one realises that Irish children are better off by a thousand fold in comparison to some of their international peers. Irish children are not shot dead on the streets by police or army hit squads as is reputed to be the case in Rio de Janeiro or experimented on by unscrupulous scientists, as was the case in other countries such as under the Nazi regime in the 1930s. They are not forced into military service as with some African countries today. There are, however, varying degrees of hostility and ambivalence shown towards what are understood to be "dysfunctional," "out-of-control," "problem" children, and Ireland does not have an unblemished record.

Over 1000 school children do not transfer between primary and post-primary education annually. This is a national scandal given the fact that Ireland introduced the concept of the Celtic Tiger to economists the world over with our supposedly wondrous economic system that made the cover of Time magazine. At the height of the Tiger's roar, the 1998 National Assessment of English Reading revealed that 10% of children still exit primary school with significant literacy problems despite the reductions in class sizes, increases in library resources, and in the availability of learning support teachers in recent years.

Some of the Limerick children and youth I first met in the summer of 1995 when I began to think about this research spent periods in Dublin, Clonmel, Cork, and Limerick, either in residential care for young offenders, in prison or on release. Some admit to being users of controlled substances. On the other hand, the majority of interviewees could be said to have broadly done well when one takes into account their family and personal histories and reasons for entering the Youth Encounter Project system in the first instance. Of course, the precise understanding and measurement of "doing well" is open to interpretation. I might point to the work on risk by Zygmunt Bauman (1991) who notes the emergence of a less probabilistic risk-taker who bets more than he can lose, uses hands that he is unsure of, and bets money he does not have. This is a useful analogy for the children and young people in this study as they are so vulnerable to adversity.

CONCLUSION

A significant percentage of the difficulties being experienced in schools at the start of the twenty-first century are largely connected with the very significant changes the Irish family is undergoing, hence the concentration on exploring the dynamics of families in this study. Coleman (1992) has argued that while locating the primary source of distress within the family, we have failed to identify the ecological embeddedness of families in the larger society. Separating at-risk children from their family and community environment and then expecting them to perform and succeed in formal school examinations is fraught with problems as predicting potential success and failure is a much more subtle, complex process. Due regard must be given to where youth live, their family circumstances and history, their peers and their expectations and ambitions if any intervention policies are to be truly effective in the long term (see Benard, 1999).

Many commentators, such as the German sociologist, Ulrich Beck (1992), and John Coates (2003), suggest that living and working in the *risk society* is fraught with potential and catastrophic danger for everyone. But is this the way children and young people from inner-city Limerick, Ireland, view the world?

Partly in an attempt to answer this, the theoretical discussion on risk in this study commences by examining the socio-political debate around risk and the "risk society." The work of such influential writers as Ulrich Beck, Anthony Giddens, and Mary Douglas suggests that trust and risk have become both politicised and radicalised. Child protection, welfare policy, and practice in the Republic of Ireland may be usefully interpreted from a perspective that Ferguson (1997) has termed a "radicalised consciousness of risk." Ireland is modernising in a late-modern world, characterised by fragmentation and polarisation, and coping with this fragmentation is surely the challenge facing young people in general and the pupils of St. Augustine's Special School in particular. We cannot be certain of anything in the risk culture that now pervades child and youth care. In Giddensian terms, we have become all too aware of risk and danger.

This book, then, examines some of these global and regional issues. I challenge the notion that we can prosper simply by taking a consumerist view of progress. I challenge the views and beliefs held by those who suggest that it is up to each child and young person to "make it on her own." The creed of individualism has a number of negative attributes that cannot go unanswered. It is the children and youth of Limerick, and cities and towns like Limerick all over the world, who end up "walking the roads." It is the teachers and child and youth care workers who intervene.

REFERENCES

Anglin, J., & Glossop, R. (1987). 'Helpers in the war over the family.' *Journal of Child Care, 3*(2), 1-19.

Anthony, J., & Cohler, B. J. (Eds.). *The invulnerable child.* New York: The Guilford Press.

Bates, B. (1996). *Aspects of childhood deviancy: A study of young offenders in open settings.* Unpublished doctoral dissertation. Dublin: University College Dublin.

Baizerman, M. (1990). *At risk students: A review of some basic issues.* Unpublished manuscript, prepared for the Texas Education Agency. Austin: Texas.

Bauman, Z. (1991). *Modernity and ambivalence.* Cambridge: Polity Press.

Beck, U. (1992). *Risk society. Towards a new modernity.* London: Sage.

Benard, B. (1999). Mentoring: New study shows the power of relationship to make a difference. In N. Henderson, B. Benard, & N. Sharp-Light (Eds.), *Resiliency in action* (pp. 93-99). Gorham, ME: Resiliency in Action, Inc.

Boyd, V. (1993). *School context: Bridge or barrier for change.* Austin, Texas: Southwest Educational Development Laboratory.

Bronfenbenner, U. (1979). *The ecology of human development: Experiments by nature and design.* Cambridge, MA: Harvard University Press.

Casas, F. (1995). Social research and policy-making. In M. Colton, H. Ghesique & M. Williams (Eds.), *The art and science of child care.* Aldershot: Arena.

Coates, J. (2003). *Ecology and social work: Towards a new paradigm.* Halifax: Fernwood Press.

Cochran, M. (1993). 'Parenting and personal social networks.' In T. Luster & L. Okagaki (Eds.), *Parenting: An ecological perspective.* Hillsdale: Lawrence Erlbaum Associates.

Coffield, F. (1983). *'Like father like son: The family as a potential transmitter of deprivation.* In N. Madge (Ed.), *Families at risk.* London: Heinemann.

Cohen, M. J. (1997). 'Risk society and ecological modernisation: Alternative visions for post-industrial nations.' *Futures, 29*(2), 105-119.

Coleman, H. (1992). Good families don't . . . *Journal of Child and Youth Care, 7*(2), 59-68.

Combat Poverty Agency. (1995). *Bridging the Divide: A Submission to Government for the 1995 Budget.* Dublin: Author.

Department of Health and Children. (2001). *National Children's Strategy.* Dublin: Author.

Donaldson, M. (1978). *Children's minds.* London: Fontana.

Dryden, J., Johnson, B., Howard, S. with McGuire, A. (1998). Resiliency: A comparison of construct definitions arising from conversations with 9-12 year old children and their teachers, *Proceedings of the American Educational Research Association Meeting,* San Diego, April 13th-17th.

Dunphy, S. (2006). *Wednesday's children.* Dublin: Gill and McMillan.

Durkheim, E. (1915). *Elementary forms of religious life.* New York: Macmillan.

Durkheim, E. (1979). *Essays on morals and education.* In W. F. F. Pickering. (Ed.). Routledge.

Durrant, M. (1993). *Residential treatment: A cooperative competency-based approach to therapy and programme design.* New York: W.W. Norton.

Egan, O., & Hegarty, M. (1984). *An evaluation of the Youth Encounter Project.* Dublin: Educational Research Centre, St. Patrick's College.

Ennis, J. (2006). *Goldcrest falling.* Dublin: Dedalus.

Ferguson, H. (1997). 'Understanding man and masculinities.' In *Men and Intimacy: Proceedings of a Conference hosted by St. Catherine's Community Services Centre, Carlow and Accord.* Carlow.

Ferguson, H., & O' Reilly, A. (2001). *Keeping children safe: Child abuse, child protection and the promotion of welfare.* Dublin: Farmer and Farmar.

Fewster, G. (1998). Introduction. *Journal of Child and Youth Care, 12*(1-2), p. vi.

Fewster, G. (1991). The paradoxical journey: Some thoughts on relating to children. *Journal of Child and Youth Care, 6*(4), v-ix.

Forkan, C. (2001). *Needs, concerns and social exclusion: The millennium and beyond.* Waterford: Centre for Social Care Research, Waterford Institute of Technology.

Garbarino, J. (1982). *Children and families in the social environment.* New York: Aldine Press.

Garbarino, J. (1992). *Children and families in the social environment* (2nd Ed.). New York, NY: Aldine de Gruyter.

Garbarino, J., & Sherman, D. (1980). High-risk neighbourhoods and high risk families: The human ecology of child maltreatment. *Child Development, 15,* 188-198.

Garfat, T. (1998). The effective child and youth care practitioner: A phenomenological inquiry. *Journal of Child and Youth Care, 12,* 1-2.

Garfat, T., & McElwee, C. N. (2001). The changing role of family in child and youth care practice. *Journal of Child and Youth Care Work.*

Garfat, T., & McElwee, N. (2004, 2007). *Effective interventions with families* (p. 1). Cape Town, South Africa: Pretext Publishers.

Garmezy, N. (1991). Resiliency and vulnerability to adverse developmental outcomes associated with poverty. *American Behavioral Scientist, 34*(4), 416-30.

Giddens, A. (1991). *Modernity and self-identity: Self and society in the late modern age.* Cambridge: Polity Press.

Giddens, A. (1992). *The transformation of intimacy.* London: Cambridge Press.

Gilles, P., Elwood, J., & Hawtin, P. (1985). Anxieties in adolescents about unemployment and war. *British Medical Journal, 291,* 383-4.

Gilligan, R. (1998). The importance of schools and teachers in child welfare. *Child and Family Social Work, 3,* 13-25.

Gilligan, R. (2000). Adversity, resilience and young people: The protective value of positive school and spare time experiences. *Children and Society, 14,* 37-47.

Hacking, I. (1982). Why are you scared? *The New York Review of Books, 29*(14), 30-3 and 41.

Hendrick, H. (1981). *The history of childhood and youth: A guide to the literature,* Oxford Polytechnic, Faculty of Modern Studies, Occasional Papers, 1, 1981.

Hill, M., & Tisdall, K. (1997). *Children and society.* UK: Addison Wesley Longman.

Hixson, J., & Tinzmann, M. (1990). *Who are the at risk students of the 1990s?* North Central Regional Educational Laboratory: Oak Brook.

Irish National Anti-Poverty Strategy. (1997). Dublin: NAPS.

Jack, G. (1998). The social ecology of parents and children: Implications for the development of child welfare services in the UK. *International Journal of Child and Family Welfare, 98*(1), 74-88.

Kasperson, R., Renn, O., Slovic, P., Brown, H., Emel, J., Gobel, R., Kasperson, J., & Langan, M. (1996). Series editor's preface. *Child protection and family support: Tensions, contradictions and possibilities.* London: Routledge.

Limerick Leader. (8.9.2001). Twilight Children Out in the Cold (p. 7).

London Borough of Brent. (1985). A child in trust (Jasmine Beckford Inquiry Report). London: Brent.

London Borough of Greenwich. (1987). *A child in mind: Protection of children in a responsible society: Report of the commission of inquiry into the circumstances surrounding the death of Kimberley Carlile.* London: Borough of Greenwich.

London Borough of Lambeth. (1987). *Whose child? The report of the panel appointed to inquire into the death of Tyra Henry.* London: Borough of Lambeth.

London Borough of Wandsworth. (1990). *Report of the panel of inquiry into the death of Stephanie Fox.* London: Borough of Wandsworth.

Luthar, S. (1991). Vulnerability and resilience: A study of high-risk adolescents. *Child Development, 62,* 600-616.

Lynch, K. (1999). *Equality in education.* Dublin: Gill and Macmillan.

Machlis, G., & Rosa, E. (1989). Desired risk: Broadening the social amplifications of risk framework. *Risk Analysis, 10*(1), 161-168.

Madge, N. (1983). *Families at risk*. Heinemann Educational Books, London.

Maier, H.W. (1979). The core of care: Essential ingredients for the development of children at home and away from home. *Child Care Quarterly, 8*(3), 161-173.

McElwee, N. (1996a). Research on crime. *The Irish Times.* 20.1.1996.

McElwee, N. (1996b). *Lone parents in the Republic of Ireland: Some sociological observations*. International Erazmus ICP Conference, University of Ulster at Jordanstown.

McElwee, N. (2000). *'Damned if you do and damned if you don't: Self-regulation or formal registration of social care workers in Ireland?'* Paper to Annual Conference of the Irish Association of Care Workers. Ennis, Ireland.

McElwee, N. (2001). *Using the creative use of self as an entry point into effective social care practice*. Paper to the Faculty and Students of the Social Care Programmes at Waterford Institute of Technology. 12.10.01.

McElwee, N. (2006). *Research with hard-to-reach populations*. Paper to the Faculty and Postgraduate Seminar, University of Victoria, Canada. 27.3.2006.

McElwee, N., & Lalor, K. (1997). *Prostitution in Waterford City: A contemporary analysis*. Waterford: StreetSmart Press.

McElwee, N., & Monaghan, G. (2005). *Darkness on the edge of town*. Athlone: Centre for Child & Youth Care Learning.

McKenna, S. (1996). *Walking the roads: The children of St. Augustine's*. Unpublished diploma dissertation. Waterford: Centre for Social Care Research, Waterford Institute of Technology.

McWilliams, D. (2005). *The Pope's children*. Dublin: Gill and McMillan.

Mid-Western Health Board. (1991). *Child care practice policy statement*. Limerick: Author.

National Economic and Social Forum Report Number 11. (1997). Dublin: Government Publications.

National Economic and Social Forum Report Number 26. (2002). Dublin: Government Publications.

National Forum for Early Childhood Education. (1998). Dublin: The National Forum Secretariat.

Nolan, B. (2000). Trends in child poverty 1999-2000. *Poverty Today, 46*, 4-5.

Parton, N. (1985). *The politics of child abuse*. London: McMillan.

Parton, N. (1991). *Governing the family: Child care, child protection and the state*. London: MacMillan Press Ltd.

Parton, N. (1996). Social work, risk and the "blaming system." In N. Parton (Ed.), *Social theory, social change and social work*. London: Routledge.

Redl, F., & Winemen, D. (1952). *Controls from within: Techniques for the treatment of the aggressive child*. New York: Free Press.

Richardson, V., Casanova, U., Placier, P., & Gulifoyle, K. (1989). *School children at risk*. New York: The Falmer Press.

Ricks, F., & Garfat, T. (1989). Working with individuals and their families: Considerations for child and youth care workers. *Journal of Child and Youth Care Work, 5*(1), 63-70.

Ritchie, J., & Spencer, L. (1994). Qualitative data analysis for applied policy research. In A. Bryman & R. Burgess (Eds.), *Analyzing qualitative data*. London: Routledge.

Russell, D.E.H. (1983). The incidence and prevalence of intrafamilial and extra-familial sexual abuse of female children. *Child Abuse and Neglect, 7,* 133-146.

Rutter, M. (1979). Protective factors in children's responses to stress and disadvantage. In M. W. Kent & J. E. Rolf (Eds.), *Primary Prevention of Psychopathology, Volume 111: Social Competence in Children.* Hanover, NH. University Press of New England.

Task Force on School Discipline. (2006). Dublin: Department of Education and Science.

Ungar, M. (2002). *Playing at being bad: The resilience of troubled teens.* Lawrence-town, NS: Pottersfield Press.

Ungar, M. (2004). *Nurturing hidden resilience in troubled youth.* Toronto: University of Toronto Press.

Ungar, M. (2005). Resilience among children in child welfare, corrections, mental health and educational settings: Recommendations for service, *Child & Youth Care Forum, 34*(6), 445-464.

U.S. Department of Education. (1997). *Educational reforms and students at risk: A review of the current state of the art.* Office of Educational Research and Improvement: Washington.

Werner, E. F., & Smith, R. S. (1992). *Overcoming the odds: High-risk children from birth to adulthood.* Ithaca, NY: Cornell University Press.

Wolin S., & Wolin, S. J. (1996). The challenge model: Working with strengths in children of substance-abusing parents. *Adolescent Substance Abuse and Dual Disorders, 5,* 243-256.

Wroe, A. (1988). Social work, child abuse and the press. *Social Work Monograph, 66.* Norwich: University of East Anglia.

doi:10.1300/J024v29n01_01

Chapter 2

From Risk to At-Risk

SUMMARY. The American economist, Frank Knight (1921), introduced risk as far back as the early 1920s with his analysis of profit legitimisation. In the profession of law, by the latter part of the 19th century risk had entered into mainstream social law in Europe (Ewald, 1991). Risk discourse seems to have regained popularity since the 1970s. Despite the voluminous work published since then with over three thousand books and articles by the end of the 1990s (Renn, 1998) there is no consensus regarding the risk construct itself, as it is approached from so many differing perspectives and disciplines. Many researchers tended, when writing about risk and children and youth, to focus on single variables such as intense interparental conflict that exacerbates maladjustment in children. This has now changed since the introduction of population health child and youth care perspectives. We are now far more interested in co-occurring adversities and the total, or whole, environment of a child. This chapter explores how and why a child or youth might be considered at risk exploring educational environments, the world of insurance, the natural world, medical discourse, and the world of the individual. doi:10.1300/J024v29n01_02 *[Article copies available for a fee from The Haworth Document Delivery Service: 1-800-HAWORTH. E-mail address: <docdelivery@haworthpress.com> Website: <http://www. HaworthPress.com> © 2007 by The Haworth Press, Inc. All rights reserved.]*

KEYWORDS. Children and youth at risk, educational disadvantage, at-risk indices, mental distress, youth work, child and youth care

---

[Haworth co-indexing entry note]: "From Risk to At-Risk." McElwee, Niall. Co-published simultaneously in *Child & Youth Services* (The Haworth Press, Inc.) Vol. 29, No. 1/2, 2007, pp. 29-56; and: *At-Risk Children & Youth: Resiliency Explored* (Niall McElwee) The Haworth Press, Inc., 2007, pp. 29-56. Single or multiple copies of this article are available for a fee from The Haworth Document Delivery Service [1-800-HAWORTH, 9:00 a.m. - 5:00 p.m. (EST). E-mail address: docdelivery@haworthpress.com].

There are a number of connections between the research problems presented in this book and the wider body of knowledge around risk and at-risk concepts. A reading of technical and non-technical literature[1] including material on children, adolescents, child and youth care, special education, resiliency, at-risk, and risk suggests that there is a notable shift from the earlier discourse on risk to at-risk to resiliency with the areas of marginalised, vulnerable, or at-risk children and youth receiving widespread attention over the past thirty years in academic literature and, particularly, in the Irish and international media over the past two decades (McElwee, 2001). Several influential factors affect the capacity for resiliency in a child attending school environments. These include but are not limited to attendance, ability, consistency, self-discipline, supervision, adequate teachers, adequate facilities, home environment, school environment, peers, and society. This chapter is, thus, organised around this view of at-risk.

This literature review illustrates that there is, in fact, no consensus regarding the risk construct itself, as it is approached from so many differing perspectives and disciplines such as the social and behavioural sciences, the physical sciences and, for a long time we relied on the supposed objectivity of science (McQuaid, 1998). In the past, many researchers tended, when writing about risk in the context of children and youth, to focus on single variables such as intense interparental conflict that exacerbates maladjustment in children. A move towards exploring mechanisms that underlie competent and healthy functioning is obvious in the international literature since the 1980s, particularly in the area of health promotion. Increasingly in North America, chronic and cumulative adversities are being studied in the context of co-occurring adversities (Coates, 2003; Garfat, 1998; Garfat & McElwee, 2001; Garmezy & Masten, 1994; Rutter, 1996; Ungar, 2002) and in Ireland (Boldt, 1994; Garfat & McElwee, 2004; Gilligan, 2000).[2]

TOWARDS AN UNDERSTANDING OF AT-RISK

Academic literature first referred to invulnerable rather than vulnerable populations acknowledging that there is a dynamic relationship between human vulnerability and the precarious character of social institutions. Researching what we now generally understand as hidden, hard to reach, elusive, vulnerable or special populations arose in the nineteenth century and several disciplines such as psychology, sociology, anthropology and, increasingly, child and youth care now have well-developed methodologies for viewing and analysing their subjects or research partners (McElwee & Monaghan, 2005).

How or why might a child or a youth be considered to be at risk? It is unfortunate that the term at-risk "is . . . particularly applied to young people whose prospects for becoming productive members of society look dim" (Hepburn & White, 1990, p. 5). We need to understand why their prospects have dimmed. Factors that can lead to problem behaviours in children and youth are typically classified within four realms: community, family, school, and individual/peer. These obviously relate to some societies and even within some cities and towns more than others.

> *Community:* The availability of drugs and weapons; an absence of community norms against drug use, weapons, and crime; media portrayals of violence; high rates of mobility into and out of the community; low neighbourhood attachment; extreme economic deprivation.

> *Family:* A family history of problem behaviour; family management issues; family conflict (such as physical and emotional abuse); ambivalent parental attitudes toward problem behaviour.

> *School:* Early and persistent anti-social behaviour; early academic failure; absence of commitment to school; engaging in problem behaviour; favourable attitude towards problem behaviour; early onset of the problem behaviour; personality factors.

> *Peer group and individual constitution:* An innate sense of rebelliousness; negative influence of peers who engage in problem behaviours; early onset of the problem behaviours.

Having obtained a generic understanding of at-risk, it is important to note that any attempt to define at-risk specifically in relation to educational intervention programmes is controversial. This is mainly because in the educational setting at-risk is most commonly related to dropping out of school. For me, it is much more complex than that and definitions must take account of differing cultures. For example, *The Goals 2000: Educate America Act of 1994* identifies an at-risk student as one "who, because of limited English proficiency, poverty, race, geographic location, or economic disadvantage, faces a greater risk of low educational achievement or reduced academic expectations" (U.S. House of Representatives Report 103-446, pp. 99-100). This understanding certainly would not have worked in an Irish context as English proficiency and race were not, until very recently, either a social or political issue.

My own understanding of educational at-risk suggests *the singular or combined characteristics of various ecological environments, in their totality, in which pupils hold a significant or, above odds, probability of failure of realising their potential.* Risk factors, then, are variables that *decrease* the probability of scholarly success for a pupil. Pupils are placed at-risk when they experience a significant mismatch between their circumstances and needs and the capacity or willingness of the school to accept, accommodate, and respond to them in a manner that supports and enables their maximum social, emotional, and intellectual growth and development.

RISK AVERSION VERSUS RISK ACCEPTANCE SOCIETY

How extraordinary! The richest, longest-lived, best-protected, most resourceful civilisation, with the highest degree of insight into its own technology, is on its way to becoming the most frightened. (Wildavsky, 1979, p. 32)

Risk calculation is big business and is seen to pervade every area of our lives from the internal (smoking, healthy eating) to the external (environment, governments).[3] The U.S. military budget request for the Fiscal Year 2006 is an incredible $441.6 billion and in 2005 it was $420.7 billion, yet the 2006 budget intends to spend only $1.9 billion for the Climate Change Science Program spread across 13 agencies. Where should one spend one's money to remain safe? Post 9/11, in the US at least, the discussion moved back and forth between what I might designate homeland (national security) and home (personal security). We are inundated in the mass media with daily stories of existing and potential doom and disaster and with the idea that life is now more fraught with risk than in the past. Issues such as whether risks are immediate or delayed, whether we can see risks and weigh them, and whether we can reduce risks in both a global and personal context dominate (Yeomans, 1984, p. 12). Just to take one example, between 1985 and 1999 14 percent of the world's weather catastrophes hit the U.S. However, these caused 58 percent of the world's insurance losses. The Insurance Services Office calculated that a hurricane-sized weather catastrophe hitting a major U.S. city such as Miami could cost insurers $50 billion and would bankrupt more than a third of American insurance companies. It is easy to see why there is such disquiet and how a sense of doom might pervade this industry. Such scenarios are not just hypothetical because

Hurricane Andrew, which hit Florida in 1992, cost insurance companies $17 billion and put several companies out of business.

Turner's (1978) nature and nurture disaster model is interesting in the global risk debate. He visualises knowledge and ignorance as being in place before the disaster and shock and surprise after the event. Humankind suffers from a failure of foresight. The concept of socio-technical systems is deliberately kept somewhat vague. Later, Turner (1994) acknowledges that one of the distracting mechanisms of postmodern existence is that the expert actors involved have different goals and strategies and are directed more by their individual agencies' theoretical and empirical models of discourse than by cooperation. At the crux of the risk debate lays a contentious problem: "How does one define risk in the first instance as risk includes a number of elements such as exposure, possibility, accident, injury and loss or profit?"[4]

Slovic et al. (1979; 1982) suggest that perceived risk is quantifiable and predictable and that people generally categorise risks in similar ways. To define something as a risk one needs to place this against something else or to use common parlance, "weigh it up." For example, a businessman rushing to work might weigh up the risk involved in potentially missing a meeting by opting for a mode of transport that has a time risk element involved e.g., a car ferry which, if all runs smoothly, will cut half an hour off his normal journey time. However, if the weather is poor it might actually add half an hour to his schedule. Our businessman must have some form of mental probability adjustment and different measures will lead to different conclusions about the perceived risk factor.

Individuals perceive risks in a somewhat insular manner (Langer, 1980; Fischhoff et al., 1981).[5] They tend to worry about future generations and future environmental degradation and engage in wonderful flights of rhetoric. Gray (1976) argued that people tend to regard risks and hazards that they believe are in their control less seriously than risks and hazards they see as extrinsic or external to their daily existence. Risks are always collective; it is only accidents that are personal (Ewald, 1991). The worst will not happen because we (think we) are in control. A useful example here is the risk involved in riding a motorcycle in Ireland (Bellaby, 1990). It has been estimated by the Insurance Federation of Ireland that one is 528 times more likely to be injured or killed on a motorcycle than in a car and yet thousands of people ride motorcycles every day. When I had a motorcycle, I tended to believe that because I was a competent rider I could limit the risks of being injured. Unfortunately, this proved not to be the case as a car that was driving the wrong way up a one-way street knocked me down. Having no protection other than a helmet, I broke several bones and became a risk statistic, because risk, in this framework, was perceived as external. The lesson was hard learned.

Studies of risk perception, then, generally fall into three categories: The first approach examines perceived risk by using groups of respondents in laboratory environments using psychometric tests. The second approach examines potential hazards of specific relevance to a subject population, within the context of a siting controversy. One regularly sees, for example, signs posted around Irish communities stating things such as "Carrick says no to dump" and "Ballina rejects Incinerator." The third approach examines potential hazards of specific relevance to subject populations such as exposure to mobile phone masts. Some twenty-five million mobile phones are in use in the UK and there a government-commissioned inquiry into mobile telephone safety warned in 2000 that children should be discouraged from using mobile telephones because of their potential health risks as children have thinner skulls, smaller heads, and their nervous systems are still developing which *could* make them more vulnerable to any potential adverse effects from the phones.

MEDICAL LITERATURE ON RISK

The latter part of the 1800s witnessed the acceptance of germ theories and contagion.[6] Ill-health became biological (Jones & Moon, 1983) with medicine turning more and more to allopathic principles (the use of large amounts of drugs to control symptoms). The early investigations in epidemiology sought largely to identify and contain disease entities of an acute and infectious nature and to view underlying processes.[7] It was only by the second half of the century that other disease determinants were located with illness increasingly seen as connected to societal, economic, cultural, and behavioural factors.

In the middle of the 20th century, Doll and Hill (1950) found links between smoking and lung cancer, which threw up the idea of risk indicators in epidemiology. A number of educational programmes for children at-risk in the United States were modelled on the famous Heart and Disease Prevention Model developed at Stanford University by Hawkins and his colleagues (1984) who focused on factors that increase the risk of heart disease such as family history, smoking, too little exercise, and a fatty diet. The authors discovered that people could prevent heart disease by reducing the risk factors in their behaviour. Their thesis was simple.

To prevent a problem from developing in the first instance, identify the factors that increase the risk of that problem and then directly address those problems by either eliminating them or their effects. Focusing on a harm approach as opposed to an uncertainty perspective in medical literature on risk, Kronenfield and Glik (1991) describe ". . . risk perception as reflecting a shift in peoples thought processes away from an emphasis on fate, luck or change, to notions of control" (p. 307).

In both medicine and the insurance industry, risk is identified by defining and measuring probabilistic outcomes and is defined in relation to a specific event. Werner (1990) noted the fact that the presence of risk factors does not guarantee a negative developmental outcome but, rather, increases the odds or the probability that problem behaviours will occur. The medical usage of the term carries with it the added implication that treatment or prevention of some kind is called for (Levine, 1990; Richardson et al., 1989). What is of particular note here is the origin of at-risk in epidemiology as this refers to the incidence, distribution, and control of disease in a population.

Because medical care is advancing steadily, attribution of injury and disease to behavioural causes (smoking, excessive alcohol consumption) inevitably arrive on the political agenda. The question then becomes which policies should the government pursue toward deliberate risk-takers? There is a strong philosophy in social policy that if one captures the market of at-risk children, one can control the spread of risk in later life or, to borrow a phrase from Giddens, "colonise the future."[8]

MORE SINNED AGAINST THAN SINNING IN THE AT-RISK DEBATE

Until recently, efforts have largely concentrated on the negative aspects of at-risk children and adolescents with generalised prescriptions leaving many questions unanswered. The participants in this study articulated a sense of being marginalised, stigmatised, and stereotyped by what they perceive as an overemphasis on their negative behaviours from police, teachers in the formal school system, and other professionals.

This focus on negativity has been identified as one of the failures of risk assessment in child protection and welfare strategic planning and in child and youth care practice more generally. Current research suggests that a majority of at-risk pupils actually go on to exhibit protective factors that shield them against failure. There is an over-concentration on non-accidental injury to children, despite the fact that genuine accidents injure more children statistically. There is also a societal fear that people with a mental illness are likely to kill other people and yet, statistically, they are more likely to kill themselves. In short, high-probability, low benefit outcomes are under explored. Such a scenario has led Bogenschneider et al. (1994) to comment that the compartmentalisation and isolation of youth from the wider ecology of family, peers, school, work settings, and community can no longer continue. Numerous social, economic, personal conditions, and circumstances can combine to place a child at-risk. Viewing childhood adversity through an exclusively deficit lens obscures seeing their resiliencies, coping mechanisms, and environmental adaptation, and yet research shows that resiliency amongst at-risk populations should not be underestimated.

The various difficulties in trying to use life stressors as effective measurement of at-risk status have been noted as their exact nature and extent is unknown (Gore & Eckenrode, 1996; Masten, Best & Garmezy, 1990). There is a significant amount of literature examining various perspectives to understanding risk as applied to educational discourse. As noted in the preceding discussion, there is general consensus that educational at-risk is inclusive of a host of factors that mitigate against a child succeeding as a productive member of society (Hepburn & White, 1990), and the language used is less pejorative than in the past. The home life of a pupil, psychological factors, personal circumstance, peer pressure, genetic predisposition (perhaps), school life, and the wider community are all understood as exerting a strong influence on the will and ability to succeed and to be resilient in the face of adversity (Farrington, 1996).

Past areas of research have tended to concentrate on eight categories of risk profiles with varying emphases in different systems: Prenatal stress and potential consequences for subsequent growth and well-being in infants and children, delinquent children and adolescents (with varying emphases on family environment as a source of stress and inadequate parenting), delinquent and criminal career paths, parental schizophrenia, affective disorders, antisocial behaviour, hyperactivity and attention deficit disorder and socially isolative behaviour.[9] At-risk may, then, be perceived as a function of deficiencies in, at least, some of these areas.

UTILISING THE TERM EDUCATIONAL DISADVANTAGE

It is worth commenting in some more detail on the term educational disadvantage as it shares some similarities in the Irish context with the more generic at-risk discourse in that there are several understandings of how it should be used and with which categories of vulnerable populations. The term educational disadvantage is continually used in Irish public discourse but to refer to differing phenomena. The Education Act (1998: 32 [9] refers to educational disadvantage as: "The impediments to education arising from social or economic disadvantage which prevent students from deriving appropriate benefit from education in schools." But how does this play out in the daily lives of those children and youth at-risk? We will return to this several times during this book.

The *Report of the Special Education Review Committee* (1993, p. 144) acknowledges that disadvantage, in the Irish context, has been mostly understood as referring to poor socio-economic environment. Therefore, the *area*, rather than the *individual*, has frequently been taken as the unit of measurement in past analyses. This is of particular importance as Rutter (1979) noted over a quarter century ago that some young people appear to be invulnerable to major life stresses because of assets in their environment that compensate for risk factors. The current Irish national policy in relation to addressing educational disadvantage covers three broad areas:

- Developing partnerships and coordinating government services.
- Targeting and restructuring resources and provision within the formal school system.
- Addressing the problem of early school-leaving and the needs of early school-leavers.

Why Use the Term At-Risk in Education?

One of the frustrating things about reading the risk literature is that a number of authors have written about the use of the term at-risk without being specific. The issue here surrounds the very understanding of risk and at-risk. Some authors tend to think of risk in terms of drug use (Mayock, 2000) and others in terms of school drop-out due to the child failing to see any relevance between its life and the school (Clancy, 1995; McElwee, 1996; Oakes, 1992). Others, still, discuss risk in terms of single moms (Byrne, 1997) or stress (Barnes, 1997) or examination failure (Ekstrom, Goertz, Pollack & Rock, 1986; Wagenaar, 1987).

The medical model assumes a mainly patient/doctor healing relationship, whereas the education model uses the pupil/teacher relationship. Both are more complex than this, as the pupil and patient may both be as reliant on environmental factors as internal coping and healing mechanisms. Pallas (1990) claims that untreated education problems can be as serious as untreated medical problems. The problem that faces the child and adolescent is one of system rather than internal control.

In Western countries, the concept of educational at-risk has been closely aligned to a conflict and, more recently, a left realist sociological perspective. *Blame* (in the context of risk and opportunity) was shifted early on in the debate by the power elites to a deficiency argument whereby the child was personally responsible for his or her failure (Goodland & Keating, 1990; Reder et al., 1993). One of the benefits of developing and using the term at-risk in an educational context is that it highlights and clarifies the general issue of students likely to have, or those currently experiencing, difficulties in the classroom.

A PERSPECTIVE ON CHILDREN AT-RISK FROM THE UNITED STATES

The official American perspectives draw on the mismatch factor, suggesting the greater mismatch, the greater level of risk for a child of dropping out of the system. North America has been struggling to meet the challenge of successfully educating all its students over the past fifty years (Hixson & Tinzmann, 1990) and it is widely acknowledged that children at-risk due to poverty, race, ethnicity and language are poorly served whilst in the formal school environment (Hilliard, 1988).

Dryfoos (1998) suggests that there are several different categories of at risk. Twenty percent of children she considers to be in the no-risk category, with 25% high risk and 10% in the very high-risk categories. Dryfoos (1998) summarizes the characteristics that are most common to high-risk youth:

- They tend to begin negative or risky behavior early (for example, purse snatching before the age of 10 or sex at 12)
- High risk youth tend to lack nurturing, caring, supportive parents
- They report high rates of physical or sexual abuse
- They tend to be failing or drop out of school
- They tend to conform to peer norms rather than society norms
- They tend to be depressed
- They tend to live in disadvantaged neighbourhoods
- Many high-risk youth do not know anyone in the work force, so they do not have role models of gainful employment.

Rutter (1979) established that the presence of one risk factor was not more likely to create dysfunction than when no risk factors were present, but with two risk factors there was four times the chance of problem behaviours and, with four risk factors, the risk increased as much as twenty times. Garmezy (1987) also suggested that having zero or even one risk factor does not denote a high level of risk but having two risk factors increases the likelihood of psychopathology by four times. Having four risk factors increases the risk by 10 times. Along with Rutter, Benson (1990) also viewed multiple risk factors and concluded that students with larger numbers of deficits are much more likely to engage in at-risk behaviours such as alcohol abuse and school truancy. Benson's study of Midwestern public school students (n = 46,799) found students with at-risk behaviours co-occurring (students using illicit drugs were also more likely to be sexually active). Similar correlations between substance abuse and increased sexual activity are found in the work of Mensch and Kandel (1988). Monk and Ibrahim (1984) found that the standardised test performances of students who regularly attended class might be negatively influenced by their classmates' truancy.[10]

UTILISING THE TERMS POVERTY AND SOCIAL EXCLUSION IN THE AT-RISK LANDSCAPE

The concept of poverty has its roots in a liberal vision of society where the lack of social resources in a competitive environment are understood as a benchmark, whereas social exclusion derives from the continental tradition where rights and obligations are located within a broad moral order (Room, 1995). Poverty may be understood as the state of being without the necessities of daily living and is understood as a relative concept in Townsend's (1979) influential study where he notes:

> Individuals, families and groups in the population can be said to be in poverty when they lack the resources to obtain the diet, participate in the activities and have the living conditions and amenities which are customary, or at least widely encouraged, or approved, in the societies to which they belong. Their resources are so seriously below those commanded by the average individual or family

that they are, in effect, excluded from ordinary living patterns, customs and activities. (p. 31)

Researchers also tend to favour the term social exclusion rather than poverty, as this is seen to be a more wide-ranging concept. The origin of the term social exclusion has been traced to Lenoirs (1974) book *Les Exclus, Un Francais Sur Dix*. Modernisation and urbanisation were the main causes of this social exclusion and the social services were understood as providing some form of solution. Kleinman (1998) acknowledges that social exclusion "used to be a term associated with French academic sociologists and worthy if impenetrable documents on Doing Good" (p. 6). Returning to an Irish context, Nolan and Whelan (1999) suggest that conceptions of cumulative disadvantage involve a number of assumptions:

- That a causal sequence over time is involved, such as from unskilled working class origins to adverse childhood circumstances, to absence of educational qualifications, to labour market failure;
- That earlier effects persist; e.g., childhood circumstances continue to have an effect when we take educational qualifications into account. Normally, this would involve the assumption that the earlier variable has both a direct impact on the outcome of concern, and an indirect one, which is mediated through later links in the causal chain; and
- The impact of earlier factors interacts with later ones. The most clear-cut example is where the consequences of early disadvantage for poverty or unemployment are exacerbated by the fact that a person is currently living in a deprived neighbourhood. (pp. 9-10)[11]

A number of themes have featured in Irish literature in relation to favouring particular terms such as poverty, on the one hand, and social exclusion on the other (Nolan & Whelan, 1999):

1. The need to move beyond a focus solely on low income and to adopt an approach that incorporates the actual experience of deprivation;
2. The importance of cumulative disadvantage and the emergence of patterns of generalised and persisting deprivation arising from the impact over the life-course of factors such as class origins, educational failure, labour market marginalisation, and household structure; and

3. The need to move from a static to a dynamic perspective, with attention being directed at the processes producing poverty or deprivation and contributing to cumulative disadvantage. (pp. 17-18)

SOCIAL CLASS AND THE AT-RISK CHILD

Schools of sociology differ as to which specific social traits are significant enough to define a class, although when sociologists speak of "class" in modern society they usually mean economically-based classes. In the early 1970s, Rawls (1972, p. 73) suggested that social class should not be a determinant in realising pupils abilities and aspirations. Nonetheless, there is a close association between lower socio-economic class and inferior outcome to a whole series of measures (when compared with more affluent groups) such as infant mortality, general health, educational attainment, or employment prospects (Gilligan, 1991). The risk of being poor (combining income and basic deprivation) rises from only one per cent at the top of the class hierarchy to about one in three for the unskilled manual class (Nolan & Whelan, 1999, p. 110).[12] Social class still continues to have an independent effect and cumulative impact on the risk of household poverty which, in turn, affects at-risk status.

POVERTY, SOCIAL EXCLUSION, STRESS AND AT-RISK

Stress is a medical term first used in 1936 by Hans Selye in the influential journal *Nature*. In common parlance, stress is associated with distress and accompanying burden, pressure, or hardship. Stress may be defined as the process of appraising events as harmful, threatening, or challenging; of assessing potential responses, and; of responding to these events. Responses may include physiological, cognitive, emotional, and behaviour changes (Lazarus, 1991; Taylor, 1991).

All Irish families are under a certain amount of stress (Garfat & McElwee, 2004; Kiely & Richardson 1995, Kiely, 2003). Demands are made on parents from so many fronts that some parents simply cannot cope because of their own poor socialisation processes. Indeed, it was suggested over a decade ago that 33% of children were in care because their parent/s were unable to cope (Gilligan, 1991) as opposed to the children being necessarily troublesome or out-of-control which is often the view amongst people within the general public.

Of course, a difficulty with young children is that they often lack the verbal skills and emotional maturity to express how they feel about stress and stressful events. Ayalon and Flasher (1993) argue that stressed children often exhibit school difficulties in the context of disruptive behaviour and excessive daydreaming. Jackson (1990) has made a connection between stress and lowered self-esteem and notes the damaging effect childhood stress can have on child parent relations.

With regard to the psychology of a family experiencing multiple stresses, such as poverty, Daly and Walsh (1988) discovered that 18% of poor households cited personal relationships as having deteriorated, with increased hostility. Twenty-one per cent admitted mental strain, and 16% felt that their children were suffering deprivation. Furthermore, as increasing numbers of women enter employment, the supply of relatives willing and able to provide child care is unlikely to keep pace with increased demand (Daly & Walsh, 1998).

TRUANCY AND YOUTH AT-RISK

The primary school day in Ireland must cover at least 5 hours and 40 minutes for 183 days per year. The secondary school year, for 167 days, may not last over 6 hours daily. Compulsory education begins at age six, but almost all fives and half the fours attend infant classes in primary school. The school-leaving age has been raised to 16 from 15. There is a great emphasis in Ireland on formal schooling.

Alongside poverty, truancy is recognised as a global problem in terms of placing young people at-risk of educational failure, although there are many definitional problems with using such a term (Task Force Report, 1981; U.S. Department of Education, 1997). Simply put, truancy refers to unendorsed absences from formal or compulsory schooling. Tyerman (1958, 1968), for example, reserves the term for children who are absent from school purely from their own initiative, but this fails to include children absent from school because their parent/guardian has asked them to not to attend.

The absence rate for schools in England was 6.83% in the 2002-3 academic year of which 6.13% were authorised absences such as illness and 0.7% were unauthorised. In Wales, overall, truancy or absences without permission rose from 1.6% to 1.7% in the school year of 2003-4. Wales' two biggest cities recorded the highest levels, with Cardiff pupils skipping 3% of sessions and Swansea young people 2.4%. In the UK, as a whole, some 55,000 children a day play truant from schools (The Times, 19.1.2006).

Three questions increasingly asked in research on truancy in the UK are (a) how many school students play truant? (b) what kind of students play truant? and (c) why do they play truant? (Stoll & O Keefe, 1989).[13] Some researchers prefer to use terms such as selective and serious truancy based on hours spent away from school (Gray & Jesson, 1990), whilst others still prefer terms such as blanket and post-registration (Stoll & O Keefe, 1989). Measuring truancy is also problematic. The most common measurements used globally are records from school daily attendance roles, but this form of measurement has been challenged because of inconsistencies in recording amongst teachers.[14]

THE IRISH RESPONSE:
THE SCHOOL ATTENDANCE/TRUANCY REPORT 1994

We also have a significant truancy problem in Ireland, which was one of the main reasons behind the establishment of the Youth Encounter Projects. In 1994, the Irish House of Parliament was informed by the Minister for Education that there were an estimated 30,000 children between 6 and 15 absent per day nationally. The *School Attendance/ Truancy Report* issued by the Minister for Education in 1994 studied the phenomenon of the non-attendance of children of compulsory school age on the "streets of cities" during formal school hours. As with the earlier Egan and Hegarty study (1984), the Working Group (as with the Department of Education's observations in 1979) was of the opinion that truancy is linked to problems in the family, peer pressure, and juvenile crime. The group also felt that truancy is premeditated. The group suggests that a truant category can include children who are out of the control of their parents, children who may have emotional problems, or those who refuse to attend for a variety of reasons such as "difficulty in keeping up," disciplinary problems, bullying, school phobias, or the inability to participate in school activity for financial reasons.[15]

Let us look to an early report for a moment as it influenced the Youth Encounter Project formulation. *The School Attendance/Truancy Report* (1994) specifically noted the need for a welfare service that would take better account of the ecosystem and included an emphasis on health and social and community aspects of a child's experiences. The Report also noted that the phrase "minimum education" used in the Irish Constitution of 1937 had "proved problematic over the years and had caused tensions between some families and the State as the Constitution also acknowledges that the family is the primary and natural educator of the child." Nonetheless, between 90% and 93% of primary school children attended school on a daily basis (p. 6) although the figure for disadvantaged schools is 4% lower than ordinary schools.

Again, one sees a correlation between what are termed disadvantaged areas and lower school attendance/truancy (p. 7) and this is mirrored by the experience nationally of school attendance officers. One of the more directly relevant observations of the Working Group for this study is in relation to the Youth Encounter Projects where they comment that the children come from disadvantaged families where there is often a lack of parental control or competence (School Attendance/Truancy Report, 1994, p. 10). This was supported in the findings of this study. Crucially, the Report acknowledges that official material on school attendance such as the Green Paper on Education mask drop-out rates in disadvantaged areas and there is no central database on non-attendees for attendance enforcement authorities to access.

A further important point the 1994 Report makes is that the complex and succinct differences between truancy and non-attendance are often ignored or overlooked by social commentators and policy analysts. The Working Group prefers a definition of truancy that *differentiates between these ends of a continuum.* It suggests that truancy is merely the visible side of non-school attendance and much needed attention may be deflected away from the root causes of truancy by focusing on the manifest and externalised problem behaviour of truants.[16]

The Working Group (1994) recommended the following:

> 4.4. In the case of persistent truants, the court should have the power to make an education supervision order aimed at re-establishing regular attendance at school. Moreover, detailed discussions should be held with the Departments of Health and Justice with a view to determining appropriate powers for school enforcement officers to investigate the circumstances and take action in the case of unsupervised children of compulsory school-going age found in public places without good cause, during school hours, having regard to the respective responsibilities of health board personnel and the Gardai in such situations. (pp. 9-10)

CONNECTING TRUANCY AND DELINQUENCY
IN "AT-RISK" CHILDREN AND YOUTH

In the majority of literature on at-risk children and youth we note that truancy and delinquency (however we want to define these) feature significantly. Indeed, as early as 1925, Burt claimed such an association. Truancy is closely linked to disruptive and delinquent behaviour in more recent research (Bates, 1996; McElwee, O Connor, & McKenna, 2006). A point of concern is that there is evidence to suggest that persistent truants tend to marry each other and then encourage truancy in their children (Robins et al., 1979). This was also the case with my own findings in this study.

A criminological interest in risk may be seen as early as 1851 in the work of Carpenter, who assessed the "dangerous classes" of juveniles in prison. A sociological comprehension of risk has entered the criminology debate also although risk, in this context, has been undertheorised (Ferraro, 1995; Hollway & Jefferson, 1995; Priest, 1990). The major interests of criminologists in the risk debate lay around the stigmatising effects of predicting high risk, injustices resulting from (inevitable) cases of false prediction, and ignoring the results of controversial research findings (Farrington & Tarlington, 1985). It has been argued that the entire academic and political debate about fear of crime in Britain is driven by the relationship between risk (of victimisation) and fear (Holloway & Jefferson, 1995, p. 2). There is a level of disagreement between the official position of the state (Hough & Mayhew, 1985) and the new realist position articulated by Jones et al. (1986) in determining levels of risk and fear.

In the United States, Ferraro and LaGrange (1987) and Bursik and Grasmick (1987) have also commented on the lack of consensus in "fear of crime" analyses. Distinctions between types or dimensions of fear of crime are crudely made in research literature with the result that the public is misinformed on important points. Rountree and Land (1996) have examined perceived risk versus fear of crime and observe that, "at the individual level, the effect of gender is different across models, and routine activities variables are somewhat better predictors of burglary-specific fear in comparison to risk perception" (p. 1353). Priest (1990) argues that the court system in the United States looks more and more for the contribution to the occurrence of harm in its deliberations than it does to causation and, for Beck (1995; 1995a), the individual gets caught up in the social and becomes regulated by the group.

Farrington et al. (1995) also found that if one takes a snapshot of just one area of risk behaviour, that of juvenile crime, one notes that dominant predictors of juvenile delinquency include family criminality, poverty, and poor parental child-rearing behaviour (Farrington et al., 1995). In a Canadian study, sound educational achievement was identified as being one of four protective factors against re-offending (Hoge, Andrews & Leschied, 1996), a point also mirrored in a UK study on vulnerability and delinquency carried out by Farrington (1996). A Hawaiian study on risk and resiliency noted the benefit teachers can have on a population (Werner & Smith, 1992) and Glover et al. (1998) observed the connections between motivation, emotional well-being, and academic performance. In an Irish context, Gilligan (1996, 1998, 2000) has outlined the importance of a positive school environment as a potential risk negator for children experiencing adversity.

CHILDREN, YOUNG PEOPLE, AND MENTAL ILLNESS

International epidemiological evidence suggests a prevalence of mental illness among children and adolescents ranging from 8% to 21% with higher rates in adolescence than childhood.[17] In Carr's analysis of three major epidemiological studies of psychological disorders amongst children, he suggested there are between 100,000 and 160,000 young people in Ireland with psychological problems (Carr, 1993, p. 557). There were 105 children under the age of 15 and 704 between the ages of 15 and 19 admitted to Irish psychiatric hospitals/units in 1996. More recently, out of a sample of 187 children in residential care in Ireland, Scotland, Finland, and Spain, the EUROARRCC Report (1998) says that over 60% had *clinically significant* emotional and behavioural problems [italics mine] (p. vii). The Eastern Health Board has recently established a number of Special Care Units whose emphasis is therapeutic work with children so seriously does it perceive the problem of "psychologically disturbed" youngsters to be.

The newspaper of record in Ireland, *The Irish Times* (8.11.2005), ran a front page headline in November 2005 titled "26% of teens have mental problems–survey." It presented findings from a study completed by the Health Service Executive in the South East area of Ireland with a sample group of 4,500 children between the ages of 1 and 18. Seventeen percent of the children under age five were reported as suffering from mental health problems. Ten percent of the 12-18 year olds surveyed said that they had suicidal thoughts during the previous six months and 7% had engaged in deliberate self harm.

Another study from Northern Ireland, with a total of 64 children across five childcare teams in Craigavon and Banbridge indicated that more than 60% of 4-10 year olds assessed may have had a diagnosable psychiatric disorder with the presence of such a disorder probable in almost 50%. Among the 11-16 year olds assessed, the proportion likely to have a diagnosable disorder is slightly higher at almost two-thirds of the sample group. A significant number of children appeared in more than one diagnostic category, indicating the complexity of their presentation and probable co-morbid diagnoses (Teggart & Menary, 2005).

POVERTY AND MENTAL ILL-HEALTH

One outcome of poverty is resultant inequalities in health. Mortality and morbidity rates are closely linked with socio-economic status, and there is a clear gradient in health status with those of lowest such status carrying a disproportionate burden of ill health (Balanda & Wilde, 2004). Where this becomes hugely important is in the recognition that health status in early years is one of the determinants of ill health, educational achievements and employability later in life. In the United States at least 20% of all adolescents suffer some emotional problem, and one third of adolescents under professional help suffer depression (Wright, 1997, p. 1). Adolescents from minority and/or ethnic backgrounds are over-represented in all studies of psychological disorders (Rutter et al., 1976; Carr, 1993).

There are a number of global commonalities in relation to family adversity and psychological disorder (risk predictors) which include maternal depression, single parent families, marital discord, maternal dissatisfaction with parental role, large family size, lack of social support, financial problems, and poor educational attainment. All of these features are closely corelated with poverty. Gomm (1996) writes succinctly:

> For nearly every kind of illness, disease or disability, "physical" and "mental," poorer people are afflicted more than richer people: more often, more seriously and for longer–unless of course, they die from the condition, which they do at an earlier age. (p. 110)

As some of the parents of the children in this study have unmet requirements, their mental health is a predictor of risk in the mental health of their children. For example, research by Weissman (1990) indicates that children of depressed parents are at-risk for anxiety disorders and depression themselves, and Orvaschel, Walsh-Allis, & Ye (1988) note that attention deficit disorders in children may have roots in (their) parental depression. Thus, we can see a possible connection to the truancy debate as noted earlier.

CONCLUSION

The Southwest Educational Development Laboratory (retrieved January, 2006, from http://www.sedl.org) notes that the conceptual origin of the term at-risk as it is applied in education is somewhat optimistic, because it generates a sense of urgency for pupils. It seems to me that simply viewing a child as at-risk simply because he or she does not fit the formal educational system is to place the emphasis for intervention in the wrong place. It is also my experience that some pupils who exhibit none of the more obvious identified risk factors will still drop out of school, while others who are characterized by several predictors succeed quite well in school with little or no targeted interventions.

The concept of risk includes both an objective component (a perceived probability) and a subjective component (a perceived danger). Risk factors may exist before a problem or disorder; may be time-limited or continue over time; may derive from the individual, the family, the community or the more general environment, and may play a causal role. Risk is not certain. It is inaccurate to automatically assume a direct cause and effect relationship between a risk factor and a specific outcome. We also know that risks interact, multiplying the potential effects.

The at-risk discourse generally centres on descriptive, prescriptive, unilateral, and school factor models. Sociological understandings of risk and risk behaviours map these out as social action(s), full of meaning and continually negotiated within a social environment. The social relationships between the child or young person and family, peers, and school become increasingly important.

The North American organisation, *Pathways* (http://www.ncrel.org/sdrs/areas/at0cont.htm), begins its discussion on risk by focusing on three facts it considers integral to the at-risk debate:

- Students are not at-risk but are placed at-risk by adults.
- Building on student strengths (e.g., knowledge, experiences, skills, and talents, interests), rather than focusing on remediating, real or presumed deficiencies are the key.

- It is the quality of the entirety of the school experience, rather than the characteristics of the students, that will determine success or failure. The two can never be separated.

What researchers do generally agree upon is that students are placed at-risk when they experience a significant mismatch between their individual and structural circumstances and needs and what resources are available (McElwee, 2006; Ungar, 2006). The capacity or willingness of the school to accept, accommodate, and respond to them in a manner that supports and enables their maximum social, emotional, and intellectual growth and development whilst paying attention to their cultural and familial backgrounds plays a key role in deciding whether or not the children will become resilient in the face of risk. How, then, is resiliency understood in the literature?

NOTES

1. Technical literature includes reports of research studies and theoretical or philosophical papers characteristic of professional and disciplinary writing. Non-technical literature includes biographies, diaries, documents, manuscripts, records, catalogues and other materials that can be used as primary data or to supplement interviews and field observations (Strauss & Corbin, 1990, p. 48).

2. It is also worth noting that an overemphasis has been on the family at the expense of the individual child in the risk and resiliency debate.

3. The Environmental Protection Agency in the United States published over 5,000 pages on risk assessment guidance between 1985 and 1995.

4. Perils may be divided into three categories: Natural perils: acts or events beyond human control, e.g., catastrophic weather, disasters, disease. Human perils: action, inaction, or irresponsibility of person or group, e.g., theft, homicide, negligence, incompetence, dishonesty. Economic perils: actions of governments or large groups that impact or threaten organisational stability or operations, e.g., market factors, strikes, and technological advances.

5. This is apparent in the work of the anthropologist Willett Kempton (1991) who argues that his research respondents often failed to understand technical issues around issues such as global warming and, instead, related to concrete, personal experiences in defining their concerns.

6. One notes here the pioneering work of Koch, Erlich, and Pasteur.

7. An awareness of the importance of environmental and social factors in human disease etiology dates back to the time of Hippocrates (circa 460-377 AD).

8. UNICEF established global goals by the mid-1990s which included the elimination of neonatal tetanus, a reduction in the measles morbidity by 90%, reduction of measles mortality by 95%, achievement of 80% ORT use for diarrhoeal disease, eradication of polio in certain designated countries, the elimination of iodine deficiency disorders, success of the baby-friendly hospital initiative, elimination of vitamin A deficiency, elimination of guinea worm, and the achievement of 80% immunisation in

all countries (UNICEF, 1994, p. 56). The organisation views these as risk factors predictable, treatable and curable.

9. On a more micro-level, many of the parents, pupils, and ex-pupils in this study have indicated to me that they feel there is a notable breakdown between levels of expectations and the ability of the child, family, school, community and State to meet their expectations.

10. Of course, many at-risk behaviours co-occur due to cause and effect. Children who miss school are more likely to miss out on education and instruction and be at a loss later when it comes to examinations.

11. Commins describes social exclusion as a failure on the part of several structures:

  a. the democratic and legal system, which promotes civic integration;
  b. the labour market, which promotes economic integration;
  c. the welfare state system promoting what may be called social integration;
  d. the family and community system which promotes interpersonal integration (Commins, 1993, p. 4).

12. It is interesting to note that, by far, childbirth in Ireland took place in a hospital environment with the majority of babies being bottle fed (McSweeney, 1986), but despite this structured start, many children were at-risk even prior to birth at hospital because of factors such as one (or both) of their parents ill health, alcohol abuse, drug abuse, and lack of pre-parenting skills.

13. One intentional category of truancy during the Battle of Britain (1940) was somewhat encouraged by a safety edict that children returning to school at lunchtime should make their way to the nearest air raid shelter and stay there until the "All Clear" was signalled before making their way back to school–sensible advice, which was often debased by children staying outside to watch the overhead air battles (http://en.wikipedia.org/wiki/Truancy).

14. This was my experience with the St. Augustine's teaching staff. When the school records over the nineteen-year period were assessed, I quickly realised that there were various inconsistencies in information recorded.

15. Non-attendance in school is often associated with delinquent behaviour and truancy is one of the main reasons for referral to the Youth Encounter Projects.

16. It is an indictment of Irish child care services that vacant posts for School Attendance Officers have not been filled due to financial and staffing cut-backs in the local authorities. The Working Group has noted the School Attendance Officers becoming more and more involved in rescuing children at risk in the wider community in a wider context (1994, p. 23).

17. Fifteen per cent of the adolescents in Peterson's (1987) study experienced serious turmoil. In 1993, 7.3% of the population of the United States were young adolescents (19 million), with 20% of these living below the federal poverty line.

REFERENCES

Ayalon, O., & Flasher, A. (1993). *Chain reaction: Children and divorce.* London: Kingsley Publishers.

Balanda, K., & Wilde, J. (2004). *Inequalities in perceived health. A report on the all-Ireland social capital and health survey.* Dublin/Belfast, Institute of Public Health in Ireland.

Barnes, S. (1997). *Childhood stress.* Unpublished diploma dissertation. Waterford: Centre for Social Care Research, Waterford Institute of Technology.

Bates, B. (1996). *Aspects of childhood deviancy: a study of young offenders in open settings.* Unpublished doctoral dissertation. Dublin: University College Dublin.

Beck, U. (1995a). Freedom for technology: A call for a second separation of powers *Dissent, Fall,* 503-507.

Beck, U. (1995b). *Ecological politics in an age of risk.* Cambridge: Polity.

Bellaby, P. (1990). To risk or not to risk. Uses and limitations of Mary Douglas on risk-acceptability for understanding health and safety at work and road accidents. *The Sociological Review, 38*(3), 465-483.

Benson, P. L. (1990). *The troubled journey: A portrait of 6th-12th grade youth.* Minneapolis, MN: Search Institute.

Bogenschneider, K., Small, S., & Riley, D. (1994). An ecological risk-focused approach–youth at-risk issues. In A. C. Wagenaar & C. L. Perry (Eds.), *Study of resilient children and youth.* New York: McGraw Hill Book Company.

Boldt, S. (1994). *Listening and learning: A study of the experiences of early school leavers from inner city of Dublin.* Dublin: Marino Institute of Education.

Bursik, R., & Grasmick, H. (1993). *Neighbourhoods and crime: The dimensions of effective community control.* Lexington Books.

Burt, C. (1925). *The young delinquent.* London: University of London Press.

Byrne, A. (1997). Single women In Ireland. A re-examination of the sociological evidence. *Women and Irish society. A sociological reader* (pp. 415-431). Dublin: Beyond the Pale Publications.

Carr, A. (1993). The epidemiology of psychological disorders in Irish children. *Irish Journal of Psychology, 14*(4), 546-560.

Clancy, P. (1995). *Access to higher education: A third national survey.* Dublin: Higher Education Authority.

Coates, J. (2003). *Ecology and social work: Towards a new paradigm.* Halifax: Fernwood Press.

Commis, P. (Ed.). (1993). *Combating exclusion in Ireland 1990-1994: A midway report.* Dublin: The European Programme to Foster the Social and Economic Integration of the Less Privileged Groups.

Daly, M., & Walsh, J. (1988). *Moneylending and low income families.* Dublin: Combat Poverty Agency.

Doll, R., & Hill, B. (1950). Smoking and carcinoma of the lung: Preliminary report. *British Medical Journal, 11,* 739-748.

Dryfoos, J. (1998). *Safe Passages: Making it through adolescence in a risky society.* New York: Oxford University Press.

Egan, O., & Hegarty, M. (1984). *An evaluation of the Youth Encounter Project.* Dublin: Educational Research Centre, St. Patricks College.

Ekstrom, R. B., Goertz, M. E., Pollack, M., & Rock, D. A. (1986). Who drops out of high school and why? Findings from a national study. *Teachers College Record, 87,* 357-373.

EUROARRCC. (1998). *Care to listen: A review of residential child care in four european countries.* Dublin: Centre for Social and Educational Research.

Ewlad, F. (1991). Insurance and risk. In G. Burchell, C. Gordon, & P. Miller (Eds.), *The Foucault effect: Studies in governmentality* (pp. 197-210). Chicago: University of Chicago Press.

Farraro, K. (1995). *Fear of Crime: Interpreting victimisation risk.* New York: SUNY Press.

Farrington, D. (1996). *Understanding and preventing youth crime.* York: York Publishing Services.

Farrington, D., & Tarling, R. (1985). Criminological prediction: An introduction. In D. Farrington & R. Tarling (Eds.), *Prediction in criminology* (pp. 2-33). Albany, New York: State University of New York Press.

Ferraro, K., & LaGrange, L. (1987). The measurement of fear of crime. *Sociological Inquiry, 57,* 70-101.

Fischoff, B., Lichenstein, S., Slovic, P., Derby, S. L., & Keeney, R. L. (1981). *Acceptable risk.* New York: Cambridge University Press.

Garfat, T. (1998). The effective child and youth care practitioner: A phenomenological inquiry. *Journal of Child and Youth Care, 12,* 1-2.

Garfat, T., & McElwee, N. (2001). The changing role of family in child and youth care practice. *Journal of Child and Youth Care Work, 15,* 236-248.

Garmezy, N. (1987). Stress, competence, and development: Continuities in the study of schizophrenic adults, children vulnerable to psychopathology, and the search for stress-resistant children. *American Journal of Orthopsychiatry, 57*(2), 159-174.

Garmezy, N., & Masten, M. S. (1994). Chronic adversities. In M. Rutter, E. Taylor, & L. Hersov (Eds.), *Child and adolescent psychiatry* (3rd edition, pp. 191-208). Oxford: Blackwell.

Gilligan, R. (1991). *Irish child care services: Policy, practice and provision.* Dublin: Institute of Public Administration.

Gilligan, R. (1996). The role of teachers and schools in protecting children at risk of abuse or neglect, *Oideas* (Journal of the Irish Department of Education), *44,* 26-45.

Gilligan, R. (1998). The importance of schools and teachers in child welfare. *Child and Family Social Work, 3,* 13-25.

Gilligan, R. (2000). Adversity, resilience and young people: The protective value of positive school and spare time experiences. *Children and Society, 14,* 37-47.

Glover, S., Burns, J., Butler, H., & Patton, G. (1998). Social environments and the well being of young people, *Family Matters, 49,* 11-17.

Goodlad, J., & Keating, P. (1990). (Eds.), *Access to knowledge: An agenda for our nations schools.* New York: The college entrance examination board.

Gore, S., & Eckenrode, J. (1996). Context and process in research on risk and resilience. In R. Haggerty, L.R. Sherrod, N. Garmezy, & M. Rutter (Eds.), *Stress, risk, and resilience in children and adolescents: Processes, mechanisms, and interventions* (pp. 19-63). Cambridge, England: Cambridge University Press.

Gray, E. (1976). *Remarks on the problem of nuclear waste management. Proceedings of the 1976 Conference on Public Policy Issues in Nuclear Waste Management* (pp. 195-202). Washington, DC, National Science Foundation.

Gray, J., & Jesson, D. (1990). *Truancy in secondary schools amongst fifth year pupils.* Sheffield University: QQSE Research Group Educational Research Centre.

Hawkins, D. (n.d.). *Risk-focused prevention: Prospects and strategies.* Invited Lecture at the Co-ordinating Council on Juvenile Justice and Delinquency Prevention.

Hepburn, L., & White, R. (1990). *School dropouts: A two generation problem.* Public Policy Research Series. Athens, Georgia: The University of Georgia, Carl Vinson Institute of Government.

Hilliard, A. (1988). Public support for successful instructional practices for at-risk students. In Council of Chief State School Officers (Ed.), *School success for students at risk.* Chicago: Harcourt Brace Jovanovich.

Hixson, J., & Tinzmann, M. (1990). *Who are the at risk students of the 1990s?* Oak Brook, IL: North Central Regional Educational Laboratory.

Hoge, R., Andrews, D., & Lescheid, A. (1996). An investigation of risk and protective factors in a sample of youthful offenders. *Journal of Child Psychology and Psychiatry, 37*, 419-424.

Holloway, W., & Jefferson, T. (1995). *The risk society in an age of anxiety. Situating fear of crime.* Paper presented to the 1995 British Criminology Conference, Loughborough University. July 18th-21st.

Hough, M., & Mayhew, P. (1985). *Taking account of crime.* London: HMSO.

House of Representatives Select Committee on Children, Youth and Families. (1989). *Barriers and opportunities for Americas young black men.* Washington DC: Author.

Institute of Public Health in Ireland. (2001). *Report of the working group on the national anti-poverty strategy and health.* Dublin/Belfast: Institute of Public Health in Ireland.

Jackson, A. (1990). *Stress control through self-hypnosis.* Australia: Doubleday.

Jones, K., & Moon, G. (1987). *Health disease and society.* London: RKP.

Jones, T., Maclean, B., & Young, J. (1986). The Islington crime survey. Aldershot: Gower.

Kempton, W. (1991). Public understanding of global warming. *Society and Natural Resources, 4*(4), 331-345.

Kiely, G., & Richardson, V. (1995). Family policy in Ireland. In I. Colgan-McCarthy (Ed.), *Irish family studies: Selected papers.* Dublin: Family Studies Centre, University College.

Kiely, G. (2003). The situation of families in Ireland, 1996-2001. *The European Observatory on the Social Situation, Demography and Family.* Retrieved April 2003 at: *http://www.europa.eu.int/comm/employement_social/eoss/index_en.html*

Kleinman, M. (1998). Social exclusion and underclass. New concepts for the analysis of poverty. In H. J. Andreb (Ed.), *Empirical poverty research in comparative perspective.* Aldershot, UK: Ashgate.

Knight, F. (1921). Risk, uncertainty and profit. *London School of Economics and Politics.* New York: Kelley.

Kronefeld, J. J., & Glick, D. C. (1991). Perceptions of risk: Its applicability in medical sociological research. *Research in the Sociology of Health Care, 9*, 307-34.

Langer, E. (1980). The psychology of chance, In J. Dowie & P. Lefrere (Eds.), *Risk and chance. Selected readings.* London: The Open University.

Lazarus, R. (1991). Psychological stress in the workplace. *Journal of Social Behavior and Personality, 6*, 1-13.

Lenoir, R. (1974). *Les Exclus: Un Francais Sur Dix.* Paris: Le Seuil.

Levine, R. et al. (1990). Breast feeding saves lives: An estimate of breastfeeding-related infant survival. Maryland, US: Centre to Prevent Childhood Malnutrition.

Masten, A. S., Best, K. M., & Garmezy, N. (1990). Resilience and development: Contributions from the study of children who overcome adversity. *Development and Psychopathology, 2,* 425-444.

Mayock, P. (2000). *Choosers or losers?* Dublin: The Childrens Research Centre, Trinity College.

McElwee, N. (1996). *Children at risk.* Waterford: Streetsmart Press.

McElwee, N. (2001). *Perspectives from the Canadian child and youth care landscape.* Paper to the National Council for Educational Awards 2nd Working Party on Social Care.

McElwee, N. (2006). *Irish Society & Travellers: A child & youth care commentary.* Seminar to Faculty and Postgraduate Students at the University of Victoria, BC, Canada. March.

McElwee, N., & Monaghan, G. (2005). *Darkness on the edge of town: An exploratory study of heroin misuse in Athlone and Portlaoise.* Athlone: Athlone Institute of Technology.

McElwee, N., O'Connor, M., & McKenna, S. (in press). St. Xaviers boys home: Aftercare commentary. *Journal of Child and Youth Care Work.*

Mcquaid, J. (1998). The future of risk research. *Journal of Risk Research, 1,* 3-6.

McSweeney, M. (1986). *National survey of infant feeding practices.* Dublin: HEB.

Mensch, B. S., & Kandel, D. B. (1988). Dropping out of high school and drug involvement. *Sociology of Education, 61,* 95-113.

Monk, D. H., & Ibrahim, M. A. (1984). Patterns of absence and pupil achievement. *American Educational Research Journal, 21,* 295-310.

Nolan, B., & Whelan, C. (1999). *Loading the dice. A study of cumulative disadvantage.* Dublin: Oak Tree Press/Combat Poverty.

Oakes, J. (1992). Grouping students for instruction. In M. C. Alkin (Ed.), *Encyclopedia of Educational Research* (6th ed.) (pp. 562-568). New York: McMillan.

Orvaschel, H., Walsh-Allis, G., & Ye, W. (1988). Psychopathology in children of parents with recurrent depression. *Journal of Abnormal Child Psychology, 16,* 17-28.

Pallas, A. (1990). Who is at risk? Definitions, demographics and decisions. In W. Schwartz & C. Howley (Eds.), *Overcoming Risk: An Annotated Bibliography of Publications Developed by ERIC Clearinghouse* (pp. 1-25). Charleston, WA: ERIC/CRESS at AEL.

Priest, G. (1990). The new legal structure of risk control. *Daedalus, 119*(4), 207-228.

Rawls, J. (1972). *A theory of justice.* Oxford: *Oxford University Press.*

Reder, P., Duncan, S., & Gray, M. (1993). *Beyond blame–Child abuse tragedies revisited.* London: Routledge.

Renn, O. (1998). Three decades of risk research: Accomplishments and new challenges. *Journal of Risk Research, 1,* 49-71.

Report of the Special Education Review Committee. (1993). Dublin: DoES.

Richardson, V., Casanova, U., Placier, P., & Gulifoyle, K. (1989). *School children at risk.* New York: The Falmer Press.

Robins, L., Ratcliffe, K., & West, P. (1979). School achievement in two generations: A study of black urban families. In S. Shamsie (Ed.), *New directions in children's mental health.* New York: Spectrum.

Room, G. (1995). Poverty and social exclusion: The new European agenda for policy and research. In G. Room (Ed.), *Beyond the threshold*. Bristol: Policy Press.

Rountree, P., & Land, K. (1996). Perceived risk versus fear of crime: Empirical evidence of conceptually distinct reactions in survey data. *Social Forces, 74*(4), 1353-1376.

Rutter, M., & Madge, N. (1976). *Cycles of disadvantage*. London: Heinemann Educational Books.

Rutter, M. (1979). Protective factors in childrens responses to stress and disadvantage. In M. W. Kent & J. E. Rolf (Eds.), *Primary Prevention of Psychopathology (Volume 111): Social Competence in Children*. Hanover, NH: University Press of New England.

Rutter, M. (1996). Autism research: Prospects and priorities. *Journal of Autism and Developmental Disorders, 26*, 257-275.

Slovic, P. et al. (1982). Why study risk perception. *Risk Analysis, 2*, 83-89.

Slovic, P., Fischhoff, B., and Lichtenstein, S. (1979). Rating the risks. *Environment, 21*, 14-20, 36-39.

Stoll, P., & O Keefe, D. (1989). *Officially present: An investigation into post-registration truancy in nine maintained secondary schools*. London: Institute of Economic Affairs.

Task Force on Child Care Services, Final Report. (1981). Dublin: Stationary Office.

Taylor, S.E. (1991). *Health psychology*. New York: McGraw-Hill.

Teggart, T., & Menary, J. (2005). An investigation of the mental health needs of children looked after by Craigavon and Banbridge health and social services trust, *Child Care in Practice, 11*(1), 39-51.

The School Attendance/Truancy Report. (1994). Dublin: Government Publications.

Townsend, P. (1979). *Poverty in the United Kingdom*. Harmondsworth: Penguin.

Turner, B. (1978). *Man-made disasters*. London: Wykeman Publications.

Turner, B. (1994). The future for risk research. *Journal of Contingencies and Crisis Management, 2*, 146-156.

Tyerman, B. (1958). A research into truancy. *British Journal of Educational Psychology, 28*, 217-25.

Tyerman, M. (1968). (Ed.). *Truancy*. London: University of London Press.

Ungar, M. (2002). *Playing at being bad: The resilience of troubled teens*. Halifax: Pottersfield Press.

U.S. Department of Education. (1997). *Educational reforms and students at risk: A review of the current state of the art*. Washington: Office of Educational Research and Improvement.

Wagenaar, T. C. (1987). What do we know of dropping out of high school? In R. G. Corwin (Ed.), *Research in the Sociology of Education and Socialisation* (pp. 161-190). Greenwich, CT: JAI.

Weismann, M. M. (1990). Evidence for comorbidity of anxiety and depression: Family and genetic studies of children. In J. D. Maser & C. R. Cloninger (Eds.), *Comorbidity of mood and anxiety disorders* (pp. 349-365). Washington DC: American Psychiatric Press.

Werner, E. E. (1990). Protective factors and individual resilience. In M. Kessler & S. E. Goldston (Eds.), *A decade of progress in primary prevention* (pp. 205-234). Hanover: University Press of New England.

Werner, E., & Smith, R. (1992). *Overcoming the odds: High risk children from birth to adulthood.* New York: Cornell University Press.
Wildavsky, A. (1979). No risk is the highest risk of all. *American Scientist, 67,* 32-37.
Wright, P. (1987). The social construction of babyhood: The definition of infant care as a medical problem. In A. Bryman, B. Bytheway, P. Allatt & T. Keil (Eds.), *Rethinking the lifecycle.* London: McMillan.
Yeomans, L. (1984). Uncertainties in risk estimation and implications for risk management in industry. In L. Zuckerman (Ed.), *Risk in society.* John Libbey & Company Limited.

doi:10.1300/J024v29n01_02

Chapter 3

A Focus on the Personal and Structural: Resilience Explored

SUMMARY. It may be said that risk and resilience lie at two ends of a spectrum co-dependent on each other for existence. This chapter explores the concept of resiliency noting that it is used interchangeably within and between discourses and that there remains much disagreement around which factors constitute vulnerability and invulnerability. Gordon and Song (1994), for example, found that "the conditions we label as resiliency, resistance, invincibility and so forth, are relative, situational and attributional" (p. 31). This confusion has resulted in practitioners focussing too much on individual psychopathology (Lesko, 2001; Ungar, 2004; Wolin & Wolin, 1995). For the individual young person, her sense of personal and social empowerment can be dragged underneath the veil of expert lens which, I argue, is unhelpful as the focus moves to stated dysfunction and away from promise with an onus on the young person to, somehow, demonstrate exceptional outcomes or invulnerability in the face of risk and adversity. My own research and involvement with the St. Augustine's Project in Limerick City leads me to support Rutter's (1979) thesis that protective mechanisms operate as critical turning points in a child's life and can redirect his or her development. Those of us working with children and their families must be culturally sensitive in all of our attempts to make sense of their world. And it is their world. doi:10.1300/J024v29n01_03 *[Article copies available for a fee from The Haworth Document Delivery Service: 1-800-HAWORTH. E-mail address:*

[Haworth co-indexing entry note]: "A Focus on the Personal and Structural: Resilience Explored." McElwee, Niall. Co-published simultaneously in *Child & Youth Services* (The Haworth Press, Inc.) Vol. 29, No. 1/2, 2007, pp. 57-69; and: *At-Risk Children & Youth: Resiliency Explored* (Niall McElwee) The Haworth Press, Inc., 2007, pp. 57-69. Single or multiple copies of this article are available for a fee from The Haworth Document Delivery Service [1-800-HAWORTH, 9:00 a.m. - 5:00 p.m. (EST). E-mail address: docdelivery@haworthpress.com].

Available online at http://cys.haworthpress.com
doi:10.1300/J024v29n01_03

<docdelivery@haworthpress.com> Website: <http://www.HaworthPress.com>
© 2007 by The Haworth Press, Inc. All rights reserved.]

KEYWORDS. Resiliency, protective factors, youth work, child and youth care, resilience

There are many narrative accounts of resilience coming to the fore in Irish popular literature such as Frank McCourt's Pulitzer Prize winning *Angela's Ashes* (1996), Fergal Keane's *Letter to Daniel* (1996) and in child and youth care literature such as Susan McKay's *Sophia's Story* (1998) and Bernadette Fahy's *Freedom of Angels* (1999). We can go back to Anne Frank's *Diary of a Young Girl* to read harrowing accounts of survival despite significant odds being stacked against the narrators. How can one child thrive and another fail to thrive when living with the same family in the same neighbourhood? How can one child in a family remember a series of events with such vivid recollection, whilst a sibling has no memory of these events? Surely an answer lies in the individuality of each child, in how each child makes sense of and engages with the world with the perceived "barrage of hazards" (Anthony, 1987) or meaning-making (Garfat & McElwee, 2004). This is a resiliency approach. It is at the heart of understanding and practicing child and youth care and it is expressed so beautifully in the Youth Encounter Projects.

MAKING THE CASE FOR A RESILIENCY PERSPECTIVE

Resiliency is a term that is frequently thrown about in conversation so I am going to attempt to aid the reader in this chapter by limiting myself to thematic discussions with less than *four* points in each sub-discussion (because this is the number chosen by the youth in my study as meaningful). A plant is said to be resilient if it survives a harsh winter, a bird is said to be resilient if it breaks a wing but lives on and is eventually to fly away, and a trash can is said to be resilient if it does not break when one overfills it with heavy rubbish. Can all these different things be *resilient?*

In fact, resiliency derives from Latin roots meaning "to jump or bounce back" and may be defined, in a child and youth care context, as the ability to build and strengthen protective factors in families, schools, and communities. Werner and Smith suggested resiliency was a child's "capacity to cope effectively with the internal stresses of their vulnerabilities" (1982, p. 4). So, despite the many stresses heaped on a child, if the child survives and prospers, she may be said to be resilient. There is now a focus on prevention strategies in child and youth care and *being* resilient incorporates many dynamic, responsive elements.

The research on resiliency focuses on the perceived, potential and existing positive attributes of the child or youth which is crucial as it moves us away from a loss lens. Resiliency concerns itself with the ability to adapt to changes and to approach difficult problems and situations. It is suggested that resilient youth possess a set of qualities that foster a successful process of adaptation and transformation, despite significant risk and adversity in their lives.

There are dozens of definitions of resiliency from numerous sources. One of the leading commentators on resiliency, Garmezy (1991) defines resiliency as "the maintenance of competent functioning despite an interfering emotionality" (p. 466).[1] Rutter (1990) describes resiliency more abstractly as "the positive pole of the ubiquitous phenomenon of individual difference in people's responses to stress and adversity" (p. 181). Linquanti (1992) defines it as "that quality in children who, though exposed to significant stress and adversity in their lives, do not succumb to the school failure, substance abuse, mental health and juvenile delinquency problems they are at greater risk of experiencing" (p. 2), and Masten (2001) defines resilience as a "class of phenomena characterised by good outcomes in spite of serious threats to adaptation or development" (p. 228).

The nature of resilience has been conceptualised in four distinct ways, including good coping, opportunities for growth, beating the odds, and inoculation against future stress. There are two types of resilience: unhealthy and healthy. "Healthy" resilience is expressed through pro-social, compassionate, harmonious, adaptive behaviours. In contrast, "unhealthy" resilience is seen in the use of aggressive, controlling, withdrawing, or self-destructive behaviours. It is often the latter that presents itself in schools and projects for at-risk children and youth.

Protective factors may be broadly grouped into three categories: (1) individual characteristics (i.e., high IQ, high level of resilience, flexibility and a positive social attitude), (2) social bonds (notably warm, supportive, and affective relationships with parents and other adults), and (3) social support including positive social skills and socially acceptable pattern of behavioural norms. In the United States, researchers estimate that between 50% and 70% of children coming from at-risk environments actually grow up to become "confident, competent and caring persons"

(Werner & Smith, 1992) and this is significantly more than might have been expected. Further international research data suggests that assets are inversely related to risk behaviours, with assets appearing to be additive (Benson, 1990; Rutter, 1987). Also, each increment of assets is accompanied by a reduction in the number of risk behaviours. It seems reasonable to argue that a problem-focused approach has been only of limited value to researchers and practitioners in the prevention field, as not all young people are equally affected when confronted with the same risk factors. Far less research has concentrated on assessing the variables that can offset risk factors or enhance protective mechanisms than has on viewing risk factors in themselves (McDonald & McDonald, 1999; McElwee, 1996; Rutter, 1993). It is certainly the case that resilience is a source of strength in young people that is sustained or nurtured by caring and effective parents or other adult caregivers, positive learning environments in schools and access to community resources.

THREE STRANDS IN RESILIENCY LITERATURE

The concept of resilience has a fairly recent but well-established history in both theoretical and empirical studies with three strands in resiliency research having been identified. The first includes authors who viewed successful adaptation in the face of threatening or challenging circumstances (Masten, Best, & Garmezy, 1990). A second trend looked at how children and young people acquire resiliency traits, described by Flach (1988) as a disruptive and reintegrative process. A third wave builds on the second approach and focuses on critical disruptions that would result in the acquisition of protective factors. Resiliency is sometimes referred to as "retained competence" (Garmezy, 1996).

Resiliency is understood in some Canadian literature as consisting of a balance between stress and adversity, on the one hand, and the ability to cope and availability of support on the other (Mangham, McGrath, Reid, & Stewart, 1995). In this view, resiliency is a dynamic process and can strengthen an individual's coping mechanisms over time. Resilience has been referred to as "bouncebackability."

IS THERE SLIPPAGE IN USE OF THE TERM RESILIENCY?

It is suggested by Martineau (2001) that the origins of the term resiliency lie with child psychologists in the 1940s discussing "invulnerability to trauma." Martineau argues that there has been a "slippage" in the understanding and use of the term resiliency in relation to children and young people as the term more correctly refers to children who experienced extreme trauma but later exhibited successful social skills and school performance. Such resilience was then measured by various psychology tests. Martineau (2001, p. 2) notes three points of slippage; where the meaning moved from one of being "invulnerable" (Anthony, 1997) to being successful in dominant society, where research moved focus from small groups to larger at-risk and disadvantaged populations and, finally, to where children's symptoms of severe trauma were misinterpreted.

Other researchers suggest that resilience research began in the 1950s with those dissatisfied with the prevailing deficit model and that this is really only beginning to influence educational thinking with a paradigm change taking place (Howard, Dryden, & Johnson, 1999). Most commentators agree that children and youth can overcome the most horrendous circumstances if there are protective mechanisms in place, *or* if effective protective mechanisms are introduced and utilised. Partly because of this, Moskovitz (1983) terms resiliency "the quality of stubborn durability" and "the affirmation of life." In her follow-up study of survivors of Nazi concentration camps (a sure example of extreme trauma), she provides an example of resiliency:

> Despite the severest deprivation in early childhood, these people are neither living a greedy, me-first style of life, nor are they seeking gain at the expense of others. None express the idea that the world owes them a living for all they have suffered. On the contrary, most of their lives are marked by an active compassion for others. (Moskovitz, 1983, p. 233)

Such a perspective is echoed a decade later by Freiberg (1993) who defines resiliency as a multifaceted process by which individuals or groups exhibit the ability to draw the best from the environment in which they find themselves. Finally, Werner and Smith (1992, p. 4) note that a number of researchers prefer to employ the term resiliency (to risk) because it "implies a track record of successful adaptation ... and it also implies an expectation of continued low susceptibility to future stressors." The property of the family system that enables it to maintain its established patterns of functioning after being challenged and confronted by risk factors is termed *elasticity*. Therefore, resilience also includes the family's ability to recover quickly from some kind of trauma or transitional event, which is termed *buoyancy*.

THREE STATES IN RESILIENCY:
A CLOSER LOOK

Garmezy (1985) identified three *stages* in the search for understanding resiliency. Stage one identifies children at-risk who have good coping capabilities. Stage two involves searching for individual, familial and extrafamilial correlates of these abilities and stage three identifies the mediating processes. Later, Masten, Best, & Garmezy (1990) defined three *kinds* of resiliency. The first is an ability to "overcome the odds," which is an inner strength of some kind. The second type of resiliency involves an ability to incorporate a sustained, competent functioning in the face of serious trauma or stress, and the third involves the ability to recover from trauma.

As was noted earlier, the majority of literature around resiliency tends (a) to view it from an individual's perspective (Masten, Best, & Garmezy, 1991; Rutter, 1990, 1993) and (b) to adopt a long-term view of behaviour (Rutter, 1993), but there are four emerging research strands within this:

1. Longitudinal research on resilience in children (McElwee, 2000; Werner, 1984; Werner & Smith, 1982).
2. The study of resilience in inner-city children (Luthar, 1991; McElwee, 1996).
3. The study of children at-risk to adverse developmental outcomes (Garmezy, 1991; Rutter, 1979; Rutter, 1987; Rutter, 1990).
4. The investigation on children's competencies as protective factors in the face of risky situations (Garfat & McElwee, 2004; Luthar & Dornberger, 1993; McElwee, 2001).

It seems to me that what makes a child resilient is the *relative strength* of individual characteristics and external protective processes (supports provided by school staff, communities and families) compared to the influence of risks and vulnerabilities in the external environment (see Winfield, 1994, p. 2). There is a range of mechanisms influencing risk factors, and the features that constitute resilience will vary according to the risk mechanism (Rutter, 1993, p. 626). Rutter outlines the major protective processes that foster resilience as:

1. Reducing negative outcomes by altering the risk or the child's exposure to risk.
2. Reducing negative chain reaction following risk exposure.

3. Establishing and maintaining self-esteem and self-efficacy.
4. Opening up opportunities (cited in Winfield, 1994, p. 5).

In his influential article, *Resilience: Some Conceptual Considerations* (1993), Rutter notes that one of the predisposing risk factors to heart disease in infancy is being underweight, but the exact opposite is true when one reaches middle age if one becomes overweight. The manner in which an individual perceives life events differs from person to person and this can have a significant impact. Although weight itself is not a perception, some people, such as anorexics, simply cannot come to terms with their real weight (i.e., physical weight as measured). Rutter sums up by suggesting that we "focus on the specific processes that operate in particular circumstances for particular outcomes" (Rutter, 1993, p. 627). He observes that some people, due to their individual behaviour rather than family circumstance, create a range of risk experiences for themselves that are known to lead to psychopathological outcomes. Issues of control are important in predicting later risk vulnerability. Positive relationships with family, peers and authority figures are clearly important in assisting and promoting resiliency (Elder, 1986) as are positive experiences within environments (Rutter, 1993). Rutter concludes by stating, that we have some appreciation of *indicators* of risk and protective factors, a little understanding of the processes that they seem to reflect, but substantially less knowledge about how to influence those processes in order to increase resilience (p. 631).

IMPLICATIONS FOR CHILD AND YOUTH CARE RESEARCH

The implications of the findings of this review for research into children and young people at-risk are multiple. We have seen that it is not always helpful to adopt an epidemiological perspective as an ecological human-developmental approach may better suit research in discrete areas of child and youth care. Certain childhood risk factors create a vulnerability which gives greater effect to later, disorder-related risk factors (Health Canada, 1995). The emotional availability of parents, the school, and community are crucial to reaching children and young people and letting them see that there is another way of navigating relationships, choosing role models, and seeing a future for themselves (Benard, 2004).

In general, three particular resiliency approaches to designing programmes are favoured in the at-risk school climate:

- Universal programmes are aimed at the general population but in a
  defined setting such as all students in a school at a given time.
- Selective programmes aimed at target groups within the general
  population that research has identified as at-risk such as children
  of drug abusers and poor school achievers.
- Indicated programmes designed for children already designated as
  at-risk such as children coming from multi-agency families and
  children with psychiatric illness in their families.

We could reasonably argue that all children and young people are at-risk
from a number of internal and external sources but, clearly, some children
and young people could be considered more at-risk than others (McElwee,
2001; Ungar, 2004). This seems to have much to do with personal factors allied to familial and support factors (Garfat & McElwee, 2004;
Mangham *et al.*, 1995). However, we should also note that neither risk
nor resiliency are certain nor easily determinable and we must develop
more sophisticated tracking systems (Ferguson & O'Reilly, 2001;
Martineau, 2001). Research could usefully focus on those children and
youth that have not succumbed to risk and adversity. Furthermore, protective factors have strong cumulative effects in individual children's
lives with relationship construction across all three areas (family, school
and environment) identified as critical variables throughout childhood
and adolescence (Pence, 1988).

CONCLUSION

It is accepted that for resilience to be present there must be exposure
to risk. The literature on resilience varies greatly in its estimate of how
many children and youth "survive and thrive" (Ungar, 2004) with some
commentators suggesting about 10% of at risk children will grow up to
be resilient (Higgins, 1994) whereas Wolin and Wolin (1995) estimate
as much as 66% and even all at risk youth can be expected to beat the
odds and we see this in a later chapter. Discourse on educational risk and
resiliency is heavily influenced in more recent years by concentrating
on children's strengths, their family backgrounds and prior experiences,
varied teaching strategies, collaborative learning, school-wide restructuring programmes, creating schools within schools, and interdisciplinary

teaching teams. Benard (2004), in her review of the resiliency literature, notes the evidence that resiliency prevails in most cases by far–even in extreme situations, such as those caused by poverty, troubled families, and violent neighborhoods.

The deficits approach focuses on tracking practices, grade retention, pull-out programmes, ability grouping, high achievement learning environments and special education (Letgers et al., 1993; Levin, 1988).[2] A resiliency perspective can reframe they way in which we think about and engage with youth and their families because, "resiliency research offers a more positive and a more accurate perspective. It offers hope based on scientific evidence that many, if not most, of those who experience stress, trauma, and risks in their lives can bounce back. It challenges educators to focus more on strengths instead of deficits. Most important, it indicates what must be in place in institutions . . . for resiliency to flourish" (Henderson & Milstein, 1996, p. 3).

Maintaining a broader social focus on resilience targets our interventions in three ways: (1) risk prevention or reduction; (2) asset enhancement; and (3) facilitating protective mechanisms in youth (e.g., avoiding risk behavior) and in the family, school, and the community (Hawkins et al., 1992; Masten & Coatsworth, 1998). Let us celebrate a resiliency approach because the meaning that children and youth construct around their riskness and resiliency profiles is all too often overlooked. Egan and Hegarty (1984, p. 16), for example, note that the single most striking difference between children in the Youth Encounter Projects around Ireland as a whole and their counterparts in the local primary school, is in the *quality* of their home life. Simply put, family atmosphere, rather than family composition, is more likely to predict children at-risk of dropping out of school. This is an important point.

The importance of the total family environment is crucial in resiliency literature and I return to this in the analysis of interview data later. The link between a negative and chaotic home environment where a child cannot thrive because it is born into poverty, socially excluded, and discriminated against, and being at-risk becomes obvious early in the educational context.[3] Ungar (2004) makes the point that high-risk youth choose their pathways to resilience from within the various structures in which they find themselves.

Finally, a resiliency approach to marginalised or vulnerable children and young people can focus on the inner strengths of families, children, and their teachers within and outside the school environment. Understood in this manner, Lee and Bobko (1994) suggest that those individuals with a strong sense of self-efficacy "will try harder and persist longer"

(p. 364) if presented with protective measures. High expectations from school-teachers and child and youth care workers can assist in the promotion of resiliency in children and young people who daily struggle with adversity. I will return to these issues.

NOTES

1. Garmezy (1976) was one of the first authors to consider the line of protective factors and his interests have tended to center around research on families where there is mental illness or families where the situation might best be described as chaotic.

2. The Irish Government's *White Paper on Education* (1995) adopts a resiliency perspective in noting the importance of tackling educational disadvantage for pupils by ensuring "continuity and consistency of interventions . . . throughout their educational lives."

REFERENCES

Anthony, E. J. (1974). The syndrome of the psychologically vulnerable child. In J. Anthony & B. J. Cohler (Eds.). *The invulnerable child* (pp. 103-148). New York: Guilford Press.

Benard, B. (2004). *Resiliency: What have we learned?* US: Wested.

Benson, P. L. (1990). *The troubled journey: A portrait of 6th-12th grade youth.* Minneapolis, MN: Lutheran Brotherhood.

Egan, O., & Hegarty, M. (1984). *An evaluation of the Youth Encounter Project.* Dublin: Educational Research Centre. St. Patrick's College.

Elder, G. H. (1986). Military times and turning points in men's lives. *Developmental Psychology, 22,* 222-233.

Fahy, B. (1999). *Freedom of angels: Surviving Goldenbridge Orphanage.* Cork: The O'Brien Press.

Ferguson, H., & O'Reilly, A. (2001). *Keeping children safe: Child abuse, child protection and the promotion of welfare.* Dublin: Farmer and Farmar.

Flach, F. (1988). *Resilience: discovering a new strength at times of stress.* New York: Fawcett Columbine.

Freiberg, H. J. (1993). A school that fosters resiliency in inner-city youth. *Journal of Negro Education, 62,* 364-376.

Garfat, T., & McElwee, N. (2004). *Effective interventions with families.* Cape Town: Pretext.

Garmezy, N. (1971). Vulnerability research and the issue of primary prevention. *Journal of Orthopsychiatry, 41,* 101-116.

Garmezy, N. & Neuchterlien, K. (1972). Invulnerable children: The facts and fiction of competence and disadvantage. *American Journal of Orthopsychiatry, 42,* 328-329.

Garmezy, N. (1974). The study of competence in children at risk for severe psycho-pathology. In E. J. Anthony & C. Koupernik (Eds.), *The child in his family: Children at psychiatric risk, international yearbook* (Vol. 3). New York: Wiley.

Garmezy, N. (1976). *Vulnerable and invulnerable children: Theory, research and intervention.* Washington, DC: Journal Supplement Abstract Service, APA.

Garmezy, N. (1983). Stressors of childhood. In N. Garmezy & M. Rutter (Eds.), *Stress, coping and development in children* (pp. 43-48). New York: McGraw Hill.

Garmezy, N. (1985). Stress resistant children: The search for protective factors. In J. E. Stevenson. *Recent Research in Developmental Psychopathology. Journal of Child Psychology and Psychiatry.* (Book Supplement No. 4). Oxford: Pergamon Press.

Garmezy, N. (1987). Stress, competence and development: Continuities in the study of schizophrenic adults, children vulnerable to psychopathology, and the search for stress resistant children. *American Journal of Orthopsychiatry, 57*(2), 159-174.

Garmezy, N. (1991). Resilience in children's adaptation to negative life events and stressed environments. *Pediatric Annals, 20*(9), 462-466.

Garmezy, N. (1991). Resiliency and vulnerability to adverse developmental outcomes associated with poverty. *American Behavioural Scientist, 34*(4), 416-430.

Garmezy, N., & Masten, A. (1994). Chronic adversities. In M. Rutter, L. Hersov, & E. Taylor. (Eds.), *Child and adolescent psychiatry* (3rd edition, pp. 191-208). Oxford: Blackwell Scientific Publications.

Garmezy, N. (1996). Reflections and commentary on risk, resilience and development. In R. Haggerty, L. Sherrod, N. Garmezy, & M. Rutter. *Stress, risk and resilience in children and adolescents: Process, mechanisms and interventions* (pp. 1-18). Cambridge, England: Cambridge University Press.

Gordon, E. W., & Song, L. (1994). Variations in the experience of resilience. In M. C. Wang & E. W. Gordon (Eds.), *Educational resilience in inner-city America: Challenges and prospects* (pp. 27-43). Hillsdale, NJ: Lawrence Erlbaum and Associates.

Hawkins, J. D., Catalano, R. F, Morrison, D. M., O'Donnell, J., Abbot, R. D., & Day, L. E. (1992). The Seattle social development project: Effects of the first four years on protective factors and problem behavior. In J. McCord & R. E. Tremblay (Eds.), *Preventing antisocial behavior: Interventions from birth through adolescence* (pp. 139-161). New York: Guilford Press.

Health Canada. (1995). Resiliency: Relevance To Health Promotion-Discussion Paper. http://www.hc-sc.gc.ca/ahc-asc/pubs/drugs-drogues/resiliency-ressortpsycholoique/index_e.html.

Henderson, N., & Milstein, M. M. (1996). *Resiliency in schools: Making it happen for students and educators.* Thousand Oaks, CA: Corwin Press.

Higgins, G. O. (1994). *Resilient adults overcoming a cruel past.* San Francisco: Jossey Bass.

Hixson, J. (1993). *Redefining the issues: Who's "at-risk" and why.* Revision of a paper originally presented in 1983 at "Reducing the Risks," a workshop conducted by the Midwest Regional Center for Drug-Free Schools and Communities.

Howard, S., Dryden, J. & Johnson, B. (1999) Childhood resilience: review and critique of the literature, *Oxford Review of Education, 25*(3), 307-323.

Keane, F. (1996). *Letter to Daniel.* London: Penguin.

Lee, C., & Bobko, P. (1994). Self efficacy beliefs: Comparison of five measures. *Journal of Applied Psychology, 79*, 364-369.

Legters, N., McDill, E., & McPartland, J. (1993, October). Section II: Rising to the challenge: Emerging strategies for educating students at risk. *Educational reforms and students at risk: A review of the current state of the art* (pp. 47-92). Washington, DC: U.S. Department of Education, Office of Educational Research and Improvement. Available on-line: http://www.ed.gov/pubs/EdReformStudies/EdReforms/chap6a.html.

Lesko, N. (2001). *Act your age: A cultural construction of adolescence.* New York: Routledge & Falmer.

Levin, H. (1984). *Costs and cost-effectiveness of computer-assisted instruction.* Stanford, CA: Stanford University, California Institute for Research on Educational Finance and Governance.

Levin, H. (1988). Accelerated schools for disadvantaged students. *Educational Leadership, 44*(6), 19-21.

Linquanti, R. (1992). *Using community-wide collaboration to foster resiliency in kids: A conceptual framework.* San Francisco: Western Regional Centre for Drug Free Schools and Communities.

Luthar, S. (1991). Vulnerability and resilience: A study of high-risk adolescents. *Child Development, 62,* 600-616.

Luther, S., Dornberger, C. H., & Zigler, E. (1993). Resilience is not a unidimensional construct: Insights from a prospective study of inner-city adolescents. *Development and Psychopathology, 4,* 287-299.

MacDonald, K. I., & MacDonald, G. M. (1999). Perceptions of risk. In P. Parsloe (Ed.), *Risk assessment in social care and social work.* London: Jessica Kingsley Publishers.

Mangham, C., McGrath, P., Reid, G., & Stewart, M. (1995). *Resiliency: Relevance to health promotion: Discussion paper.* Ottawa: Alcohol and Other Drugs Unit, Health Canada.

Martineau, S. (1999). Critical discourse analysis of childhood resilience and the politics of teaching resilience to "kids at risk" in inner-city schools. Unpublished Dissertation. Canada: University of British Columbia.

Martineau, S. (2001, Winter). The risky business of translating resiliency research into advocacy practice. *BE Institute against Family Violence Newsletter,* 1-6.

Masten, A. S. (2001). Ordinary magic: Resilience processes in development. *American Psychologist, 65,* 227-238.

Masten, A. S., Best, K. M., & Garmezy, N. (1990). Resilience and development: Contributions from the study of children who overcome adversity. *Development and Psychopathology, 2,* 425-444.

Masten, A. S., & Coatsworth, J. D. (1998). The development of competence in favorable and unfavorable environments: Lessons for research on successful children. *American Psychologist, 53,* 205-220.

McCourt, F. (1996). *Angela's ashes: A memoir.* New York: Scribner.

McElwee, N. (1996). *Children at risk.* Waterford: Streetsmart Press.

McKay, S. (2004). *Sophia's story.* Dublin: Gill and McMillan.

Moskovitz, S. (1983). *Love despite hate.* New York: Schocken Books.

Pence, A. R. (Ed.). (1988). *Ecological research with children and families: From concepts to methodology.* New York: Teachers College Press.

Rutter, M., & Madge, N. (1976). *Cycles of disadvantage.* London: Heinemann Educational Books.

Rutter, M. (1979). Protective factors in children's responses to stress and disadvantage. In M. W. Kent & J. E. Rolf (Eds.), *Primary Prevention of Psychopathology: Social Competence in Children* (Vol. 3). Hanover, NH. University Press of New England.

Rutter, M., Maughan, B., Mortimore, P., & Ouston, J. (1979). *Fifteen thousand hours: Secondary schools and their effects on children.* Cambridge: Harvard University Press.

Rutter, M. (1980). *Changing youth in a changing society.* Cambridge, MA: Harvard University Press.

Rutter, M., & Giller, H. (1983). *Juvenile delinquency. Trends and perspectives:* Penguin.

Rutter, M. (1987). Psychosocial resilience and protective mechanisms, *American Journal of Orthopsychiatry, 57,* 316-331.

Rutter, M. (1988). *Developmental psychiatry.* Cambridge: Cambridge University Press.

Rutter, M. (1990). Psychosocial resilience and protective mechanisms. In J. Rolf, A. S. Masten, D. Cicchetti, K. H. Nuechterlin, & S. Weintraub (Eds.), *Risk and protective factors in the development of psychopathy* (pp. 181-214). New York: Cambridge University Press.

Rutter, M., & Rutter, M. (1993). *Developing minds.* Harmondsworth: Penguin.

Ungar, M. (2002). *Playing at being bad: The resilience of troubled teens.* Lawrencetown, NS: Pottersfield Press.

Ungar, M. (2004). *Nurturing hidden resilience in troubled youth.* Toronto: University of Toronto Press.

U.S. Department of Education. (1994, June). *Roosevelt Renaissance 2000* [On-line]. Available: gopher://gopher.ed.gov:10001/00/OVAE/school2work/promise/exam3.txt.

Werner, E. E. (1984). Research in review. *Young Children, 39*(9), 68-72.

Werner, E. (1990). Protective factors and individual resilience. In S. Meisels & J. Shonkoff (Eds.), *Handbook of early childhood intervention* (pp. 97-116). New York: Cambridge University Press.

Werner, E. E., & Smith, R. S. (1982). *Vulnerable but invincible: A longitudinal study of resilient children and youth.* New York: McGraw-Hill.

Werner, E., & Smith, R. (1992). *Overcoming the odds: High-risk children from birth to adulthood.* New York: Cornell University.

White Paper on Education, (1995). Dublin: Government Publications.

Winfield, L. F. (1994). *Developing resiliency in urban youth.* NCREL Monograph. http://www.ncrel.org/sdrs/areas/issues/educators/leadrsho/leOwin.htm.

Winnicott, D. W. (1965). *The maturational processes and the facilitative environment.* New York: International University Press.

Wolin, S., & Wolin, S. J. (1995). Resilience among youth growing up in substance abusing families. *Pediatric Clinics of North America, 42*(2), 415-429.

doi:10.1300/J024v29n01_03

Chapter 4

Riding the Juggernaut in the Risk Society

SUMMARY. There are irreconcilable and contested positions taken around the definition and understanding of risk. The purpose of this chapter is to locate risk discourse more solidly in a social scientific framework by providing an historical analysis of literature dealing with risk drawing from the fields of risk assessment and, later, the social sciences where two major families of theory have been developed by social scientists: the Psychometric Paradigm and Cultural Theory. "Risk society" is the term used by social scientists to describe modern society–one where tradition has broken down and scientific advances rather than nature dominate our lives. The consequences of human actions across a range of areas have introduced new sources of risk and uncertainty which serve to emphasise the risk(s) involved in making everyday decisions, and a central paradox to the risk society is that these risks are generated by the processes of modernisation trying to control them. In a risk society, traditional certainties and securities can no longer be assumed. Fundamental to this understanding of risk society is the connected breakdown in expert systems and this is particularly relevant to the world of child and youth care. doi:10.1300/J024v29n01_04 *[Article copies available for a fee from The Haworth Document Delivery Service: 1-800-HAWORTH. E-mail address: <docdelivery@haworthpress.com> Website: <http://www. HaworthPress.com> © 2007 by The Haworth Press, Inc. All rights reserved.]*

KEYWORDS. Risk and the social sciences, risk assessment, unmasking of science, risk and the moral order, the risk society

[Haworth co-indexing entry note]: "Riding the Juggernaut in the Risk Society." McElwee, Niall. Co-published simultaneously in *Child & Youth Services* (The Haworth Press, Inc.) Vol. 29, No. 1/2, 2007, pp. 71-101; and: *At-Risk Children & Youth: Resiliency Explored* (Niall McElwee) The Haworth Press, Inc., 2007, pp. 71-101. Single or multiple copies of this article are available for a fee from The Haworth Document Delivery Service [1-800-HAWORTH, 9:00 a.m. - 5:00 p.m. (EST). E-mail address: docdelivery@haworthpress.com].

Available online at http://cys.haworthpress.com
© 2007 by The Haworth Press, Inc. All rights reserved.
doi:10.1300/J024v29n01_04

For the purposes of this chapter I am going to concur with Rosa's definition of risk as "a situation or event where something of human value (including human themselves) has been put at stake and where the outcome is uncertain" (Rosa, 1998, p. 28). One view of risk includes a personal, private assessment of danger, whilst the other is a more public articulation of monumental risks which are pervasive, all around us, and cannot be effectively managed (see Coates, 2003). The latter acknowledges that the central feature of our dangers is that they are rapidly changing. Risks, essentially, are an attempt to make the incalculable calculable, and risk assessment literature accepts that some levels of risk can be deemed acceptable and manageable resulting in what may be termed a risk-benefit balance.

Humanity's restructuring of the Earth during the past two centuries may well exceed changes to the planet over the last billion years, and new boundaries of risk are increasingly (re)defined in the social sciences, with risk occupying that murky territory between private and social fears. Risks have become social events rather than an individual experience (Beck, 1995, p. 21). Here I explore and critique the work of some of the leading global voices in theoretical risk discourse such as Giddens, Beck, Lash, and Douglas. Then I discuss the question, "Has the emphases on threat and danger intensified the sociological awareness of risk?" On the one hand, Giddens argues that while social knowledge is no longer stable, it is, nonetheless, possible to create functional versions of knowing that can be reflexively adapted as circumstances change. Beck, on the other hand, argues more pessimistically that the disastrous consequences of unanticipated knowledge must be fundamentally challenged.

TRACING THE ORIGINS OF RISK

> Our public fears are endlessly debated in terms of probabilities: chances of meltdowns, cancers, muggings, earthquakes, nuclear winters, AIDS, global greenhouses, what next? There is nothing to fear (it may seem) but the probabilities themselves. (Hacking, 1990, pp. 4-5)

It is interesting to look back to the origins of the use of the term risk and one can trace a societal understanding of risk as far back as Hippocrates (circa 460-377 AD). Literature on risk is littered with historical references to early humans attempting to weigh up the possibilities of engaging in behaviour that was in some ways dangerous but in others potentially rewarding. Is it safe to leave the cave to hunt for animals? Is it safe to bathe in water where there might lie crocodiles? Is it safe to eat certain insects and flowers? How does one know if it is risky? More recently we have become interested in such questions as whether nuclear fusion is a safe option. Is it risky to let my child use a cell phone? Is it safe to consume genetically modified foods?

It may be suggested that the world's first risk assessors were the Asipu who lived in the Tigris-Euphrates valley about 3200 BC. These people acted as what we might understand, today, as risk consultants for the various peoples that might come to them. If a decision needed to be made concerning a forthcoming risky venture, such as a proposed marriage arrangement or a suitable building site, one could consult with a member of the Asipu who would identify the important dimensions of the problem, identify alternative actions, and collect data on the likely outcomes of each alternative (Oppenheimer, 1997). Admittedly, they were highly influenced by the gods and deeply influenced by magical and mysterious stellar signs; nonetheless they did embark on studies for their fellows which involved them taking measurements and crude data in order that they could predict the potential success or failure of a proposed venture The term risk has been conventionally defined as *something that can be ascribed a numerical value of some kind* (see Covello & Mumpower, 1985) and we see this particularly in environmental science, banking, and engineering today.

Other tribes were also active in risk assessment. The Naskapi, for example, were the most north-easterly of the Algonquian tribes, occupying parts of Quebec and Ungava peninsula, north of the Gulf of St. Lawrence and extending from the vicinity of lake Mistassini to Ungava bay on the North. Refinements from the Naskapi Indians' practice of using cracked animal bones to determine possible tribal strategy were made in professional risk assessment, and by the 16th to 18th centuries the basis for the current approach to risk assessment were well established. This included, for example, an appreciation of exposure and response as separate phenomena. Risk was understood now as the *probability* of an event occurring, combined with an accounting for the losses and gains that the event would represent if it came to pass.[1]

Giddens (1990) suggests that the word risk found its way into the English language in the 17th century and derives from a nautical term meaning to run into danger or to go against a rock. It replaced what was known as *fortuna* (fortune or fate). This thesis is supported by Ewald (1991) who states that risk developed from a neologism of insurance and was derived from the Italian word *risco*, which meant "that which cuts," hence "reef" and, consequently, "risk to cargo on the high seas." *Fortuna* was used alongside the French word *risque*.[2] About the history of the word risk, Slovic (1992, p. 119) writes with a jaundiced eye that "Human beings have invented the concept of 'risk' ... there is no such thing as 'real risk' or 'objective risk.'" Tell that to the hundreds of thousands of inner city children, but more of this later.

ASSESSING RISK ASSESSMENT

Risk was understood as being neutral because it took account of the probability of losses and gains. Curiously, where risks are greatest (imminent or imaginary) *fortuna* tends to return. It is in such a context that "notions of probability became embedded in modern ways of thinking" (Parton et al., 1997). Probably, the major shortcoming of risk assessment as an academic discipline is that ultimately it can be really only considered as subjective. Put simply, everyone has something to lose or win depending on the perceived risk and perceived resultant opportunity (one man's loss is another man's gain, so to speak). This is particularly the case when one looks to the world of consumer science where it is often articulated that scientists sell out to their sponsors in terms of how they present findings. One thinks here of the worlds of health care and pharmaceuticals where one continually is faced with what is euphemistically designated misinformation.

The scientists themselves do not agree on mathematical theories for risk. One UNESCO definition, for example, reads: *risk = hazard x vulnerability x potential loss* whilst another United States Department of Environment definition reads, *scenario risk = likelihood x consequences*. Still another definition from the business world reads *risk = threat x vulnerability x impact*. Ultimately, a hazard is something bad that might happen whilst risk is the likelihood that a bad thing will happen. Confusing, eh?

At the heart, then, of the "new" understanding of risk lies Starr's (1969) "revealed preference" approach to uncovering what risks might be considered acceptable by society. His major finding was that people will accept risks 1,000 greater if they are voluntary (e.g., driving a car) than if they are involuntary (e.g., a nuclear disaster). Later research in the 1980s by Slovic et al. reported the opposite where people generally saw most risks in society as being unacceptably high. They also found that the gap between voluntary and involuntary risks was not nearly as great as Starr claimed. There is opinion and counter opinion throughout the risk literature.

One attempt to be practical in the risk debate is the field of risk assessment which may be approached from a number of perspectives. Thompson (1986), for example, distinguishes between three types of risk assessment:

- Real Risk: The combination of chance and negative consequence that exists in the real world.
- Observed Risk: The evaluation of the combination of chance and negative consequence as measured by a theoretical model of the physical world.
- Perceived Risk: The estimate of real risk made in the absence of a theoretical model of the physical world.

Risk assessment remained somewhat crude until the incorporation of complex quantitative exposure assessment during the 1980s and 1990s.[3] Risk assessment has now entered mainstream discourse as a distinct intellectual discipline and is now understood as a scientific process which includes: (1) hazard identification, (2) hazard characterisation, (3) exposure assessment, and (4) risk of characterisation.

Rayner and Cantor (1987) argued that risk managers should no longer ask themselves, "How safe is safe enough?" but, rather, "How fair is safe enough?" They argued that the public was fearful of three separate dimensions in terms of social policy: how decisions are made, the acceptability of principles employed to apportion costs and benefits of such decisions, and whether the public should invest trust (when it comes to funding) in those who make, manage, and regulate technologies. This has percolated down to child and youth care and human services.

SCIENCE CAN NO LONGER BE TRUSTED?

So we have seen that risk has been problematised and is no longer seen by either the scientists or the public as a pre-given objective reality that exists "out there" but is actively constructed through social and cultural processes and frameworks of analyses. Risk is associated both with personal fate and with a complex political debate concerning power, governance, and the nature of personal freedom (Culpitt, 1999). Risk evaluations cannot, in their entirety, be performed as "expert" assessments divorced from the political decision making process and from social values in general.[4] Science is increasingly perceived to be the cause of modern environmental and health problems rather than a solution. We know that scientists have tended, in the past, not to disclose in public misgivings around environmental issues supposedly to "avoid unnecessary social conflicts before some conclusive policy measure is taken" (Morioka, 1987). And yet society has experienced a greater awareness of collective and individual risk (with)in the personalised context of living i.e., how we understand and see ourselves in the greater scheme of things and risk acceptance or rejection has become highly personalised because these very decisions scientists make affect us on every level (Rowe, 1977).

Disagreement amongst scientific and technical experts creates a vacuum that encourages a rampant individualism where risk is encapsulated in not only danger but also opportunity if short lived. The relationship between cause and effect, so central to scientific rationality, is suspended in the risk society where scientists and experts compete for public credibility and where knowledge is externalised. Within the framework of what sociologists term "reflexive modernisation," scientific knowledge is forced to face itself within the public arena. I will return to this concept later in this chapter.

Scientific credibility itself is a major issue. Allegations of misconduct by research scientists in the United States, to take but one example, reached record highs in 2004 where the Department of Health and Human Services received 274 complaints, 50 percent higher than 2003 and the most since 1989 when the federal government established a programme to deal with scientific misconduct. Indeed, research suggests this is but a small fraction of all the incidents of fabrication, falsification, and plagiarism, and a survey published in the journal *Nature* reported that 1.5 percent of 3,247 researchers admitted to falsification or plagiarism. (Las Vegas Sun, July 10, 2005). This has mainly to do with researchers saying they feel under pressure to deliver results and/or researchers wanting to make a name for themselves–but without the rigour in research one should expect.

A SOCIOLOGICAL CRITIQUE OF RISK:
A CAREERING JUGGERNAUT

The emergence of risk society focuses politics on the protection and securing of individual autonomy and not on social obligation or cohesion. Various disjunctions between how individual success will be protected, and escalating social need denied, has significantly altered our contemporary politics. (Culpitt, 1999, p. 40)

Since the 1970s, a number of social scientists such as Douglas (1973; 1982; 1985; 1992), Beck (1986; 1987; 1989; 1992; 1995, 1997; 1998) Ewald (1991), Luhmann (1979; 1988; 1993), Giddens (1990; 1991;1992; 1994;1995; 2006) and Lash (1993; 1994) have contributed to the social scientific discourse on risk. These commentators are interested mainly in the rise of social movements and the environment, the situation of the individual, and related discourses around politics.[5] Understanding risk is a central concern for living in any democratic system, because detailed scientific and technical information is essential to policy formulators and governments. As is noted in the analysis of the data in this study, the people who have to trust these expert scientists and technicians are the people who have to live with the outcome of decisions that have far reaching consequences. This includes service users and professional child and youth care workers and social workers.

IT'S RISKY TRYING TO AGREE ON A DEFINITION OF RISK

There are few agreed definitions of risk between and amongst the academic disciplines of sociology, social theory, anthropology, and economics. Fischoff et al. (1981) define risk as "the existence of threats" (p. 2) to life or health . . . as a chance of some kind of adverse outcome. Yates and Stone (1992) suggest that three elements of the risk construct include (a) potential losses, (b) the significance of those losses, and (c) the uncertainty of those losses (p. 4). In economic terms, the risk implications differ significantly when increasing the chance of liability from 1% to 5% if considering sums of $2,000,000 as opposed to $2,000 (Yates & Stone, 1992).

More formally, the Oxford English Dictionary defines risk as: "To hazard, endanger; to expose to the chance of injury or loss," and the Webster Comprehensive Dictionary defines risk as "a chance of encountering harm or loss; hazard, danger . . . to expose to a chance of injury or loss; hazard."[6] Alaszewski and Manthorpe (1991) define risk as "the possibility that a given course of action will not achieve its desired outcome but instead some undesirable situation will develop" (p. 277). Social and behavioural scientists have viewed demographic and contextual factors that influence perceptions of risk in society, which involve personal and societal value judgements.

Bilton, Bonnett, Jones, Skinner, Stanworth and Webster (1996) cast their net much wider and interpret risk as "a term encapsulating the distinctiveness of people's experiences of danger in late modernity" (p. 41). Increasingly, the threats we face are of global proportion and are side effects of social development. Risks, as opposed to older dangers, are consequences that relate to the threatening force of modernisation and to its global of doubt. They are politically reflexive (Beck, 1992, p. 21). Risk has become the chance of encountering loss or harm, but increasingly on a global level.

GIDDENS AND RISK

It is not that day-to-day life is inherently more risky than was the case in prior eras. It is rather that, in conditions of modernity, for lay actors as well as experts in specific fields, thinking in terms of risk and risk assessment is a more or less ever-present exercise (Giddens, 1991, pp. 123-4).

Giddens, who has been influential in the thinking of New Labour in the U.K., sees Britain as living in a post-traditional society in which the Risk Society is the context of politics. Giddens considered the concepts of modernity, late modernity, trust, opportunity and risk in his book, *The Consequences of Modernity* (1990), where he suggested that a number of factors are responsible for modernity being so fraught with risk. Giddens argued that we are forced to "ride the Juggernaut," because all of us are (merely) lay persons in a global society bound together by expert systems of knowledge. These systems of knowledge and control are difficult to question because many of them are complex to deconstruct and analyse in the first instance. Giddens develops the point that experts make mistakes, which *may* be catastrophic, and we cannot predict the fluid running of any expert system (italics my emphasis).

What is mostly assumed to be natural is, in fact, social. For him, the consequences of modernity include "the dissolution of evolutionism, the disappearance of historical teleology, the recognition of thoroughgoing, constitutive reflexivity, together with the evaporating of the privileged position of the West–moves us into a new and disturbing universe of experience" (p. 53). Risk can be divided into two types. External risk originates from events that happen frequently enough to be broadly predictable. It is something experienced as a cause derived from the fixities of tradition or nature experienced in earlier times as bad harvests, floods or the plague. Manufactured risk is created by the very progression of human development, especially science and technology. It is an unknown quantity because there are no historical parameters against which to judge it, and it makes managing risk difficult. No one can rely on answers from science because of the conflicting definitions of risk produced by the experts (Giddens, 2006).

Giddens is more hopeful of risk resolution (or reduction) than Beck, and his theory of risk includes a presumption "that risk reducing elements seem substantially to outweigh the new array of risks" (Giddens, 1991, p. 116). Later, Giddens (1994) argues that manufactured uncertainty does not necessarily ". . . mean that our existence on an individual or collective level is more risky than it used to be" (p. 21).

In his work, Giddens discusses risks and dangers to the environment and potential nuclear war and sees risk as an inevitable consequence of late modernity, as does Niklas Luhmann (1979; 1988) who looks to the separation of risk and danger. Indeed, Luhmann attempts a critical understanding of sociology where we should look beyond the surface for an understanding of risk from an historical and social change perspective involving the society's construction of reality itself. He refers to 'resonance' and constructs a theory of risk communication. Luhmann (1988) suggests that crucially, post-industrial societies have failed to solve "the problems of the natural environment" as "nature does not speak."

Giddens acknowledges that the sheer number of risks in respect of socialised nature is quite daunting, and both Luhmann and Giddens perceive (post)modern risk as a movement away from God and Godlike dangers to human created and controlled risks on massive environmental scales. They differ, however, in their *emphasis* on risk. Giddens (1990) claims that people react in different ways to threat of disaster. He delineates four different patterns of reaction: "pragmatic acceptance," "sustained optimism," "cynical pessimism," and "radical engagement" (p. 134). I return to these later in this study in the context of children and youth.

THE GLOBAL STAGE OF RISK

Our very existence is vastly influenced by the global stage. The oil crisis in the Middle East in the 1970s, for example, had severe economic repercussions in Ireland and the price of petrol rocketed with many people simply unable to use their cars to travel to work. We abandoned the fixed financial exchange system. There is, as Hafting (1996) suggests, an implication to think in *whole terms* now and we live in a condition marked out by anxiety and insecurity. Since 9/11 in the US, petrol and gas prices in Ireland have fluctuated between €1 and €1.30 a litre on the forecourts and any economic change in the US is immediately felt in Ireland.

Giddens (1990) contends that increased scientific knowledge does not infer an accompanying sense of control over our fate, individual or collective, national or international and, much as in the past, the physical world is full of hazards (real and imaginary). He elaborates: "By a risk profile I mean the particular portmanteau of threats or dangers characteristic of modern social life" (p. 110). We are pawns in the greater scheme of things. Luhmann (1988) asserts that refraining from action means that there will be less risk, but Giddens believes even *inaction* can be risky as forces external to us control our destiny. What is the ordinary person to think?

TRUST IN EXPERT SYSTEMS

Giddens (1990) elaborates on the concept of risk in a general sense mentioning, for example, the risk of getting into a car and travelling in it where risk is left to the expert system. Modern post-industrial lives are lived according to a set of assumptions and beliefs, such as roads and bridges will not collapse because they are structurally sound and have been well designed. Giddens tends to view these experts as (sometimes) hiding risks from the general public, the technically redundant person on the streets, who has to believe to an extent. The ordinary person in the street is forced to *trust* in an expert system outside his or her control, because this is one of the very constructs on which expert systems are based in the first instance. We can only hope to be expert in some areas of life, and it is in all the other areas that risks abound. He links trust and risk, "For the lay person . . . trust in expert systems depends neither upon a full initiation into these processes nor upon mastery of the knowledge they yield. Trust is inevitably, in part, an article of faith" (Giddens, 1990, p. 29).[7] Thus, when I power up my laptop each morning, I expect it to work and the anti-virus system I purchased on the internet at my home in Galway from somewhere in India will work to protect my all-important files. This is life in post-modernity or what is increasingly being called "hyper-modernity."

The connections between trust (which he sees as inter-linked with modernity) and risk occur where:

- Trust is basically bound up, not with risk, but with contingency.
- What risk presumes is precisely danger (not necessarily awareness of danger).
- There are some circumstances in which patterns of risk are institu- tionalised, within surrounding frameworks of trust.
- Risk is not just a matter of individual action. (Giddens, 1990, pp. 33-35).

In his discussion of risk, Giddens alludes to "globalising of risk" and returns to his familiar theme, that of nuclear war, although he cites Beck's idea (1986, p. 7) that certain risks transcend socio-economic sta- tus. The supply of risks follows most directly from the construction of human made environments.

SCIENCE DEMYSTIFIED

Only when medicine opposes medicine, nuclear physics opposes nuclear physics . . . can the future that is being brewed up in the test-tube become intelligible and evaluable for the outside world. (Beck, 1992, p. 234)

Lash and Wynne (1992) make the point that "in the public domain, science inexorably tends to refute itself as its culture of scientism cre- ates false claims and expectations in society at large" (p. 2), and Freudenberg (1993) has argued that due to the increased dependency on technical expertise, specialisms have come to dominate. The public evaluates and judges risk-related matters on whether or not it trusts those with power and responsibility for decision taking in a socially responsible way. Freudenberg's concept of "recreancy" denotes the failure of institutional actors to live up to the expectations the public has of them. This is particularly apparent in the area of child protection and welfare.

Increasingly, applied science is asked to mediate between expert systems. Indeed, Beck (1995) suggests that ". . . only with the help of complicated, and usually expensive, measuring instruments and methods can the nature and degree of the threat be determined" (p. 313). The problem now is that despite claims to rigorous and flawless methodology, a significant minority of the public no longer trusts applied scientists.[8] This extends into popular culture.

A POPULIST EXAMPLE

One of the highest earning films of the last two decades is Michael Crichton's *Jurassic Park* in which applied scientists and technologists have sold the public out for their own monetary rewards. The key players are all scientific doctors. In their attempt to promote science as God, they fail to think out fully the consequences of their actions. The results of their genetic coding are unpredictable and they fail to factor in chance in their risk analysis. This manipulation of science is a frequent theme in Hollywood where rogue or ignorant scientists and experts populate all professions.

The constant push and pull between humankind and the environment becomes important because the consequences of late-modern mistakes are global. We see this in the mistake of extracting resources from the Earth where, for example, within the lifetime of a child born today, petroleum, mercury, copper, nickel, lead, zinc and tin will disappear (New Road Map Foundation, 1991, pp. 8-9).

RISK, ONE-ARMED SCIENTISTS, EXPERTS AND MAD COW DISEASE

Science, Popper says, is built upon shifting sand; it has no stable grounding at all. Yet today it is not only scientific enquiry but more or less the whole of everyday life to which this metaphor applies. (Giddens, 1994, p. 87)

In the United States, Senator Muskie once famously called for one-armed scientists who do not respond, "On the one hand, the evidence is so, but on the other hand" when asked about the health effects of pollutants (cited in David, 1975). Scientists and experts claim to deal only in factual, logical argument and they do this by referring to abstract, external systems. They engage in issues of fact and correctness and are not necessarily interested in "appropriateness" or "goodness" (Glicken, 1996). This is where the public often diverges from the expert systems as the public is most interested in making sense of it all and does not generally wish to be bombarded by statistical data generated by what are seen to be detached scientists.

When mad cow disease came to the attention of the Irish public in 1996, we were inundated with various experts from the disciplines of veterinary science, microbiology, medicine, and nutrition informing us of what we should and should not eat. Mad cow disease has been linked to Creutzfledt-Jacobs disease in humans. In terms of Beck's risk discourse, what is so potentially catastrophic about BSE is that one infected cow could potentially infect 400,000 people according to a European Union scientific committee (Ahlstrom, 2000). Indeed, a number of countries banned Irish beef products and the Irish Minister for Agriculture was publicly ridiculed for his reaction to the scandal. In 1999, there were 95 cattle infected with BSE in Ireland, an increase of twelve from the preceding year. Those of us who transferred our allegiance to poultry have now to look elsewhere as a condition known as Newcastle disease is threatening to damage the poultry business. Finally, we can no longer reliably eat bacon as the experts recently informed us that studies completed on Irish bacon suggest that the bacon has a plus 15% antibiotic content above the European average which is potentially dangerous to one's health. What is one to do? The views of these experts will mean a change in the culinary habits of the Irish.

In effect, what happened was that a pervasive risk climate developed in both the UK and Ireland where scientific experts publicly disagreed on what, to the layperson, appeared to be very fundamental points such as, was it safe to hill-climb and play golf as leisure activities without the fear of spreading the virus? Was it safe to travel between Ireland and the UK? Was it safe for animals to be kept in enclosed areas with no access to public walkways?

The Irish government reacted very quickly in the initial stages of this scare. The perceived risks of foot and mouth disease entering into this country were taken very seriously and resulted in the Government banning many events, asking that national sporting and cultural associations defer events to a later date, placing mats with disinfectant at all points of public access to buildings, running advertisements across all media outlets, and having police checks on all border crossings (see Irish Times, 16.3.01).

The authorities in the UK adopted a different stance toward potential risk, believing that the risk of spreading the virus was far less than the Irish government feared. The government there refused to call for social and sporting events to be postponed and allowed greater mobility of travel for farmers with their livestock over the first thirty days after confirmation of the original case. The result of this is that cases exceeded over 1000 in mid-2001 and over 5000,000 healthy sheep had to be slaughtered. Once again, the public in both systems watched nightly as various expert biologists, virologists, and veterinary scientists argued in the media over potential risks to animals and humans.

An even more recent example relates to the infamous bird virus flu. The H5N1 virus, alone, has killed 50 people since its resurgence in Southeast Asia in late 2003. In March, 2005, the North Korean government admitted its first outbreak and that "hundreds of thousands" of chickens had been culled and their carcasses burned. However, the official news agency refused to state which particular strain of virus was involved, claimed that only "two or three" chicken farms were involved, and that the outbreak was "recent." This partial knowledge, or partial truth, contributes to a degree of fear amongst the public. It should be obvious at his stage that there are a number of actors in the risk debate as illustrated in various discussions above. For example, in areas of high-risk, Zebroski (1975) noted that fear sells and the media tend to dwell on potential catastrophes, not on day-to-day success.

Scientists themselves are largely to blame for disseminating misinformation to the public. This is partly to do with the fact that science is supposed to be exact (Giovacchini, 1984), but the scientific community continually identifies new products (related to the commercial environment), new illnesses (related to the medical environment), new substances (related to the industrial environment) and new ways of enumerating the risks of the above to us all. There are conflicting demands and expectations on the different streams of science and the results are often not compatible with one another's disciplines.

Some sociologists perpetuate the myth of science as power and the language used by scientists is often full of densely packed jargon that the public cannot access (of course, one might argue that this is the intention). Giovacchini (1984) observes, "We (the scientists) were bogged down in data and found a different answer from almost every expert. The lay people only had summary information from the press and media. Thus, they saw the issues in black and white, a simple yes or no. Perhaps they saw things more clearly" (p. 70). Of course, the public is, once again, left out of this process, and this has a damaging effect whereby the public then has to rely on a series of *versions* of the truth or what is euphemistically termed disinformation.

It could be argued that science empowered itself to determine and measure safety. The notion of "absolute safety" was popular for decades in risk literature and has now been deconstructed, but in accumulating knowledge science found even more risks for us to worry about so that nothing is safe (Giovacchini, 1984). Goulding (1984) makes the point in relation to the problems of the sciences in this area: "Toxicology unfortunately lends itself to political polarisation, expressed as the innocent, exploited public workers on the one hand and the multinational capitalist corporations inspired by cupidity on the other" (p. 47).

The news, however, is not all bleak. Lowrance (1976) believes that humankind may now actually be in a position to *manage* aspects of tragedy (in the risk debate) as this tragedy occurs. This point is crucial, as there is one theorist who rejects the idea of risk management in his highly influential risk society thesis. Beck (1995) acknowledges that there are two approaches to decontamination through science, "on the one hand, wholesale condemnation of any criticism of technology; on the other hand, obstruction of any new advance" (p. 503). His fear is that decision-making takes place in "a twilight zone where politics, science, and industry meet" (p. 506). The consequence of this is that decisions may be compromised by political agendas and not taken for the "right" scientific reasons.

BECK AND THE RISK SOCIETY

Environmental literature since the 1970s has become fragmented and, in many senses, contradictory. Hajer claims that radical environmentalism became supplanted in the latter part of the 1970s by "ecological modernisation"–a theme made popular by Giddens.[9] The power elites have successfully integrated with the eco-modernisation discourses.

Ulrich Beck, who draws heavily from the work of philosophers such as Martin Heidegger, Jacques Ellul, Theodore Adorno and Herbert Marcuse, is part of the European social ecology movement where social constructivism reigns supreme. Beck's (1992) *Risk Society* is written in a metaphorical style and questions the validity of risk society, high modernity and/or the transition to post-modernism (cf. Bauman, 1992; 1997).[10] At its heart, *Risk Society* is concerned with risk and reflexive modernisation.

BEING FEARFUL OF THE PRESENT AND THE FUTURE

Beck suggests that people used to be afraid of the past but are now, ironically, deeply fearful of both the present and the future.[11] He terms this "Risikogessellschaft" or "risk society." Beck's essential point is that both science and technology have turned society into a laboratory (an example being the release of genetically modified organisms into the environment and food chains) where nature is a historical product of human action (the "death of nature" as an independent entity from humans with the advent of global warming causing the "humanisation of nature"). Beck suggests that the threats we currently experience are fundamentally different from those that existed in earlier eras for three reasons: (1) They are undetectable by direct human sensory perception; (2) they are capable of transcending generations, and (3) they exceed the capacity of current mechanisms for compensating victims (Beck cited in Cohen, 1997, p. 107). The distinction is now between (safe) civilisation and (dangerous) nature.

What then are the causes of risk in Beck's risk society? First, modernisation itself, secondly technology and, thirdly, globalisation. Relations of definition as opposed to relations of production structure politics in the risk society. The environmental risks discussed by Beck are largely invisible and socially disputable, and it is difficult to compile a list of risks or a set of possible control strategies. We occupy a period of transition "not towards modernity but towards a second modernity in which the logic of industrial production and distribution (i.e., wealth) is becoming increasingly tied to the logic of the social production of risk" (Carter, 1993).

Beck's theories are beginning to change the understanding of risk itself "from a purely technical term to a socially defined state" (Glicken, 1997). Beck attempts to create a new theory of modernity and is most interested in the effects of industrialism and the potential effects on social and cultural spheres. The risk society lies somewhere between industrial and post-industrial society where the dominant focus of politics becomes the distributions of costs and risks of societal development.

DEFINING, RECORDING AND MAKING SENSE OF RISK

Beck's theory engages with defining and recording risks and how individual people make sense of risk in their lives. Insecurity and uncertainty pervade our lives as we have conflicting information from experts explaining technological progress and how it may or may not affect us. In many ways, risk in late modernity is invisible because, in the past, danger was tangible; one could see flames from a fire, see the enemy approach, or hear a raging waterfall and avoid such danger, but this is no longer the case. The five senses are no longer enough to protect us (Beck, 1992) and threats are all around us. Indeed, the character of modern risks are consequences of "decisions that focus on techno-economic advantages and opportunities and accept hazards as simply the dark side of progress" (Beck, 1992).[12]

Beck controversially calls for a complete refusal to accept any increase in the dangers that face us with regard to acceptable levels in the omission of poisons and toxins. Societies are characterised by "organised irresponsibility," whereby risk producers are protected at the expense of risk victims where no one can be sure of one's roles as to who will be the aggressor and who will be the victim.

AN AWARENESS OF COLLECTIVE RISK

Risks can be changed, adapted, ". . . magnified, dramatised or minimised within knowledge; and to that extent they are particularly open to social definition and construction" (Beck, 1992, pp. 22-23). The optimism of the last century has been largely replaced by an awareness of collective risk, and profound social, political, and economic changes have brought in unforeseen and (risk filled) potentials that create a sense of global scepticism. These profound changes will inevitably result in a challenge to the legitimacy of the very systems that created the risk society, as no one is sure whom to trust anymore. There is little doubt a risk sensitivity is developing in Western politics with the increasing number of environmental scandals over which the public has no control. The costs of modernisation are beginning to outweigh the alleged benefits.

The term risk society encapsulates risk as a central analytical tool for understanding social forms characteristic of modernisation and late modernity or reflexive modernity. Beck develops the proposition that while the classic social issue of early modernisation is the distribution of wealth and thus the division of society along very visible class lines, today's world is one in which the central issue will increasingly become the distribution of risk. Beck crucially argues that risk society has swept away the possibility of class consciousness as a trigger for political mobilisation. Beck charts a move from the first modernity characterised by the distribution of wealth to the risk society (a more complex modernity) characterised by the distribution of risks.

THE PROFOUND RISKS OF THE RISK SOCIETY

Although not as dominant in the public psyche as in the 1960s, the threat of nuclear war looms large in terms of potential ecological disaster. At the end of the last millennium, it was estimated that Russia has some 2,500 nuclear warheads poised to launch at any one time. The real fear is that nuclear warheads cannot be primed to self destruct once launched and will, inevitably, strike their intended targets.

Local electricity suppliers in Russia have switched off power sources due to non-payment of bills in nuclear weapons installations. Two thirds of Russia's early warning radar systems are thought not to work, and there are problems around the deployment of personnel to very diverse locations including, for example, the Ukraine, Azerbaijan and Kazakhstan.

Now, our fear has moved from the former Soviet Bloc to renegade ex-military personnel who have access to sensitive information and materials. We are aware of nuclear submarines lying idle with reactors churning over. There is a recognised international trade in uranium which, if it falls into the wrong hands, could be truly and indiscriminately horrific.

Chemical pollution causes long-term invisible damage, and we must rely on expert scientific data. One might cite the supposed size of the hole in the ozone layer, the supposed harmful effects of pesticide spraying, and the recent scares on the dangers of genetic testing and cloning with the now infamous Dolly the Sheep. This process Beck (1992) calls "scientism," and "the consequences of scientific and industrial development (are) a set of risks and hazards which are no longer limited in time and space and for which no one can be held accountable" (Beck, p. 2). The Irish Doctors Environmental Association under Article 3 of its Paris Appeal document (2004) recently noted that, "As our own health, that of our children, is under threat, the human race itself is in serious danger." The threat of chemical pollution is pervasive. Perhaps what worries Beck most is that, ironically, knowledge leads to risk consciousness: "Sources of danger are no longer ignorance but *knowledge*, not deficient but a perfected mastery over nature; not that which eludes the human grasp, but the system of norms and objective constraints established with the industrial epoch" (p. 181).

BECK AND REFLEXIVE MODERNISATION

Reflexive modernisation implies coming to terms with the limits and contradictions of the modern order. A complex theory, reflexive modernisation can focus on either the self-monitoring of individuals or on the self-monitoring of a social system. With reflexive modernisation, public risk consciousness and risk conflicts will lead to forms of scientization of the protests against science" (Beck, 1992, p. 161). Beck's typology of modernities includes reflexive modernisation, with an axial principle embracing production of risks and distribution of "bads." His understanding of reflexive modernisation recognises that "the risk epoch of modernity occurs unintentionally, unseen, compulsively, in the course of a dynamic of modernisation which has made itself autonomous" (Beck, 1996, p. 28). In Beck's understanding of reflexive modernisation, institutions now have to confront and engage with the side-effects of modernisation processes. It is argued that they are forced to examine the side effects of side effects. Institutions have to minimise negative consequences generated by modernisation.

Turner (1994) suggests that "the reflexive self is a core feature of the general progress of detraditionalisation in high modernity" (p. 187). Earlier, in his *Risk Society*, Beck (1992) suggests that "risks become the motor of the self-politicisation of modernity in industrial society" and that reflexive modernisation means "the possibility of a creative (self)-destruction for an entire epoch: that of industrial society" (p. 2).

The source and attribution of hazards is a by-product of techno-industrial development. Beck divides society into three epochs: pre-industrial society, industrial society and "global risk society" (Beck, 1994, p. 7). Beck (1992) identifies Western society's current phase of development "reflexive modernization" because it is characterized by the way industrial society's technological and institutional processes of modernization make their mark on today's risk society. There is a correlation between social class and risk with toxic waste dumping in third world countries, the location of incinerators and factories emitting major pollutants in inner-city areas. Beck seems to assume that one cannot approach the post-modern world objectively in a third-person manner. One is inevitably caught up in the world and included even if one attempts to resist this process.

Beck analyses the contribution of influential social and political institutions, economics (private property, industrialisation) and law (administrative law and private law). All of these institutions produce risks we are forced to live with and live under, but these institutions seek to reassure the ill-informed public and make the risks disappear. Rational calculations are no longer possible or, perhaps, reliable. Nonetheless, he sees hope for the future in the capacity of humankind to re-invent social (inter)communication by mobilising peoples across the globe against environmental disaster in a common life mission. This will actively challenge moral and political will and a new moral consciousness will come into being.

Critiquing Beck's Risk Society

Several authors have argued that Beck takes a rather optimistic view of the ability of the State to re-invent itself. Risk society can present opportunities for democratisation and institutional innovation. "Progress can be understood as legitimate social change without democratic political legitimation" (Beck, 1992, p. 214). Culpitt (1999) asked whether Beck's risk society mark a major rupture with modernity. Criticism of Beck's risk society includes his inadequate representation of the past to the fact that his theories display no awareness that risks may be willingly chosen for personal reasons. Carter (1993) suggests that Beck's use of the term risk becomes overloaded with a number of meanings ranging from the colloquial to the scientific. The book suffers, then, from a lack of clarity.

J. R. Hall (1994) takes Beck to task for his analysis of depoliticisation which, he suggests, is vague and has a tendency to generalise. Nonetheless, although Beck's vision of the future is apocalyptically threatening, it also offers the opportunity to plan for and hedge against risk. Cohen (1997) argues that the concept of risk society has currency because it confronts three issues, "namely, the liabilities of economic growth, the pervasiveness of hazardous technology, and the inadequacies of reductionist scientific research" (p. 107).

THE RISK EXPERTS ENGAGE IN DIALOGUE

The desired + the familiar = new modernity (Beck, 1994, p. 4).

In *Reflexive Modernisation: Politics, Tradition and Aesthetics in the Modern Social Order* (1994) Beck, Lash and Giddens come together to produce some additional debate around reflexivity and late modernity. Lash is particularly interested in modernisms and "the complex of cultural institutions that provide the value systems of the modern world" (cited in Braun, 1996, p. 752). The central thesis of the book is that the western world and postmodernity no longer reign supreme as the entire globe is in transition and progress is no longer guaranteed. The authors are concerned with the cost of progress. How much cost can society, and the individual, subsume for progress to be made and when do the costs outweigh the benefits?

THWARTING THE BEST MADE PLANS

There is intentional and unintentional change caught up with risks of change itself from the old accepted order to a new order of power and knowledge. The authors acknowledge the number of common threads in each other's writings, which could usefully be analysed as part of a cohesive approach to risk. The whole thrust of modern life is lived "as if" (p. 7); something could happen to thwart the best made plans. We cannot rule out something bad because the threat of the expert systems and trust hangs over us like a dark cloud. Even attempts at controlling risk create new risks, which may be uncontrollable. Abstraction causes the risk society.

BECK'S VIEW

Beck notes the year 1989 as the symbolic end of an epoch, when the Communist world fell apart. According to his analysis, we must rethink and reinvent industrial civilisation. Beck terms reflexive modernisation a new stage where ". . . progress can turn into self-destruction, in which one kind of modernisation undercuts and changes another" (p. 2). He is critical of sociologists who have tended to ignore new ways of collecting data about a new age with Beck suggesting "reflexive modernisation encompasses the conflict dynamism of risk society in the narrower sense (Beck, 1994, p. 4)." The modern information highway is no longer self-reflecting, rather it spews out information overload.

Risks are a controlling principle in that they act to stop us from engaging in pursuits that we would engage in if we were not fearful of the potential consequences. We cannot choose or reject the risk society. Beck acknowledges that someone who depicts the world as wholly risk-driven will ultimately become incapable of action (Beck, 1994, p. 9). Risk society then becomes an intensely self-critical society. The state, itself, creates confusion. Beck accords certain institutions zombie status, where they are unable to live or die but exist in a clinical haze, perpetually trying to reinvent themselves. As examples, one could take class parties without classes, armies without enemies or a governmental apparatus which in many cases claims to start and keep things going which are happening anyway. The individual has not become trapped by circumstance and the individual, nor groups, nor governments can extricate him from his unhappy lot. Braun (1996) argues that this view embraces "traditional sociological determinism of both the left and right" (p. 753).

A problem Beck sees with attempting to live in the risk society is that one has competing and mutually exclusive global and personal risks and one can become obsessed with risk avoidance and, ultimately, incapable of action. His is the most pessimistic vision of both the present and future of the three authors. He writes, ". . . people are not being released from feudal and religious-transcendental certainties into the world of industrial society into the turbulence of the global risk society. They are being expected to live with a broad variety of different, mutually contradictory, global and personal risks (p. 7).

Sica (1997) notes that the book's central argument lies around the possible creation of a new order of politics by an informed people that was not (it seems) possible before. This new departure would embrace a definite set of aesthetic awareness and, "here, the punch line–make standard political-economy power theories, and semiotics quite out of date" (p. 112).

GIDDENS' VIEW

Giddens examines the "disinterring and problematising of tradition" (1994, p. 57) and illustrates that reflexivity is a modern, not post-modern, collection of attitudes and cultural practices (whilst Beck concentrates on rejuvenating the public sphere in Germany). Giddens argues that it is not exclusively the West that is in flux. He notes the processes of intentional change as processes of *evacuation* (italics original). Decisions are reshaped and reorganised in the global and local. Giddens argues that risk moves through two stages: risk as "given," "a part of an essential calculus, a means of sealing off boundaries as the future is invaded," and risk as "a new type of uncalculability" such as global warming. In this we are offered a series of "scenarios" and "it is like a *dangerous* adventure, in which each of us has to participate whether we like it or not" (p. 59, my emphasis).

Later, Giddens argues that reflexive modernisation is marked by the "twin processes of globalisation and the excavation of most traditional contexts of action . . ." (p. 95). Braun (1996) suggests that Giddens "concretizes" reflexive modernisation by discussing addictive lifestyles as social as well as biological. Obsessions are needed in the modern world to a degree as feelings are in constant danger of being lost and we are left with the effect of looking at ourselves in a fun house mirror. Distortions of reality (the truth?) become the norm. Table 1 outlines the central differences between Beck and Giddens.

TABLE 1. Stated Differences in Understandings of Reflexivity Between Giddens and Beck

Giddens	Beck
A shift in trust relations	Growing freedom from expert systems
Trust in expert systems	Growing critique in expert systems
Problem of order	Problem of change
Problem with psychic hazards	Problem with environmental hazards
Expert systems are instruments	Expert systems are obstacles

Source: Extrapolated from Lash, S. (1994, pp. 116-117).

LASH'S VIEW

In the third chapter, Lash takes up the theoretical baton and develops his proposition that the aesthetics of culture creation need to be nurtured. Mutual validation and mutual concern are explored in the context of the patterns of everyday life. Lash contends that reflexive modernisation is "a theory of the ever-increasing powers of social actors, or 'agency,' in regard to structure . . . the theory as formulated by Beck and Giddens presupposes that reflexivity is essentially 'cognitive' in nature . . . the theory of reflexive modernisation is a very strong programme of individualisation" (p. 111). Two types of reflexivity, structural- and self-reflexivity, are proposed by Lash. In Lash's scheme of things, Giddens and Beck are agreed on "the bracketing of the life-world to arrive at individualised, subject-object forms of social knowledge" (p. 156) and that we live in a fundamental sense for the first time in a post-traditional society (p. 212).

Lash's view of reflexive modernisation, then, includes the replacement of earlier social structures by information and communication structures. Whilst accepting the validity of Lash's practical insights on corporatism and markets, Braun (1996) criticises Lash for being overly simplistic in his analysis of reflexive modernisation and empowerment and for neglecting to raise certain social issues that could usefully have been examined in the wider context of his argument.

THE AUTHORS DISCUSS THEIR COLLECTIVE VIEWS

Beck concludes that the interests of sociologists are not whether the world will fall, but, rather, the threat of downfall. The side effect of scientization is "becoming the motor of social history" (p. 181). Giddens acknowledges that the growth in human knowledge has meant the origins of unpredictability have changed.

Active trust becomes more and more important in the risk society, but Giddens recognises the irony in this as "increasing freedom for some regularly goes along with, or is even the cause of, greater oppression for others" (p. 187). This is a point supported by Lowi (1990) who argues that all action by an individual can potentially cause harm to others. In reply to the fragile-flower theory of democracy, Giddens offers a sturdy-flower thesis where systems can reinvent themselves very quickly (he cites post-world war Japan and Germany as examples).

Finally, Lash argues that there has been a shift in the work of Beck and Giddens from an emphasis on the transformation of modernity at the beginning of the 1990s to one to the realm of politics. The pivotal importance of Beck and Giddens on reflexive modernity is placed in the context of postmodernism and social relations. Cognitive knowledge is based on technical expertise and is resolved by reference to external, abstract systems (science). This is developed in the work of Mary Douglas over the years as we will see in more detail in a later chapter.

CONTESTING THE CLAIMS
OF SCIENTIFIC RATIONALITY AND CERTAINTY

Douglas (1982; 1985; 1992; 1992a) and Wildavsky (1979) also connect risk with opportunity but make more of a connection with *blame*, which is interesting when one connects this to what has happened in the human services and child and youth care landscape over the past two decades.

Douglas is seen by many as, perhaps, the greatest living anthropologist (see Douglas, 1973). In her work she speculates that the physical body is a microcosm of the social body and that symbols grounded in the human body are used to express social experience, and vice-versa. By understanding how the body works, we understand how society works.

More specifically, Douglas is interested with how society is organised through its understanding of risk to protect its way of life, and she asks (amongst many other things), is risk really a modern phenomenon? Why are some fears ignored whilst others are emphasised? How is it that different groups look at the same risks in different ways?[13] "Opportunity" presents potential reward but also "failure," and the larger the undertaking the greater the risk therein. Douglas teases out how blame is accorded and notes that all risks are morally and politically charged.

She sees risks as being culturally biased, meaningful, being based around a society's way of life (the total culture) and influenced by socially embedded values and beliefs.

Douglas (1992) makes the point that what most people mean by risk in technologically advanced societies has little to do with probability calculations, *but much more to do with concepts of danger, avoidance and prevention* (Douglas, 1992, p. 24, emphasis mine). She argues that risk has emerged as a key idea for modern times because of its many uses as a forensic resource and because it "is invoked for a modern-style riposte against abuse of power" (1990, p. 3). In short, high risk means a lot of danger.

Douglas (1970) described hazard controversies in an early essay: "Credibility for any view of how the environment will react is secured by the moral commitment of a community to a particular set of institutions" (p. 241). In her later work, Douglas (1985; 1992) assesses the risk consciousness debate and suggests the politicisation of risk is a feature of late modernity where the universe is moralised and politicised.

Douglas (1992) views risk as fitting into the late modernity debate simply because it is so strongly connected with the global culture. Risk, for Douglas, is characterised by an association with new technologies and a public consciousness-raising in the 1960s when the environment became a highly politicised phenomenon. The word risk has evolved to mean danger:

> Now risk refers only to negative outcomes. The word has been pre-empted to mean bad risks. The promise of good things in contemporary political discourse is couched in other terms. The language of risk is reserved as a specialized lexical register for political talk about the undesirable outcomes. (1992, p. 24)

CONCLUSION

The now voluminous work of social and behavioural scientists since the 1970s has illustrated that research on risk has located a number of similarities and concerns across a variety of disciplines (Dean, 1999; Lash, 1993; Renn, 1998; Short, 1994). Risk has become the explanatory paradigm of the 21st century. Advances in technology and science have precipitated a new public risk awareness and the perceived threat of invisible risks is very powerful, and a concern for future generations is apparent in the literature on risk, trust, opportunity and uncertainty amongst all of the major commentators.

A point of interest is that we live in societies obsessed with mass production and consumption yet we want little or no risks to us as individuals. In all of this, we tend(ed) to rely on science and scientists, but a key finding in early psychometric research was that the experts were not necessarily any more scientific or better at estimating probabilities than were lay people. Indeed, experts were often overconfident in the exactness of their estimates, and put too much stock in limited data sets.

Democracy allows for an open display of distrust in institutions, and this has found a voice in a number of influential organisations such as Greenpeace, Save The Earth, One Planet and Campaign for Nuclear Disarmament and in individuals such as Beck, Giddens, Douglas and Lash (albeit to varying degrees). A recognition of the limits and boundaries of post-modernity, late-modernity, hyper-modernity or high-modernity, depending on one's preference, and a willingness to share both positive and negative outcomes of social and technical experiments will temper the distrust of the public.

This chapter has discussed some of the literature on risk and sets the scene for the following section on how risk pervades the lives of professionals involved in child protection and welfare, child and youth care, and special education. It is clear that an understanding of risk and uncertainty has percolated down to the micro-level of discourse and their daily lived lives but to what extent? (Bernstein, 1998). How professionals cope with risk has a range of implications for children and youth in care of these experts as the more traditional paternalistic and regulatory framework that governed practice has started to crumble. The globalisation and politicisation of risk-consciousness affects children designated as at-risk in terms of prevention and intervention programmes and, I argue, that it has done this at the expense of a resiliency focus.

But risk certainly pervades the child and youth care provision terrain and the compartmentalized, competing and, at times, antagonistic paradigms are as confusing as they are confused. Perhaps the strongest connection worth making at this juncture is that the duality in the sometimes vigorous debate over the very definition of risk (Fischoff et al., 1984) with, on the other hand, the silence about defining risk at all (Douglas & Wildavsky, 1982; Giddens, 1990; 1992) is mirrored in child and youth care.

NOTES

1. Probability theory dates back to the seventeenth century with its inception in the analysis of games of chance. Philosophical debate has been divided between two schools of thought: the frequentist interpretation (Fisher and Neyman) and the subjectivist, or Bayesian interpretation (Savage).

2. For most of its history, the idea of unpredictable future events was articulated in the notion of chance, from the Greek *aos* meaning "the first state of the universe, a vast gulf or chasm, the nether abyss, empty space" (Oxford English Dictionary, 1991).

3. In the United States, over 300 of 5,000 chemicals routinely used have been acknowledged to be and are labelled as carcinogens due to results of animal testing. The difficulty with this, of course, is that some animal carcinogens vary dramatically in their carcinogenic and/or mutagenic potency for humans. Four hundred chemicals have been discovered in animal studies that produce tumours but fewer than 20 of these are accepted human carcinogens.

4. Many risk assessment experts argue that attempts to standardise assessment methods for the sake of public safety have actually introduced unmanageable layers of conservatism into the process.

5. The legislative emphasis (in terms of risk assessment) in Europe has been on chemical safety, pesticide residues, food additives and occupational exposure (Paustenbach, 1995).

6. The Webster International Dictionary (1981) defines risk as, "the possibility of suffering loss, injury, disadvantage, or destruction."

7. Moving away from Giddens for a moment, it is worth commenting on Barber's (1983) understanding of trust which includes expectations of technical competence, expectations that fiduciary obligations will be discharged properly and the expectation that the natural and moral social orders will be preserved.

8. Part of this new distrust is the sense of discomfort the public has with science being allied to major financial corporations, academic institutions engaging in applied scientific research as opposed to theoretical pursuits, and governments willingness to selectively call on experts when it suits them to do so.

9. At the core of this social scientific and policy-oriented approach is the view that contemporary societies have the capability of dealing with their environmental crises. Experiences in some countries demonstrate that modern institutions can incorporate environmental interests into their daily routines. Elsewhere, economic and political interests singularly dominate development trajectories, and environmental deterioration continues, challenging the premises of ecological modernisation.

10. In the first five years of publication, *Risk Society* sold over 60,000 copies making it one of the most popular books from a European social scientist.

11. Bauman (1991, p. 16) argues that it matters little whether the present is conceptualised as late or postmodernity as the most important feature of the human condition is "the great modern campaign against ambivalence."

12. Ecological Risks: global warming, biodiversity loss, ecosystem destruction. Health Risks: health risks of genetically-altered food stuffs, skin cancer, BSE, pollution, asthma. Economic Risks: decline in job security. Social Risks: personal safety, crime and breakdown of community, divorce/separation.

13. What is considered radical about Douglas's analysis is that instead of classifying human societies into different categories that require different analysis criteria she applies the same principles to all societies.

REFERENCES

Ahlstrom, D. (2000, January 6). One BSE cow can infect 400,000 people, says report. *Irish Times.*

Alaszewski, A., & Manthorpe, J. (1991). Literature review: Measuring and managing risk in social welfare. *British Journal of Social Work, 21,* 277-290.

Barber, B. (1983). *The logic and limits of trust.* NB: Rutgers University Press.

Bauman, Z. (1991). *Modernity and ambivalence.* Cambridge: Polity Press.

Bauman, Z. (1992). *Intimations of postmodernity.* London: Routledge.

Bauman, Z. (1992, November 13). The solution as problem. *The Times Higher Educational Supplement,* p. 43.

Bauman, Z. (1997). *Postmodernity and its discontents.* New York: New York University Press.

Beck, U. (1986). *Risikogesellschaft: Auf dem Weg in eine andere Moderne.* Frankfurt: Suhrkamp.

Beck, U. (1987). The anthropological shock: Chernobyl and the contours of the risk society. *Berkeley Journal of Sociology, 32,* 153-165.

Beck, U. (1989). On the way to industrial risk-society? Outline of an argument. *Thesis Eleven,* 86-103.

Beck, U. (1992). *Risk society. Towards a new modernity.* London: Sage.

Beck, U. (1995). *Ecological politics in an age of risk.* Cambridge: Polity.

Beck, U. (1995, Fall). Freedom for technology: A call for a second separation of powers, *Dissent,* 503-7.

Beck, U. (1995). *Ecological enlightenment: Essays on the politics of risk society.* Atlantic Highlands, NJ: Humanities Press International.

Beck, U. (1996). Risk society and the provident state. In S. Lasyh, B. Szersynski & B. Wynne (Eds.), *Risk, environment & modernity: Towards a new ecology* (pp. 27-43). London, Sage Publications.

Beck, U. (1997). Politics of risk society. In J. Franklin (Ed.), *The politics of risk society* (pp. 9-22). Cambridge: Polity.

Beck, U. (1997a). *The reinvention of politics: Rethinking modernity in the global social order.* Cambridge: Polity.

Beck, U. (1997b). Capitalism without work. *Dissent, 44*(1), 51-6.

Beck, U. (1998). Politics of risk society. J. Franklin (Ed.), *The politics of risk society* (pp. 9-22). Cambridge: Polity.

Beck, U., Giddens, A., & Lash, S. (1994). *Reflexive modernisation: Politics, tradition & aesthetics in the modern social order.* Cambridge: Polity.

Bernstein, P. (1998). *Against the Gods: The remarkable story of risk.* New York: John Wiley & Sons.

Bilton, T., Bonnett, K., Jones, P., Skinner, D., Stanworth, M., & Webster, A. (1996). *Introductory sociology.* London: MacMillan.

Braun, J. (1996). Review of Beck, U., Giddens, A., & Lash, S. Reflexive modernisation: Politics, tradition and aesthetics in the modern social order. *Theory and Society, 25,* 752-760.

Carter, S. (1993). Risk and the new modernity. *Postmodern Culture, 3*(3). Retrieved August 2006 from http://infomotions.com/serials/pmc/pmc-v3n3-carter-risk.txt.

Coates, J. (2003). *Ecology and social work: Towards a new paradigm.* Halifax: Fernwood Press.

Cohen, M. J. (1997). Risk society and ecological modernisation: Alternative visions for post-industrial nations. *Futures, 29*(2), 105-119.

Covello, V., & Mumpower, J. (1985). Risk analysis and risk management: An historical perspective. *Risk Analysis, 5,* 103-120.

Culpitt, I. (1999). *Social policy and risk.* London: Sage.

David, E. (1975). One-armed scientists? *Science, 189,* 891.

Dean, M. (1999) Risk, calculable and incalculable. In D. Lupton (Ed.), *Risk and sociocultural theory: New directions and perspectives* (pp. 131-159). Cambridge: Cambridge University Press.

Douglas, M. (1970). *Natural symbols.* London: Pantheon.

Douglas, M. (1973). *Rules and meanings: the anthropology of everyday knowledge: Selected readings.* Harmondsworth: Penguin Books.

Douglas, M. (Ed.) (1982). *Essays in the sociology of perception.* London: Routledge & Kegan Paul and Russell Sage Foundation.

Douglas, M. (1982). *Risk and culture: An essay on the selection of technical and environmental dangers.* Berkeley, CA: University of California Press.

Douglas, M. (1985). *Risk acceptability according to the social sciences.* New York: Russell Sage Foundation.

Douglas, M. (1992). *Risk and blame: Essays in cultural theory.* London; New York: Routledge.

Douglas, M., & Wildavsky, A. (1983). *Risk and culture. an essay on the selection of technological and environmental dangers.* University of California Press.

Ewald, F. (1991). Insurance and risk. In G. Burchell, C. Gordon, & P. Miller (Eds.), *The Foucault effect: Studies in governmental rationality* (pp. 197-210). Hempstead, UK: Harvester Wheatsheaf.

Fischoff, B., Lichenstein, S., Slovic, P., Derby, S, L., & Keeney, R. L. (1981). *Acceptable risk.* New York: Cambridge University Press.

Fischoff, B., Watson, S., & Hope, C. (1984). Defining risk. *Policy Sciences, 17,* 123-39.

Freudenberg, W. (1993). Risk and recreancy: Weber, the division of labor and the rationality of risk perceptions. *Social Forces, 71,* 909-971.

Giddens, A. (1990). *The consequences of modernity.* Cambridge: Polity Press.

Giddens, A. (1991). *Modernity and self-identity.* Cambridge: Polity Press.

Giddens, A. (1992). *The transformation of intimacy.* Cambridge: Polity Press.

Giddens, A. (1992). *Human societies.* Cambridge: Polity Press.

Giddens, A. (1994). *Beyond left and right.* Cambridge: Polity Press.

Giddens, A. (1994). *Reflexive modernisation.* Cambridge: Polity Press.

Giddens, A. (2006). *Frequently Asked Questions.* Retrieved January 2006 at http://old. lse.ac.uk/collections/meetthedirector/faqs.htm.

Giovacchini, R. (1984). The acceptable risk. Does it exist? An overview of the problem. In L. Zuckerman (Ed.), *Risk in society.* John Libbey and Company Ltd.

Glicken, J. (1996). Establishing effective dialogues with interested parties: Process for reviewing draft ecological risk assessment guidelines for chemical exposures. *California Environmental Protection Agency.* Ep&t Document No. 96-0034.

Glicken, J. (1997). *Risk management: What, who and why?* Presentation to Risk Management for Critical Infrastructures. New Mexico: TechnoScience. AL.

Goulding, R. (1984). Risk from chemicals. Medical priorities: The place of chemicals. In L. Zuckerman. (Ed.), *Risk in society.* John Libbey and Company Ltd.

Hacking, I. (1990). *The taming of chance.* Cambridge. Cambridge University Press.

Hafting, T. (1996). *Complexity and natural disasters: The failure of foresight and hindsight.* UCLA: SCOS Conference.

Hall, J. (1994). Review of risk society: Towards a new modernity. *The Sociological Review, 42*(2), 344-346.

MacConnell, S., & Millar, F. (2001, March 16). Walsh Expected to Relax Controls on Some Events. *Irish Times.*

Lash, S. (1993). Reflexive modernisation: The aesthetic dimension. *Theory, Culture & Society, 10,* 1-23.

Lash, S. (1994). Reflexivity and its doubles: structure, aesthetics, community. In U. Beck, A. Giddens & S. Lash. (Eds.), *Reflexive modernisation.* Cambridge: Polity.

Lash, S., & Wynne, B. (1992). Introduction. In U. Beck (Ed.), *Risk society: Towards a new modernity* (pp. 1-8). London: Sage.

Lash, S., & Urry, J. (1994). *Economies of signs and spaces.* London: Sage.

Lowi, T. (1990). Risks and rights in the history of American governments, *Daedalus, 119*(4): 400-3.

Lowrance, W. (1976). Of acceptable risk: Science and the determination of safety. Chicago, IL: William Kaufmann.

Luhmann, N. (1979). *Trust and power.* Chichester: Wiley.

Luhmann, N. (1988). Familiarity, confidence, trust: Problems and alternatives. In D. Gambetta. (Ed.), *Trust: making and breaking cooperative relations.* Oxford: Blackwell.

Luhmann, N. (1993). *Risk: A sociological theory.* New York: Aldine de Gruyter.

McElwee, N. (2006). *Irish society & travellers: A child & youth care commentary.* Seminar to Faculty and Postgraduate Students at the University of Victoria, BC, Canada. March.

Morioka, T. (1987). Risk acceptance and risk management in Japan. *Proceedings of the 2nd Japan–USA Workshop on Risk Assessment and Management.*

Natural Hazards and Risk Assessment. Retrieved January 2006 from http://www. woodrow.org/teachers/esi/1997/53/risk.htm

New Road Map Foundation (1991). http://www.ecofuture.org/pk/pkar9506.html

Oppenheimer, L. (1997). *Ancient Mesopotamia.* Chicago, IL: University of Chicago Press.

Parton, N., Thorpe, D., & Wattam, C. (1997). *Child protection: Risk and the moral order.* London: MacMillan Press Ltd.

Paustenbach, D. (1995). Retrospective on U.S. health risk assessment: How others can benefit. *Risk: Health, safety and environment* (pp. 283-332). Franklin Pierce Law Centre.

Raynor, S., & Cantor, R. (1987). How fair is safe enough? The cultural approach to societal technology choice. *Risk Analysis, 7*(3), 1-3.

Renn, O. (1998). Three decades of risk research: Accomplishments and new challenges. *Journal of Risk Research, 1,* 49-71.

Rosa, E. (1998). Metatheoretical foundations for post-normal risk, *Journal of Risk Research, 1*(1), 15-44.

Rowe, W. (1977). *An anatomy of risk.* New York: Wiley.

Short, J. F. (1994). *Trace substances, science and the law: Perspectives for the social sciences.* Paper to American Association for the Advancement of Science Symposium on Trace Substances: Impact of Recent Instrumental Advances on Regulatory Affairs, February 23.

Sica, A. (1997). Review of reflexive modernisation: Politics, tradition and aesthetics in the modern social order. *Social Forces, 75*(3), 1119-1121.

Slovic, P. (1992). Perceptions of risk: Reflections on the psychometric paradigm. In S. Krimsky & D. Goulding (Eds.), *Social theories of risk* (pp. 117-52). Westpoint: CT: Praeger.

Starr, C. (1969). Social benefits versus technological risks: What is our society willing to pay for safety? *Science, 165*, 1232-1238.

Thompson, P. (1986). The philosophical foundations of risk. *S. J. PHIL*, 273.

Turner, B. (1994). The future for risk research. *Journal of Contingencies and Crisis Management, 2*, 146-156.

Wildavsky, A. (1979). No risk is the highest risk of all. *American Scientist, 67*, 32-37.

Yates, J. F., & Stone, E. R. 1992. The risk construct. In J. F. Yates (Ed.), *Risk taking behavior* (pp. 239-272). West Sussex, England: John Wiley and Sons.

Zebroski, E. (1975). Attainment of balance in risk-benefit perceptions. In D. Okrent (Ed.), *Risk-benefit methodology and application: Some papers presented at the Engineering Foundation Workshop* (pp. 633-644). Asilomar, CA: Report ENG-7598, School of Engineering and Applied Science, UCLA.

doi:10.1300/J024v29n01_04

Chapter 5

Putting the Study Together

SUMMARY. This chapter outlines the research design including the nature of the research strategy, tools, respondents, and theoretical and methodological concerns in a child and youth care qualitative study. doi:10.1300/J024v29n01_05 *[Article copies available for a fee from The Haworth Document Delivery Service: 1-800-HAWORTH. E-mail address: <docdelivery@haworthpress.com> Website: <http://www.HaworthPress.com> © 2007 by The Haworth Press, Inc. All rights reserved.]*

KEYWORDS. Methodology, child and youth care relational research, adapted frameworks analysis, child and youth care, at-risk youth

The aim of methodology, according to Kaplan (1973), is understanding of the process of scientific enquiry through description and analysis of methods used. Methodology represents "the particular ways the sociologist acts on his environment" (Denzin, 1970, p. 5), whilst Sacks refers to methodology as, "A most remarkable, inventive and productive account of how to study human sociality" (Sacks, 1992, p. xii). The opportunity to be immersed in a subject, thereby gaining a general understanding of the area, is crucial before defining a specific question. Methodology refers to the philosophical framework, underlying assumptions and orientation towards research (Garfat, 1998).

A qualitative approach seeks to *understand* rather than to *know*. Garfat (1998), in discussing the varying approaches to undertaking

[Haworth co-indexing entry note]: "Putting the Study Together." McElwee, Niall. Co-published simultaneously in *Child & Youth Services* (The Haworth Press, Inc.) Vol. 29, No. 1/2, 2007, pp. 103-127; and: *At-Risk Children & Youth: Resiliency Explored* (Niall McElwee) The Haworth Press, Inc., 2007, pp. 103-127. Single or multiple copies of this article are available for a fee from The Haworth Document Delivery Service [1-800-HAWORTH, 9:00 a.m. - 5:00 p.m. (EST). E-mail address: docdelivery@haworthpress.com].

Available online at http://cys.haworthpress.com
© 2007 by The Haworth Press, Inc. All rights reserved.
doi:10.1300/J024v29n01_05

research in the general area of child and youth care, notes that it is not uncommon to encounter phrases such as "quantitative versus qualitative" in relation to research methodologies whilst Patton (1980, p. 20) recognises simply that "different approaches are appropriate for different situations." This is a key point.

Marshall and Rossman (1989) identify qualitative methodology as useful when seeking to explore where and why policy, folk wisdom and practice do *not* work (my emphasis). Earlier, they also note that there is wide variation between various qualitative approaches which concern themselves with levels of intrusiveness, the nature of the documentation, the appropriateness of questioning interviewees and data analysis issues (Marshall & Rossman, 1989, pp. 10-11). A qualitative methodology requires a research problem involving people's constructions of meanings which have not been previously explored (Hassard, 1990). In terms of this particular study, VanderVen (1993) argues qualitative methodology's "mission is to tie as closely as possible to the lived experience of our client group; children, youth and families" (p. 5) and is, therefore, considered to be particularly appropriate.

The Irish literature was selected from a number of hard copy sources identified in a 1995 publication on research, from electronic data base sources and from the relevant government departments and voluntary agencies involved in child and youth care/social service and educational provision for children (Iwaniew & Pinkerton, 1998; Pinkerton & Gilligan, 1995). The international literature was selected by engaging in a comprehensive literature search of leading journals, books and postgraduate studies. I am a member of several discussion groups on the Internet in the areas of risk and resiliency and child and youth care and colleagues in the United States, Canada, South Africa, Australia and the UK were kind enough to send me materials and the "threads section" of CYC Net is invaluable (see www.cyc-net.org).

DISPLAYS OF PERSPECTIVES

This study employs a number of methodological approaches that are based on diverse theoretical principles (Gannon, 2005). Although recognising implicit dangers with qualitative styles, Silverman (1993) suggests that it is sometimes the aim of qualitative researchers to empathise with people and "turn ourselves into mirrors of other people's experiences" (p. ix). We need not be so concerned with labelling responses from respondents as true or false reports on reality and, "Instead, we can treat such responses as *displays of perspectives* and moral forms (Silverman, 1993, p. 107–my emphasis).

The Youth Encounter Projects in Ireland have not been given adequate attention in either academic or social policy contexts and this is surprising given their important remit for disadvantaged youth. They richly deserve to have their social history recorded and their overall contribution to working with children and young people "at-risk" assessed. This should take into account their individual narratives. A clear social analysis would greatly assist in developing criteria against which the success of the projects could be measured. Alongside this, a richness of detail could evolve from listening to, recording and analysing the deliberations of the young people for whom the projects were developed in the first instance. The lives of the children and young people could be amplified through their own accounts.

METHODS OF DATA COLLECTION

This research took place during a time when Ireland was beginning to emerge from a history of covert neglect towards vulnerable populations of at-risk children and youth, one where the very survival of the Youth Encounter Projects could not be guaranteed. The context of this research was that of the Youth Encounter Projects, established in the latter part of the 1970s in Ireland to cater for at-risk children and youth. The Limerick Youth Encounter Project was well known to me in a professional capacity as I was a practicum supervisor based in a college environment. Over a period of some years I had become friendly with the Director of this project and greatly admired his way of working with the children and youth in his care. Although he was employed as Director of the project, he saw his own role as much more than a teacher or an administrator. His was, and remains, a "child and youth care way of intervening" (Garfat & McElwee, 2004; McElwee & Monaghan, 2005). I chose to interview seventeen youths who had taken part in a summer programme in which I worked in a voluntary capacity during the summer of 1995 when they were in their early adolescence.

DATA SOURCES AND PROCESSES

Direct in-depth interviews and participation with the interviewees in their various educational and leisure environments (the project, a church parlour, a hotel, a family home and a social services centre) led to a greater mutual understanding between us. My goal was to occupy their life space. More specifically, the research comprised:

- Documentary research of the project's records and data from 1977-2006;

  - local, national and international scholarly material related to childhood, education, and, specifically the Youth Encounter Projects;
  - local and national newspapers, journals and reports;
  - in-depth qualitative semi-structured interviews with seventeen of the ex-pupils of the school;
  - in-depth interviewees with the Director between 1995-2006
  - direct work with youth (in conjunction with a child and youth care practitioner) during their 1995 summer school programme commencing in an attempt to construct relationships with the pupils;
  - visits to the five residential special schools located in Clonmel and Dublin over a five year research period;
  - visits to a number of child care/community development projects in Limerick city over the five year research period;
  - numerous consultations with child and youth care agencies in Limerick between 1995-2000;
  - visits to Limerick Prison during 1999 and 2000.

NEGOTIATING GATEKEEPERS

The potential power base of "gatekeepers" may prove to be problematic in applied research as studies involving children and young people necessarily involve access to them and adult care providers (see McElwee & Monaghan, 2005). As identified by Thomas and O'Kane (1998), it remains a concern that not all pupils were allowed to participate in this study because various adults decided that it might not be in their best interests. Hood, Kelly and Mayall (1996, p. 126) remark that adults tend, sometimes, to assign priority to protecting children from external researchers at the expense of children's rights to participate in a piece of research. It would appear from the literature that accessing children and young people is a universal difficulty. Nonetheless, it should be noted that, ultimately, children and young people make their own decisions about whether they will include themselves in a research study when given a choice and some of their stated reasons for inclusion or, indeed, exclusion can be as complex as reasons proffered by adults.

In relation to access, Mauthner (1997) makes the point that schools often prove more fertile grounds for study than homes because of difficulty of access, but I am not, at all, sure that this was the case in this study. The homes of the interviewees proved to be welcoming environments, whilst the school presented several difficulties such as an inability to move classes around to facilitate interviews because of space restrictions and a physical environment that did not allow for one-to-one sessions with interviewees. Many times the excuse was given that "every room was needed for one purpose or another." Indeed, for some of the interviews, the local Social Services Centre in Limerick City was booked in advance by the project director. We were thus guaranteed access to a private room where the interviewees would not be disturbed.[1]

DEVELOPING RESEARCH QUESTIONS

When formulating a research question, the majority of qualitative researchers consider the definition of the topic and associated variables, selection of the methodological framework, exploration, operationalization and formulation of hypotheses (Sarantakos, 1991, p. 111). Added to this is the process of isolating key themes and issues for the researcher referred to by Lofland (in Mischler, 1983) as "puzzlements." With these considerations in mind, I developed research questions around "risk" and "at-risk," as essentially, how the interviewees made sense of risk, opportunity, and danger in their lives and how they coped with perceived risk as of significant interest.

A RATIONALE FOR QUALITATIVE METHODOLOGY IN THIS RESEARCH PROJECT

A qualitative rather than a quantitative approach was chosen for this research study. Garfat (1998; 2001) and McElwee and Monaghan (2005) note that the former approach is preferable to the latter given certain conditions. These include when there is a need to "capture reality as it is," that is, in interaction, when the researcher wishes to present data and analysis verbally and in detailed form rather than in a numeric and formulaic context. It is also useful when the researcher wishes to capture the *meaning* and the regularities of social action and when the researcher wishes to understand *reality* from the point of view of the subject. Glaser & Strauss (1970) likened constructions of the researcher to a newborn baby full of promise and without preconceptions.

ETHICAL CONSIDERATIONS IN THIS RESEARCH: HUMAN RIGHTS PROTECTION

Researching children and adolescents raises both methodological and analytical difficulties, primarily due to the evocative nature of childhood adversity, in general, and issues of the validity of consent from young people as research partners/participants more specifically (Leadbeater, Banister, Benoit, Jansson, Marshall & Riecken, 2006). This is particularly the case in Ireland as researching young people is such a recent activity.

Understanding children and young people as *partners* in the research process rather than simply as subjects of research is relatively new and there is an emerging body of literature around methods of communicating with children (Liddle, 1992; McAuley, 1998; Vaillancourt & Igneski, 2006). Pinkerton (1998) notes that research needs to be brought alive through creative endeavours, and Sarantakos (1991) observes that all decisions are acceptable and legitimate if justified in terms of methodological standards. One could argue that with regard to certain studies, there is no right or wrong methodological framework, only weaker or stronger methodology. Referring back to the literature review, it should be noted that the ex-pupils in St. Augustine's fit neatly into three of Hartnoll's five categorisations of hidden populations which include:

- Socially marginal/deviant groups;
- private populations;
- openly visible populations on whom nobody has bothered to collect data.

The other two categories are "Those in a population not known to formal institutions or agencies," and "Those known to individual institutions/ agencies but information is not passed on." These could be arguable to a degree as the information on these children is not shared across the social services. In relation to crime, Downes and Rock (1988) make a similar point, as does Lee (1995) discussing "hidden populations" in a more general sense. Higgins (1998, p. 146) observes that "official statistics are hampered by the reports of reportability, visibility and recordability." The fact that many of the survivors of childhood adversity actually survive into adulthood is not insignificant and is a testimony to resiliency winning out over risk.[2] There are three broad ethical issues within children's research including informed consent, confidentiality and protection. Concerns have also been expressed by various authors with the unequal power relationship between adults and children (Hammersley, 1995; Morrow & Richards, 1996; Thomas & O'Kane, 1998), unequal knowledge bases, and unequal social class origins compared with the research participants (Bates, 1996; Hill & Tisdall, 1997; McCauley, 1998; McElwee & Monaghan, 2005).[3]

Children and young people present many problems in that they have their own culture that differs implicitly to adult culture. Many of the problems researchers have trying to get into the "cultural world of children" could be likened to the kinds of problems anthropologists experience when studying other adult cultures. The main assumption that adults need to confront is that they *know* children and youth simply because they were youthful once. Depending on how adults see childhood, their ethical considerations will differ to both degree and extent.

MAKING SPACE FOR CHILDREN AND YOUNG PEOPLE

It is now common amongst social science researchers to consider school-aged children as competent to give consent to participate in research (Alderson, 1995) and it is acknowledged "when space is made for them, children's voices express themselves clearly" (Mauthner, 1997, p. 21; Roche, 1996). This is not to say that adults cannot be adultcentric and they need to genuinely listen to what children tell them. Alderson (1995) notes "… the right to consent has an impact on all other rights. Consent is about selecting options, negotiating them, and accepting or rejecting them. Beyond making a decision, consent is about making an informed choice and becoming emotionally committed to it" (p. 69).

With regard to this particular study, I was conscious to facilitate the interviewees by:

1. Ensuring that informed consent to participate in the study was obtained. The Director of the school clearly explained the research to the interviewees prior to my arrival for interviews. My research partners were, therefore, free to decide on their participation before any encounter with the researcher might influence their decision. It is recognised, however, that a relationship of power

difference did exist between the partners and the Director which might, of course, have influenced interviewees' decision to some degree. Thomas and O'Kane (1998) used a three-tiered approach in their study of looked after children in the UK by first sending out an information pack detailing, in a child friendly manner, the purpose, direction and potential outcome of the study. *Active* agreement from the children and *passive* agreement from the care-takers was sought. The parents of the children and the caretakers were also sent information. The authors informed the children that they could withdraw from the research at any stage, terminate interviews, and refuse to ask questions and refuse to be taped. Thirdly, the children were facilitated in the decision making process as much as possible in their choice of research instrument.

Although I was dealing with adolescents, this model was followed closely by ensuring that an independent witness was present at each of the interviews, consent forms were designed by three of the participants and then signed by all of the various interviewees. Respecting the interviewee's right to information was communicated in a way that he or she understood by using language appropriate to the interviewees' ages and cognitive abilities in my interviews with them. Solberg (1996) suggests that researchers need to explain to pupils that there are no right and wrong answers if the school regime is one that pushes the idea of correct and incorrect answers in the curriculum delivery (Cambell, 1995). It seems that the same rule applies to research partners. Indeed, a number of participants in my study were unable to sign their full names and elected to write (in block letters) only their Christian names.

2. Ensuring that the interviewees were comfortable in the interview setting. Garfat (1998) suggests that children and young people interview best when the interview takes place alongside an everyday activity. Thus, I chose the interview sites carefully and sought the advice of both the Director and one of the youth with whom I have enjoyed a particularly strong relationship.

3. Establishing trust with the research participants by visiting the school and Director regularly over a ten year period, talking and playing with the pupils whilst there, talking with some of the parents of the pupils in their own housing estates and generally making myself known to the pupils and ex-pupils as an "interested party to their activities." As the children grew older into teens, this necessitated me meeting the participants in more adult settings

chosen by them (other than one interviewee in prison who had no choice of interview environment).

4. Respecting the research participants' wish to confidentiality in imparting sensitive information by spending considerable time going through ethical guidelines prior to commencing with interviews. This is an important point as we will see later in the interview data in a later chapter. I was conscious that the pupils were sensitive to their addresses, family constellations, and family histories and the way in which someone might react to certain information. I spent some time explaining the purpose of the study and how it might impact on any individual and the interviewees showed considerable interest in this process. In one interview held with one of the girls, we spent over half an hour on this alone.

5. Ensuring anonymity for individual research participants when the research is completed/published/disseminated by using turn-numbers instead of their real names. This is facilitated by the particular tool used for analysing the data–Frameworks Analysis–where each piece of data is coded and then the respondent given a turn-number and a fictitious reference name.

6. Ensuring that the questions were asked in a non-threatening manner and clearly explaining the study to the research participants with either a member of school staff or a child and youth care practitioner or colleague nearby to ensure that the interview style was ethical.[4]

In all interviews, a child and youth care practitioner, or a child and youth care practitioner and a teacher from the project was present. In the interview process, I was conscious that the individual experiences of each participant could be adequately sought, expanded and recorded during the interview process. The participants were asked to evaluate their lives by using plain language in the interview and informed that the interview would be recorded so that I would not miss anything that was discussed. Some of the participants were more open than others were in talking.

Bearing this in mind, the interviewees in this study are approached as social actors in their own world, a world strange to me in many ways as I come from a two-parent family where my father always had secure employment, where all my siblings attended school regularly, where there was consistent access to food, light and heat and where my parents displayed affection between each other openly. This is not the experience for the vast majority of interviewees in this study and we could not pretend the situation to be otherwise. It was hoped that the interviewees would explain their world and that somehow I might navigate their narratives. The subject and subjective feature throughout the study as integral components of social life.

In line with current research elsewhere about at-risk populations, it is assumed that the interviewees cultural world was too complex to present them with only a pre-designed schedule (Glassner & Loughlin, 1987; McAuley, 1998; McElwee & Lalor, 1997; McElwee & Monaghan, 2005). The child and adolescent is considered as an active partner in the research process by providing them with the opportunity to modify the study, and in their own words, "These are the most important questions that should be asked about us" (McElwee, 2001). The approach follows directly from Article 12 of the United Nations Convention on the Rights of the Child, which states, "State parties shall assure to the child who is capable of forming his or her own views the right to express those views freely in all matters affecting the child, the views of the child being given due weight in accordance with the age and maturity of the child."

METHODOLOGICAL DIFFICULTIES:
PRE-RESEARCH RELATIONSHIP DEVELOPMENT

The first difficulty encountered in attempting to interview ex-pupils from St. Augustine's School was how one might access the population and encourage them to openly participate in the research. It quickly emerged that there were several notable gate-keepers in the primary school system, each with his or her own agenda vis-à-vis the youth. I had to solicit the favour of the school *bean-a-ti* (a surprisingly powerful person as she was the cook and held no formal teaching responsibilities), the woodwork teacher, the youth workers and the class teachers.[5]

A most co-operative individual from the outset of the study was the Director of the project. His desire was to have the story of the project recorded in some format because he felt that such marginalised and "at-risk" children often received an unsympathetic hearing and, as previously discussed, the Limerick project had not been formally evaluated since 1984. The pupils and ex-pupils in the school were quick to articulate whether or not they would participate. It is worth commenting on this in more detail in terms of research ethics.

The pupils and ex-pupils themselves had become used to me visiting the school regularly to supervise students on practice placement from the Waterford Institute of Technology's Applied Social Studies (Child and Youth Care) programmes since 1992–three years prior to the formal commencement of this research. As with all qualitative research with children and young people, simply gaining access to their location will not ensure co-operation or that the researcher might become part of the group. However I can claim to have been successful in that I managed to engage with the pupils in the first instance and obtain their permission to partake in this study.

Nonetheless, I had taken time out to be with and be alongside the pupils whilst visiting the school and engaged in the favourite recreational activity–playing pool as is encouraged in a child and youth care approach. Success here, ironically, was assisted by my own inadequacies as a pool player. The more I lost at pool to the children, the less I appeared to be considered a threat to them. To lose to the girls was considered even more worthy of derision and I regularly lost to two girls in particular, Siobhan and Amanda, who were the gate-keepers to the girls in the school. After several heavy losses sustained over a period of several months, most of the pupils began to talk with me on an informal basis and became trusting. Incidentally, I do not believe that I could have won at pool against any of these children, as they were all accomplished players. Perhaps the childcare practitioner summed things up best by stating, "Any fool who lost so easily to everyone could not be a threat to the children" (McKenna, 1996).

Fortunately, one of the ex-pupils of the school, Joe was employed on an informal scheme by the Director and he was an invaluable source of information, or advice, and was resourceful in winning over some of the younger pupils. I connected with Joe after we made a trip to the Burren area of County Clare on a day trip with several children. Whilst travelling on the school bus, we got to talking about music and it transpired that Joe was a great fan of the Spanish Tenor, Mario Lanza, as is my father. I was in a position to talk about the singer and his music and this greatly impressed Joe as no one else in the project had heard of Lanza.

Being Forthright in My Approach

Such an ethical issue as being forthright has been identified in ethnographic research with schoolchildren. Fine and Sandstrom (1988, pp. 20-22), for example, explore the concepts of explicit, shallow and deep cover. They suggest explicit cover occurs when the participant researcher is entirely frank about the research with the study group; shallow cover occurs when the researcher is somewhat vague about the research content and stated goals, whilst deep cover occurs when the researcher deliberately hides the research from informants.

The researchers allude to the dangers of using shallow cover, particularly when research findings are published and people may feel betrayed because they participated in something without full knowledge of the outcome (Fine & Sandstrom, 1988, p. 20). An advantage of using this cover is that one can negotiate the research problem as one gathers data.[6] One has an obligation, therefore, to explain one's own perspective when using either shallow or explicit cover with research participants. The fact that I obtained consent at the beginning of the process allowed me to engage with the partners on an up-front basis.

Explicit Cover

The approach in this study may best fit in the category of explicit cover as the interviewees were informed that I would be interacting with them, "getting their ideas on life in Limerick" and then writing a book at some stage. It was also suggested that several copies of my findings would be made available in the school library area when it was completed. I did not want the participants to limit their discussions in this study for fear of reprisal from teachers or other perceived authority figures such as the Police, School Attendance Officers, Social Workers and Youth Workers. I also did not want the interviewees to either over-exaggerate or under-exaggerate their deviant/criminal behaviour when being interviewed. A micro-culture like St. Augustine's, where most of the pupils and ex-pupils attempt to out-do each other in stated acts of bravado, can be a difficult one to gather accurate and realistic data simply because of the nature of their discourse.

In an attempt to get around this, I checked as much of the data supplied by the interviewees as possible with the files held by the Director of the project, with their family members, with child and youth care practitioners connected to the project and with media court reports and feature stories. An on-going interactive relationship between the pupils and some of their families between my time attending the summer camp and the official interviews further facilitated the research process. A number of the pupils and ex-pupils were visited in their own homes as well as the summer school environment along with a child and youth care practitioner from Barnardo's (a Child and Youth Care organisation) based in Moyross, Limerick. A deliberate attempt was made to construct an understanding of these interviewee's lives *through their own accounts and perceptions* of life in Limerick.

PROCEDURE

Over nineteen years (1977-1996), 148 families were connected to the St. Augustine's project, of which 90 were two-parent families and 58 were lone-parent families. In one academic year alone, out of 25 pupils, 7 pupils had only one parent living with them and four did not live with either parent (older siblings or grandparents providing refuge). One hundred and seventy eight parents were unemployed (in what the Director of the project called a "structured" context, i.e., working regular hours, receiving a wage and paying tax), with only sixty formally working at any time during the nineteen years. Forty-six of the families had more than five children. Eighty-nine of the males and one female in the study went on to prison. Of the 148 families, no fewer than eighteen of the children "experienced violent or traumatic/tragic deaths" through suicide, shooting and drugs in their immediate families (personal communication, John Hanna, 2004). Such figures are, of course, wholly disproportionate to the general population.

Factual information was obtained from files held by the Director and from a number of written reports by the school staff, school psychologists and other child and youth care professionals. These provided an overall identikit of St. Augustine's School pupils. Not all of the staff connected to the project maintained the pupil files in an orderly fashion, nor were they all filled in correctly or, indeed, completed over the years. The Director cited "poor administrative skills" amongst some staff members in the earlier stages of the project and "an inability to find the time to write up files fully" as reasons the files were inaccurate and/or incomplete. Quite simply, the school did not appear to see the need to maintain up-to-date files until the latter part of the 1990s.[7] Nonetheless, by cross-referencing data from several sources, I was able to construct snapshot portfolios of the pupils.

Some inaccuracy in data held by the school significantly impeded the research process and I had to rely on numerous semi-formal and formal interviews with the Director of the project between 1995 and 2006 for more complete and accurate information.

Written permission to engage in this research was sought from, and granted by, the Director of the school and the school's Management Committee. As noted above, data collection was facilitated by using a topic guide co-designed by the interviewees and through use of semi-structured interviews. This approach is supported by Seidman (1991) who suggests in-depth interviewing is a most effective method of inquiry when one seeks to explore subjective understanding and, indeed, in my own research into hard-to-reach populations (McEwee & Monaghan, 2005).[8]

The term "semi-structured" is employed here to refer to an approach that Lofland (cited in Mishler, 1986, p. 66) understood as a "flexible strategy of discovery," thus the content of the conversation is not predetermined but "develops as the conversation progresses" (Garfat, 1998, p. 48).

Seventeen interviewees were selected as they had attended the project and taken part in a series of summer programmes and summer camps and were judged to be broadly representative of the pupils of the project since the project opened in 1977. My research partners came from the four main address sites of the project and were statistically representative in terms of gender breakdown (four girls and thirteen boys), personal and familial histories and educational histories. A number of child and youth care commentators such as Lindsey (1994), Charles (1995), Garfat (1992; 1998) and McElwee (2003, 2004; McElwee & Monaghan, 2005) have addressed the issue of representation in relational qualitative research. They concur that it is more important to have interviewees that are knowledgeable about the area of study and are willing to critically evaluate experiences and their responses to experiences. As the interviewees were all placed in the project because they were "at-risk" and because they further lived out their at-risk profiles (later spending time in residential care, going to prison, having babies whilst still teens themselves, not passing State examinations), it was felt that they were representative of their peers in the project.

All seventeen interviewees were contacted between 1998 and 2000 by the Director of the project either formally writing to them once or phoning them on a number of occasions. The Director and I jointly amended my proposed topic schedule for the interviews and deleted some material as a number of questions were considered by school staff to be overly sensitive for the interviewees. Examples of such questions included specific questions on heroin use, involvement in juvenile prostitution and crimes against persons.[9] Based on this consultation, the topic guide was re-worked.

The interviewees themselves, the staff of the school and the parents I met with in addition to the review of literature informed the questions for this study. Specific questions developed included:

1. How did the interviewees conceptualise risk? This was probed by dividing my topic guide into three sections based on the literature on risk and resiliency.

2. What were their attitudes towards risk and safety? I developed this question by framing my interviews around expectations from school staff, parents and family members.
3. To what extent did the interviewees see themselves as involved in risky behaviour?
4. What types of risky behaviour were most and least commonly avoided/chosen with the interviewees?
5. What was the context of such behaviour?
6. Are there predisposing and situational developments in the actual development of behaviour amongst the interviewees?

The questions I actually asked could be called "areas" and how I framed an understanding for them are crucial to this study, e.g., "Do you know what the term risk means when it is used by a teacher?" "Well, I am curious about what it means to you? In your own words, not those of a teacher of Garda?" The assumption could be made that the interviewees must have heard the word risk repeatedly–in the social service sense, and must have a sense of what I meant in my questions. This was confirmed in the interview data as we will see later in chapter seven. Such questions were asked in an attempt to gain some understanding of how the interviewees understood risk and at-risk in the context of life in Limerick City and, more specifically, their reflections on their engagement with St. Augustine's Special School.

I approached the interviewees and provided a brief explanation of the scope of the study and a copy of the consent form to read. The school Director facilitated access to the group and the interviewees themselves permitted me to go over the allotted interview time as the need arose. Each interview commenced by me re-introducing myself with a short biographical sketch and a description of the proposed study. The interview questions were read to the pupils from the topic guide and any issues they had were clarified, such as, "Would they get into trouble for saying things? Would they be able to see the study when it was completed?" I noticed a particularised understanding of risk amongst the interviewees and grew curious as to how they understood and contextualised risk more generally. All but four of the interviewees were reluctant to allow the interviews to be video taped, so sessions were audio-taped.

A difficulty, sometimes, with informal interviewing is the potential to be manipulative and/or non-objective in the discussion in order to elicit information the researcher feels is important to the exclusion of matters that may be of more interest to the interviewees. I was conscious of this throughout the study and the social care practitioner with whom I worked was asked to assist in objectivity and impartiality during the interview process. We were careful not to engage in leading questions.

METHODS OF DATA ANALYSIS

The analytical method utilised by this study is based on "framework analysis." Framework analysis is a method of analysing qualitative data through content analysis, which involves summarising and classifying data, using a thematic framework. It was developed by the Qualitative Research Unit at the National Centre for Social Research in the UK, in the 1980s. As the material collected through qualitative research is invariably unstructured in nature the overall aim of utilising this form of analysis is to try and provide some coherence and structure to data, whilst ensuring that the original data is not skewed in any way. Framework analysis depends, to a large extent, upon the creative and conceptual ability of the analyst to determine the meaning of and connections between the data. Thus it connects back to interpretive meaning(s).

In order to illustrate how framework analysis was used in this study the stages of analysis will be divided into the four interdependent parts. Firstly, there is the "Pre-Analysis Preparatory Work" section, which describes the data transcription, respondent and turn-number labelling. Secondly, the method used in "Constructing a Thematic Framework" is explained. Third is the "Application of the Framework to the Data" and, finally, the "Mapping and Interpreting the Data."

Transcription, Respondent Labelling and Allocation of Turn Numbers

When each interview was completed, its corresponding audio-tape was transcribed verbatim. The process of transcription took an average of 10 hours of typing per 1 hour of interview. The length of time for transcription may be explained due to two factors. The first is that the particular accents and colloquialisms employed proved difficult for me to understand at times and, secondly, the participants often leaned away from the microphones and attempted to turn the volume either up or down despite frequent requests to the contrary.

When transcribed, each transcript was annotated with respondent labels, for example, F1 indicating Female number 1, M1, indicating

Male 1 and so on. This process of labelling was aided by using the video recording in some instances where there were two or more interviewees present during one interview and their accents were difficult to distinguish, as the means to identify each respondent in order of contributing to the interview. This was the case because some interviewees were nervous and "wanted company" (Yvonne). The majority of the research participants favoured only the audio-taping. Finally, each transcript was allocated a set of "turn-numbers," for example 1069-1357. Each time a different respondent added to the conversation within an interview, their piece of text was allocated a number which indicated its turn or place, within the interview. This system of numbering facilitates the analyst in tracing individual segments of data back to their origin.

Constructing a Thematic Framework: Familiarisation

To develop a framework or template for analysis, two transcripts were selected. The aim of this was to provide an overall range and view of the data set. The process of familiarisation and immersion involved reading each transcript on three occasions. The first reading allows the reader to become immersed in the data and to gain an insight into both the respondents and the major emergent themes. During the second and third readings, notes are inserted on the margins of the recurrent themes and any other topics considered important to the overall research process. Lindsey (1994) argues that this allows the reader to "gain a sense of the whole" whilst Garfat (1998, p. 63) acknowledges that this process caused him "to move back and forth between the transcripts, my ideas, the experience of the conversations, and the writing I was doing." So it was with my study. Garfat goes on to elaborate on his experience of this "panning" or "high-lighting approach" and observes that "particular meanings or segments of experience that seem to express a particular theme of experiencing began to emerge" (1998, p. 64).

Identifying a Thematic Framework

Once the familiarisation process was complete, the notes recorded on each transcript were reviewed. The aim of this part of the analysis was to construct a framework with which the key issues and concepts can be examined and referenced. The framework was constructed, through a combination of *a priori* material (research aims) and emergent issues raised by the research participants.

The development of a thematic framework can be best illustrated by practical example (see Figure 1). In the first box, an extract from the study topic guide is presented. The questions relating to perceptions of risk are listed from a-d. For the purposes of the example, I focus on the first of these questions, namely, (a) What do you understand by the term risk? The emergent themes were noted on the interview transcripts and are shown in Box 2 (Research Notes from Transcripts). These emergent themes, noted in the familiarisation stage, led to the development of Box 3, the "Index." The index provides a mechanism for labelling data in manageable pieces and allows for retrieval and exploration at a later stage. This index is structured on a thematic basis, of which there are three in total. Within each theme, there are a number of categories, which, in turn, are made up of sub-categories.

It should be noted that devising and refining the framework was not an automatic or mechanical process. Instead, a great deal of consideration and logic had to be used. As well as this fact, the original research questions had to be continually addressed. The emergence of themes and the identification of them has been described by Van Manen (1990), "More accurately, as a process of insightful invention, discovery, or disclosure– grasping and formulating a thematic understanding is not a rule-bound process, but a free act of 'seeing' meaning" (p. 79).

Application of the Framework to the Data: Indexing

Indexing is a process whereby the thematic framework shown above was systematically applied to the data. Each transcript was read and annotated according to this framework (see Figure 2). The index number or code is given on the extreme left-hand side, for example A10iii, with these codes linking back directly to the framework. The second column from the left indicates the turn number (58, 59, etc.) for each new piece of data; the respondent label is shown in the third column, for example, SF1, I etc.; the data obtained from the interview is presented in the "Text" column, with a brief summary of the main point being given in the "Details" column.

Application of the Framework to the Data: Charting

After completing the indexing process, it was then necessary to consider the range of data, relating to each theme and category, within the

FIGURE 1. Development of a Thematic Framework

Topic Guide (Extract)
Perceptions of Risk
a) What do you understand by the term risk?
b) What does your family tell you about risk?
c) Is Limerick City a "risky" place to live?
d) Provide some examples of risk?

Research Notes from Transcripts
1. Things Identified as having made a difference to the way the lives of the Research Participants have Developed
2. Things Identified as being Safe
3. Things Identified as Being Considered as Sources of Risk and Danger
4. Things Identified by the Children as not Wanting to be Discovered Doing
5. Factors Identified as Leading to the Research Participants ending up in St. Augustine's Special School

Life in Limerick
a. Stereotyping
b. Limiting life chances

2. Family life
a. Location
b. Family size
c. Relationships

3. St. Augustine's School
a. Getting there
b. Staying there
c. The curriculum

FIGURE 1 (continued)

A Personal Risk/Individual Factors

1 School

I.   Primary role is diversion
II.   Source of peer support
III. Temporarily removes children from at risk environment
IV. Sometimes acts to maintain outcast status
V.   Entry to the project
VI. Relationship with project
VII. Length of time on project
VIII. Summer camp
IX. Truancy

2 Childhood

I.   A time to do mad things
II.   A time when criminal behaviour is excused

3 Crime

I.   Opportunistic
II.   Learned familial behaviour
III. Risk acceptance

4 Having a Child

I.   Provides an individual with status
II.   Affirms male status
III. Grounds an individual
IV. Responsibility stops at giving money

framework. As a result, data relating to the same categories and sub-categories was rearranged and placed into charts. The process of lifting data and rearranging it according to the pre-designed themes is described as "charting." The charts were devised with headings and sub-headings, which were based on the *a priori* data and the thematic framework, described earlier. In this study, the charts were organised on a thematic basis across the interview sites. To further clarify the process, data relating to the "Significant Person" is presented in its "charted" or re-organised way, in Figure 3.

FIGURE 2. Indexing of Data on Transcript

Index	Turn No.	Respondent Label	Text	Comment
	57	I	Can you tell me about any one of them in particular?	–
A10iii	58	SF1	Oh, bad luck always happens to me. I think there's something following me around giving me bad luck. I remember one day I went into town with money to get clothes. It was on my communion. My mother brought me in and I lost the whole lot of my communion money.	Personal Bad Luck
	59	I	You lost it?	–
C7ii	60a	SF1	I lost the whole lot. My brother is forever having accidents. He was going down the street.	Family Bad Luck

As one can see, this is an extract from the "*A7iv*" Chart, specifically dealing with the "Significant Person–Director of the Project." This method of charting was completed for each category and theme, across all of the data set.

Application of the Framework to the Data: Mapping and Interpretation

After the completion of the charting process, the key themes and characteristics of the data were pulled together. The process of mapping and interpretation is based on the *a priori* data and the emergent themes, with the subsequent analysis being guided by both of these. Piecing together the data into a coherent piece of work was difficult and, not unlike the previous sections outlined above, it was by no means a mechanical process.

The data analysis were divided into three sections, including (a) personal risk/risk factors, (b) risk to friends and peers, and (c) risk in a familial context. Thirty-five themes were identified including 180 subthemes.

FIGURE 3. Significant Person

Index	Turn No.	Respondent Label	Text
(A7iv)	1087	EM4	I would say, he made a difference to me anyway, he did anyway, because before I went into the school I was stone mad and pure running mad around the roads like and in the school I quietened down and well stayed out of prison and if I didn't join the school, I would have got prison like, I had to do something.
(A7iv)	1089	EM4	Yeah, JH made sense to me anyway.
(A7iv)	1181	EM4	Yeah, all that like, especially what JH said.
(A7iv)	1343	EM4	They should yeah, I should have done it myself like, JH offered me to do my Junior Cert, but I think I went to the Youth Centre.
(A7iv)	1395b	FM5	Because it is a good school and that, cause it is a good school, there is a laugh in there and kids running and it is alright, you know, it is alright when you want to be, do you get me and the Headmaster, JH, he is alright, he is alright to talk to, all the people in there would know him from their own area or someone from up town or something like that, so you don't get to know nothing.

CONCLUSION

This chapter has laid an "audit trail" for the reader in terms of my application of a relational research model. The methodology used to collect the data was presented and justified and as noted by Gannon (2005, p. 8) one simply does not work with a "known population or with a good sized experimental sample" but, ultimately, with "a population of one" in relational research. Explicit references to the steps taken in deciding the research partners to be interviewed and procedures favoured were outlined. The methodology was outlined and the ethical issues were considered.

NOTES

1. This was done after consultation with the Director of the school who kindly facilitated this process.

2. In his landmark publication, *The Prison Community*, Clemmer noted that "... an adult is largely the result of what he (or she) has learned through infancy, boyhood (or girlhood) and youth. People, then, as adults, are the aggregate of their experiences. Consequently, we may assume that any environment and every social experience will contribute to changes in people" (Clemmer, 1940, p. 1).

3. As Thomas and O'Kane (1998, p. 336) acknowledge, the possibility of abuse of subjects by a researcher or exploitation by the research process is present in every research relationship.

4. Of course, one should always be vigilant with regard to accuracy in data gathering and processing, employing relevant research methodology, interpreting the data adequately, accurately reporting the data analysis and disseminating one's findings thoughtfully and in appropriate form. I will return to this point later in the study.

5. This is a Gaelic term for "Woman of the House."

6. One cannot, of course, control the media in child care issues as research data tends to assume a life of its own once it has been disseminated by academics (see Ferguson's discussion on the Kilkenny Incest case, 1995, or my own work on juvenile prostitution in Waterford City, 1997).

7. There is a link to the risk society child protection debate here. The school Director noted the changing politicised culture of this period and felt that the school could be "brought to task publicly if it was not seen to be rigorous in everything it did" (McElwee, 1999).

8. As with all instruments, there are difficulties with using questionnaires. Indeed, as long ago as 1896 in the *Educational Review* the editor bemoaned "the silly question papers sent out at haphazard to be answered by persons of little scientific training or none" (Good, 1973, pp. 196-197).

9. Although, it is interesting to note that one of the children (whilst under the age of eighteen) subsequently became involved in prostitution in Limerick city.

REFERENCES

Alderson, P. (1995). *Listening to children: Children, ethics and social research*. London: Barnardos.

Bates, B. (1996). *Aspects of childhood deviancy: A study of young offenders in open settings*. Unpublished doctoral dissertation. Dublin: University College Dublin.

Cambell, A. T. (1995). *Getting to know Waiwai: An Amazonian ethnography*. London: Routledge.

Denzin, N. (1970). *The research act in sociology*. London: Butterworth.

Downes, D., & Rock, P. (1988). *Understanding deviance*. Oxford. Clarendon Press.

Fine, G. A., & Sandstrom, K. (1998). *Knowing children: Participant observation with minors*. Newbury Park, CA: Sage.

Gannon, B. (2005). A sample of one. *Relational Child and Youth Care Practice, 18*(4), 5-9.

Garfat, T. (1998). The effective child and youth care practitioner: A phenomenological inquiry. *Journal of Child and Youth Care, 12,* 1-2.

Garfat, T., & McElwee, N. (2004). *Effective interventions with families: The EirCan perspective.* Cape Town: Pretext.

Glaser, B. G., & Strauss, A. (1970). *The discovery of grounded theory.* New York: Aldine.

Glassner, B., & Loughlin, J. (1987). *Drugs in adolescent worlds: Burnouts to straights.* New York: St. Martins Press.

Hammersley, M. (1995). *The politics of social research.* London: Sage.

Hartnoll, R. (1992). *Critical overview of existing methods. NIDA Research Monograph: Research Methods for Hidden Populations.* Proceedings from an Invited Expert Meeting in Illegal Drug Use.

Hassard, J. (1990). Multiple paradigms and organisational analysis: A case study. *Organisational Studies, 12*(2), 275-299.

Higgins, K., & Pinkerton, J. (1998). Literature reviewing: Towards a more rigorous approach. In D. Iwaniec & J. Pinkerton (Eds.), *Making research work: Promoting child care policy and practice* (pp. 93-112). London: John Wiley & Sons.

Hill, M. & Tisdall, K. (1997). *Children and society.* UK: Addison Wesley Longman.

Hood, S., Kelly, P., & Mayall, B. (1996). Children as research subjects: A risky enterprise. *Children and Society, 10*(2), 117-128.

Iwaniec, D. (1996). *The emotionally abused and neglected child.* Chichester: Wiley.

Kaplan, L. (1986). *Working with multi-problem families.* Massachusetts: Lexington Books.

Leadbeater, B., Banister, E., Benoit, C., Jansson, M., Marshall, A., & Riecken, T. (2006). *Ethical issues in community based research with children and youth.* Toronto: University of Toronto Press.

Liddle, C. (1992). *Acting for children.* London: The Law Society.

Lindsey, D. (1994). *The welfare of children.* New York: Oxford University Press.

Lindsey, E. A. (1994). Health within illness: Experiences of chronically ill/disabled. Unpublished doctoral dissertation, University of Victoria, Victoria: BC.

Marshall, C., & Rossman, G. B. (1989). *Designing qualitative research.* Beverly Hills, CA: Sage.

Mauthner, M. (1997). Methodological aspects of collecting data from children: Lessons from three research projects. *Children and Society, 11*(1), 16-28.

McCauley, C. (1998). Child participatory research: Ethical and methodological considerations. In D. Iwaniec & J. Pinkerton (Eds.), *Making research work: Promoting child care policy and practice* (pp. 163-178). London: John Wiley & Sons.

McElwee, N. (1999). Mandatory reporting and the risk society. In C. Hanly (Ed.), *Child sexual abuse and rape.* Waterford: Waterford Institute of Technology.

McElwee, N. (1999). From legislation to practice: Some observations on the 1991 Child Care Act in relation to the promotion and protection of children. *Journal of Irish Family Law, 4,* 7-10.

McElwee, N., & Lalor, K. (1997). *Prostitution in Waterford city: A contemporary analysis.* Waterford: StreetSmart Press.

McElwee, N., & Monaghan, G. (2005). *Darkness on the edge of town: An exploratory study of heroin misuse in Athlone and Portlaoise.* Athlone: Centre for Child & Youth Care Learning.

McKenna, S. (1996). *Walking the roads: The children of St. Augustine's.* Unpublished diploma dissertation. Waterford: Centre for Social Care Research, Waterford Institute of Technology.

Morrow, V., & Richards, M. (1996). The ethics of social research with children: An overview. *Children and Society, 10*(12), 90-105.

Patton, M. Q. (1980). *Qualitative evaluation methods.* Beverly Hills: Sage Publications.

Pinkerton, J. (1998). The impact of research on policy and practice. In D. Iwaniec & J. Pinkerton (Eds.), *Making research work: Promoting child care policy and practice* (pp. 25-45). London: John Wiley and Sons.

Sacks, H. (1992). *Lectures on conversation* (vol. 2). Oxford: Basil Blackwell.

Sarantakos, S. (1993). *Social research.* London: MacMillan Educational.

Seidman, I. E. (1991). *Interviewing as qualitative research: A guide for researchers in education and the social sciences.* New York: Columbia University, Teacher's College Press.

Silverman, D. (1993). *Interpreting qualitative data. Methods for analysing talk, text, and interaction.* London: Sage.

Solberg, A. (1996). The challenge in child research. From "being" to "doing." In J. Brennan & M. O'Brien (Eds.), *Children in families: Research and policy* (pp. 53-65). Falmer.

Thomas, N., & O'Kane, C. (1998). The ethics of participatory research with children. *Children and Society, 12,* 336-348.

Vaillancourt, T., & Igneski, V. (2006). The study of suicidology among children and youth: Preliminary recommendations and best practice. In B. Leadbeater, E. Banister, C. Benoit, M. Jansson, A. Marshall, & T. Riecken (Eds.), *Ethical issues in community based research with children and youth* (pp. 207-220). Toronto: University of Toronto Press.

VanderVen, K. (1993). Advancing child and youth care: A model for integrating theory and practice through connecting education, training and the service system. *Child and Youth Care Forum, 22*(4), 265-283.

VanManen, M. (1990). *Researching lived experience: Towards an action sensitive pedagogy.* London, Ontario: Althouse Press.

doi:10.1300/J024v29n01_05

Chapter 6

Now Is the Time:
A Toxic Era for Child and Youth Care

SUMMARY. The purpose of this chapter is to provide a very personal series of reflections on the current debate on risk and accountability in child protection and child and youth care as the former strives to come out of a period of volunteerism and professionalize itself (McElwee, 1998; Share & McElwee, 2005). Irish culture has grown more individualist as has the work environment. An on-going theme is that of accountability, which has emerged in child and youth care throughout the Western world (Causon, 1997; Kendrick, 1997). Whether it be accountability in terms of fiscal management, specific populations served (Charles, 2001; Maier, 2001), treatment outcomes (Waterhouse, 2000), or even accountability in terms of direct practice actions (Garfat & McElwee, 2004; Parton et al., 1997), the "age of accountability" or "risk society" has certainly descended upon us. The relationship between the risk culture, actual cases of malpractice, the scapegoating culture, the collective sense of non-responsibility, and media sensationalism is becoming more dominant and complex (Fewster, 2002; Mitchell, 1999). In the middle of it all are the families in distress and youth at risk. doi:10.1300/J024v29n01_06 *[Article copies available for a fee from The Haworth Document Delivery Service: 1-800-HAWORTH. E-mail address: <docdelivery@haworthpress.com> Website: <http://www.HaworthPress.com> © 2007 by The Haworth Press, Inc. All rights reserved.]*

[Haworth co-indexing entry note]: "Now Is the Time: A Toxic Era for Child and Youth Care." McElwee, Niall. Co-published simultaneously in *Child & Youth Services* (The Haworth Press, Inc.) Vol. 29, No. 1/2, 2007, pp. 129-164; and: *At-Risk Children & Youth: Resiliency Explored* (Niall McElwee) The Haworth Press, Inc., 2007, pp. 129-164. Single or multiple copies of this article are available for a fee from The Haworth Document Delivery Service [1-800-HAWORTH, 9:00 a.m. - 5:00 p.m. (EST). E-mail address: docdelivery@haworthpress. com].

KEYWORDS. Professionalization of child and youth care, volunteerism, Catholic Church and child and youth care, child protection and welfare, youth work, youth development

The very scepticism that is the driving force of expert knowledge might lead, in some contexts, or among some groups, to a disenchantment with all experts; this is one of the lines of tension between expertise and tradition. (Giddens, 1994, p. 87)

At the end of 2001 there were approximately 5,500 children in care in Ireland but the number of children's residential centres has decreased from 176 in 2002 to 154 in 2003. Of these centres, 89 were run by health boards, 65 by the non-statutory sector and 15 by private providers (Social Services Inspectorate, 2003).[1] Fewer males are being attracted into child and youth care and retention of staff at all grades is a particular challenge as there are currently less than 150 males studying at third level in the Higher Education and Training Awards Council and Dublin Institute Technology system out of some 3,000 students (McElwee et al., 2003). The Association that represented front-line social care practitioners in Ireland for decades, the Irish Association of Care Workers, disbanded in May, 2005, and its passing went largely unnoticed by many social care practitioners. An Association in decline for some years, its membership base had fallen from five hundred in the mid-1990s down to under one hundred and twenty care practitioners by 2005.

How did this come to pass at what might be seen as the key time since the early 1970s for child and youth care in Ireland to attempt to professionalize? What are the key influencers in child and youth care? What is this risk society and who is moving forward a risk narrative agenda? Perhaps the most appropriate location to begin is around a thorny issue in our field–that of its professionalisation.

PROFESSIONALIZATION

Child and youth care was largely the preserve of religious congregations and well-minded volunteers until the 1970s in Ireland. Since then, training and qualifications have become more and more the norm–so much so that statutory registration is due to come into effect in late 2006. Literature in the field of child and youth care is full of references to the nature of the child and youth care form of practice. At various times, writers have described the uniqueness of the field and even its "magic" (Garfat, 1988), but it must be remembered that modern child and youth care in Ireland was borne out of "serious deficiencies in the running of children's centres... and the recognition of the need for professionally trained staff" (Kennedy & Gallagher, 1997). Thus, it has been closely tied to misfortune.

Lack of regulation was the norm until very recently. For example, preschool regulations were only introduced in 1996 after decades of both public and private provision. The 1908 Children's Act provided the legislative framework for child care in Ireland for the greater part of the 20th century, but by 1991 the social and political situation vis-à-vis children at-risk had significantly changed due to a number of phenomena. The 1991 Child Care Act is in total contrast to the 1908 Act that simply imposed negative duties to rescue children who had criminal offences committed against them or who were being cruelly treated. Specifically, the Act recognises that the welfare of the child is the first and paramount consideration (Part II, section 3:2, b). The rights and duties of parents are important, but due consideration must be given to the child's wishes (McElwee, 2001, p. 7).

The Joint Committee on Social Care Professionals (2003) enumerated some 2,904 social care practitioners working across various sectors including community child care (71), staff in children's residential centres (1,214), and staff in intellectual disability services (1,619). Of these, just over 55% hold what might be termed a professional qualification, with 14% still holding no qualifications at all. This is similar to my own findings in the residential child care centre where I also enumerated 14% of staff (or 105 practitioners) with no formal qualifications. Thus, there is a considerable journey to be undertaken in the field (McElwee, 2000).

A common approach to the analysis of the professions is to compile a list of key attributes. Such a list, based on numerous studies of the professions, could be the following (Williams and Lalor, 2000, p. 77):

- ownership of a recognised body of knowledge exclusive to that profession with development of new knowledge through research
- self-government through a body that sets and monitors its own standards of practice
- control of training and recruitment
- monopoly of practice in its own field of work with registration by the state
- conformity to moral and disciplinary codes of behaviour

- autonomy of practice and greater individual accountability
- a public ideology of service to a client group

One of the well known commentators on professionalism, Freidson (1990) makes the important point that a particular profession cannot, in the contemporary world, be thought of outside of the specific and distinctive *institutions* of our society. This is a key point in relation to the risk society debate as both are inextricably entwined with Parton (1997, p. 13) commenting, "As procedures have become more complex, detailed and wide ranging, the chances of making a procedural mistake are ironically increased." Partly because of this there is a debate around whether or not child and youth care should attempt to professionalize itself *a la* other more established professions such as social work (see McElwee, 1998).

A Vignette

Recently I was teaching a child and youth care professional interventions class with Certificate students and gave them an example of planning an intervention with a male youth, aged thirteen. Let's call him Doug. I informed the students that I had taken Doug to a rugby match and used the occasion to attempt to further construct a therapeutic relationship by sitting beside him, explaining the rules of the game, and purchasing him a soft drink and popcorn. Several students took issue with the fact that this took place outside the norms of the residential unit and that I was leaving myself open to allegations. Now, the interesting thing about this for me was the way many of the students were already constructing risk. Some were thinking not of the potentially positive experience for the youth but of the way in which the activity might be used against them as future professional practitioners. A safe way to work with the youth, according to several of the students, was to limit one's exposure to him. Were I to do this, Doug might never attend a rugby game whilst in care because it is not the norm for female child and youth care workers to follow rugby. And yet, I understand why Irish child and youth care students might be thinking like this even *before* they graduate into the field to become front-line staff. It is because a risk consciousness pervades the professional environment and hangs over with a deathly pall. We are the "careering juggernaut."

We have seen in an earlier chapter how risk has been identified as moving through two stages and we are living on a ledge–in a random risk society from which nobody can escape because of a state of manufactured uncertainty (a term used by both Beck and Giddens) which now prevails (Beck, 1997, p. 12). The environment in risk literature has been re-defined as being all-inclusive i.e., workplaces, hospitals, schools, care homes and the outdoors and we have become more thoughtful of the long-term results of our present day actions. This is true in the youth at-risk debate where we witnessed a movement from institutionalisation to de-institutionalisation during the 1970s and from what I have termed in the past "control models of care" to "care models of control" during the 1980s and 1990s in Ireland. What makes their "risk situation" worse for some children and youth is the fact that, for a time, more and more children and young people were being placed in care of the State on formal court orders and had no choice over their place of stay nor of the staff that worked in these centres.[2]

A TOXIC ERA FOR CHILD AND YOUTH CARE?

The newest stage of history is defined by distributions of risks, hazards, and dangers, and "reflexive" is understood by Beck (1992) to mean both the advancement and dissolution of industrial society. Borrowing from the language of environmental risk, we might argue that this new era is a toxic era and at the crux of the discussion about the care of at-risk children and youth rests issues around defining and exploring professionalism, trust, risk and danger. Few of our State agencies have not been affected by this loss of trust. Dingwall et al. have suggested that an outlook has developed following on from several high profile scandals whereby "social workers are more concerned to make a *defensible* decision than with making the *right* decision (Dingwall, Eekelaar & Murray, 1995, p. 221). As we have seen earlier, such thinking effects even students who have yet to graduate as professionals.

There is a depressingly long list of childcare scandals and debacles since what I might term the modern era of child and youth care provision (i.e., taking 1970 as a key date). The Beckford case (1985), the Henry and Carlile cases (1987), the Cleveland case (1988) in the UK and the X case (1992), Kilkenny Incest case (1993), Kelly Fitzgerald (1994), Madonna House (1993-4), Goldenbridge Orphanage (1995), Trudder House (1996), McColgan case (1998) and the Artane Industrial School scandal (1999) here in Ireland all point to the risk environment that both children and their care staff are forced to navigate. The common feature connecting all these scandals is that one could argue that children and youth were actually placed at *further* risk whilst in designated care of supposed experts and professionals.[3]

Over the past two decades professionals working with vulnerable populations have come under intense public scrutiny and although Thorpe states, "… the patterns of child protection activity in the Republic of Ireland are exactly in line with those found in the UK and Western Australia" (1997, p. 67) as notions of risk have become central to child protection practice, this is of little comfort to those on the front lines. It is ironic but as with the environment and science, the more we think we progress, the more we set ourselves up for risk–risk of failure to intervene, risk of over-intervention, risk of public perception, risk of simply "getting it wrong."

The domain of large scale residential child care provision has been, perhaps, the one area singled out as being fraught with risk for children and youth here in Ireland, chiefly because it has a lengthy history of provision in large foreboding buildings. But to understand the present, we must look to the past.

A HISTORICAL SNAPSHOT

The *experience* of risk and danger is now a central element of what it is to do welfare work. It is not simply that notions of risk are built into the operations, systems, and activities of welfare workers, but it is *felt* as a central element of what it is to *do* welfare work at the grass roots and be a social worker. (Kemshall et al., 1997, p. 228)

As noted, the Irish State has only recently broadened its terms of risk reference with regard to children and adolescents to include physical, emotional, sexual abuse, and neglect (National Children's Strategy, 2001). Risks are increasingly defined at a systemic level and are considered so worrying by human services professionals because of their perceived unmanageability and randomness (hints here of risk *a la* nuclear war and chemical pollution?). Partly because of this, there has been a rebirth of interest in risk as it applies to child and youth care and special education over the past two decades, although this has taken some time to filter into internal policy documents.

Increasingly, the past work of residential child care workers is under scrutiny and the motivations of males, in particular, going into care work is being challenged with the result that this area of work is proving less and less attractive to them (McElwee et al., 2003; McElwee, 2005) and, as Beck suggests, "The risk society contains an inherent tendency to become a scapegoat society" (1992, p. 75).

Many times, Irish male residential child care workers have told me that they are deliberately vague when asked in social gatherings what they work at. Part of their explanation for this is because male staff are fearful that they will be further questioned about all the scandals that have been reported (and be implicated merely because of gender), another reason is that they do not want to be seen to have "too much of an interest in children and youth" (fear and blame, then, being closely equated). There is good reason for this (Dunphy, 2006). The history of child care service provision in Ireland is littered with shameful and criminal incidents, much of which has only recently surfaced and central in all of this, as noted above, has been the Catholic Church as it was, for many decades, the sole provider for children and youth at-risk in Ireland. In an era of volunteerism this is somewhat understandable as there were so few checks and balances, but not so as we professionalize. The public is no longer prepared to forgive any wrongs by those working with distressed young people.

THE CATHOLIC CHURCH, VOLUNTEERISM AND THE RISK SOCIETY

One of the first impressions of the country that marks it out as different from other Western societies is that the Catholic Church is a strong and active force in everyday life. (Inglis, 1987, p. 1)

In 1965, 282 men were ordained as diocesan priests and 377 ordained into the religious orders but by 1999 the numbers had dropped to 34 and nine respectively. Our surviving priests are an aging cohort with over 50% over the age of 55. In 1970, 227 women entered convents in Ireland but in 1999 only 21 women joined. In a twenty year period, then, from 1970-1990 there is a massive downturn in numbers. In the case of nuns it went from 18,662 to 10,987 and in the case of Orders of Brothers figures went from 2,540 to 925 (O'Grady, 2001).

When Pope John Paul II died in Easter Week, 2005, the Irish President noted "We are proud that Pope John Paul II was the first Pope in history to visit Ireland and that, in the final years of his life, it was his ambition to return to our midst. I consider it a wonderful privilege to have met him in person as President of Ireland." Our most well known training college for Catholic clergy is Maynooth University situated in

Kildare. Since its foundation in 1795, Maynooth has graduated over 11,000 priests travelling, quite literally, to the four corners of the world. But in 2004 only 15 priests were ordained out of a potential 4.2 million Catholics on the entire island. To put this figure in context, the Anglican Church of Ireland ordained 19 in the same year with a far smaller demographic base from which to draw.

In 1979, over one million people turned up to a mass in Phoenix Park in Dublin. This was about 25 percent of the population of the Republic! How times have changed in 25 years. Then 90 percent of the population claimed to go to Mass once a week, but now the figure is closer to 44 percent. It has been estimated that 684 Irish women had abortions in 1979 while 6,490 abortions were performed in 2002 (Dept. of Health and Children, 2003). Divorce did not exist in 1979. A referendum for divorce was narrowly passed in 1995 and figures for 1998 show that 2,722 applications for divorce were submitted with 1,431 granted. What has been called a la carte Catholicism has taken hold. Many young people do not go to Mass at all.

The Irish people had, historically, a profound trust in the Catholic Church but throughout the 1990s the Catholic Church experienced wave after wave of scandal with religious orders such as the Norbertine Order, the Christian Brothers, the Oblate Fathers, the Sisters of Mercy, and the Good Shepherd Sisters involved in cases of abuse. What has particularly shocked many people is the manner in which the religious superiors allegedly allowed its clergy to move from one area to another whilst under suspicion of having committed sexual and physical offences against minors.

The Catholic Church has funded programmes for the rehabilitation of religious sexual offenders and, more importantly, shielded them from State prosecution in a number of countries.[4] With the death of the Pope John Paul II in April 2005, a debate quickly ensued in Ireland around the Pontiff's perceived failure to deal with institutionalised child abuse until towards the end of his papacy when so many people had been irreversibly damaged emotionally. It also transpired that a percentage of Church Sunday collection monies were being used to pay for past indiscretions of Religious.

In response to public disquiet with regard to scandals in Ireland, the Council of Religious in Ireland established, and is providing funding for, an independent counselling service titled Foiseamh. Many young people have watched and read with disbelief the high profile cases of Catholic religious involved in past and present scandals involving the abuse of power, the ill-treatment of children in care and an apparent rejection to allay the fears of "ordinary" Catholics.

VOLUNTEERISM GONE WRONG

But alarm bells were ringing out decades earlier as noted by Paddy Doyle in his excellent Irish based website (http:www.paddydoyle.com/). As long ago as 1934 *The Cussen Report*, about industrial schools, expressed reservations about the large number of Irish children in care, the inadequate nature of their education, the lack of local support and the stigma attached to the schools but concluded that "Schools should remain under the management of the religious orders." This has now been found to have been a catastrophic mistake. In 1943 St. Josephs Industrial School in Cavan, run by the Order of Poor Clare Sisters, burnt to the ground, killing 35 girls and one elderly woman. The nuns were exonerated in the subsequent inquiry but questions have been raised about why so many children died and the context of their deaths. Just one year later in 1944, P. Ó Muircheartaigh, the Inspector of Industrial and Reformatory Schools, reported that the children are not properly fed which was a serious indictment of the system. The Resident Managers of Lenaboy and Cappoquin industrial schools, both Sisters of Mercy, were dismissed for negligence and misappropriating funds, despite Church resistance. However, there were no other changes to industrial schools (Doyle, 2005).

Two years later, Fr. Flanagan, the founder of the famous Boystown Schools for orphans and delinquents in the US, visited Irish industrial schools and described them as "a national disgrace," leading to a public debate in the Irish House of Parliament and media. Unfortunately, a combination of State and Church pressure forced him to leave Ireland. Finally, in 1947 a three-year-old toddler named Michael McQualter was scalded to death in a hot bath in Kyran's Industrial School. The subsequent inquiry found the school to be "criminally negligent," but the case was not pursued by the Irish Department of Education.

The 1950s did not fare much better. In 1955 the Secretary of the Department of Education visited Daingean Industrial School in Offaly and found that "The cows are better fed than the boys." Despite this, nothing much was done to improve the lot of the boys for another 16 years. In 1957 the Marlborough House building was condemned by the Department of Works as "a grave risk of loss of life." Incredibly, no alterations were made, and it continued unchanged for 15 years.

The shameful treatment of Irish youth in care continued in the 1960s. In 1963, the infamous Bundoran Incident occurred where eight girls who tried to escape from St. Martha's Industrial School were caught and had their heads shaved. This became a scandal when it ended up as front-page news in a British tabloid with photos and a banner headline, "Orphanage Horror." The Department of Education again failed to act meaningfully. Four years later in 1967 the Department of Health visited Ferryhouse Industrial School, Clonmel, to investigate the death of a child from meningitis and described conditions as "a social malaise" and recommended the closure of the school. It did not close.

In 1978 a child care worker at Madonna House kidnapped a boy in his care, took him to Edinburgh in Scotland, and drowned him in a bath in a hotel. The Minister for Health, Charles Haughey, rejected a call for a public enquiry into the matter, stating that it "would serve no useful purpose." The lid was still being firmly pressed on public articulation of the shameful treatment of children and youth in residential care environments. Most disturbing of all was that the overwhelming cause of committal of children to these horrific Industrial Schools was "lack of proper guardianship." Only a small number were committed for inadequate school attendance, indictable offences, and homelessness. Thus, their at-risk status was familial rather than personal, inherited rather than individual.

The start of the decade in 1970 did see a chink of light when The Kennedy Report recommended closure of industrial schools, as Justice Kennedy was "appalled" by the "Dickensian and deplorable state" of industrial schools. Daingean Industrial School finally closed in 1976, but the hurt and shame continued. Let us explore this report as it advocated a community response to dealing with children and youth at-risk.

The Kennedy Report

The special educational sector was profoundly influenced by the Kennedy Report's (1970) recommendation to close down the Industrial School sector. This left a vacuum for many children and adolescents at-risk and it was thought that a sector within the national school system could attempt to engage such children if a number of structural changes were made. In 1967 a committee was formed to conduct a survey of Reformatory and Industrial schools and published its findings three years later (Reformatory and Industrial Schools Systems Report, 1970). The objective of the study was to make recommendations to the then Minister of Education, Donagh O'Malley, who admitted that the 1908 Act was too restrictive and unsuitable to an era of changing social and political conditions. The landmark report alludes to the fact that, historically, children aged seven and above were not treated differently from adults even on pain of death. Furthermore, it noted that the Irish "child care system has evolved in a haphazard and amateurish way and has not altered radically down the years" (p. 4.1). A system that "may once have been admirable ... is now no longer suited to the requirements of our modern and more scientific age and our greater realisation of our duty to the less fortunate members of society."

The Report highlighted a number of inadequacies in child care services such as staff with little or no training, poor buildings being used to house children and staff, and under-funding by the government. This report ushered in a development model of childcare as attention was (re)focused on prevention and family support as opposed to the removal of children from "failed" families. Possibly its most important recommendation, then, was: "The whole aim of the child care system should be geared towards the prevention of family breakdown and the problems consequent on it. The committal of children to residential care should be considered only when there is no satisfactory alternative" (Kennedy Report, 1970, p. 6).

Strategies and policies should facilitate this process. Residential care was to be considered only as a last "at best, substitute, resort" (1970, p. 4.8) and group homes were favoured. The Report called for the term Industrial School to be replaced by the term Residential Home (1970, p. 4.9). Conditions in 1970 reminded one of the origins of residential care in Ireland. The Report condemned "... meeting children with so little contact with the outside world that they were unaware that food had to be paid for or letters had to be stamped" (1970, p. 4.10) and recognised that children in care were at a disadvantage compared to other children. The Committee called for "over-compensation" in working with at-risk children (1970, p. 4.13). An immediate effect of the Report was the closure of a number of the older institutions and an emphasis on community care provision.

MOVING FORWARD THE AGENDA OF AT-RISK CHILDREN IN EDUCATIONAL CONTEXTS

Chapter seven of the Kennedy Report dealt with education and it is of note that the Department of Education "has played the principal role in relation to its implementation" as this serves as a potential site for blame allocation (Task Force Report, 1981). Nonetheless, in the Kennedy Report, educational provision was roundly criticised with the Committee noting the disorganisation in tracking at-risk students and the fact that deprivation was common in the lives of at-risk children. The Report called for early diagnosis. It commented that the school experience should be as broad as possible and should attempt to engage pupils by taking into consideration the totality of the home lives of children and by providing a varied and relevant curriculum. Such an approach provided the green light for the development of community based Youth Encounter Projects with their negotiated curricula.[5] School attendance was identified as an area requiring reform. The committee noted that the School Attendance Acts should be reviewed and up-dated, that the title School Attendance Officers should be changed to School Welfare Officers, and that truancy should be investigated when detected (1970, 11.3-11.4).

Both the Kennedy Report (1970) and the Task Force on Child Care Services (1981) emphasised the importance of improving services for deprived children, disadvantaged children, and children at-risk so an evolving consciousness of vulnerability is evident in the thinking of that time. The thinking was moving away from residential care and into the community.

STATES OF FEAR AND THE DEATH OF VOLUNTEERISM: BRINGING THE STATE TO ACCOUNT

Perhaps the final nail in the coffin for the Catholic Church, so to speak, came in April and May, 1999, when R.T.E. (Radio Telefis Eireann) broadcast a three-part documentary called *States of Fear*. It was an emotionally powerful series detailing the systematic abuse suffered by generations of Irish children in various State institutions and religious-run schools established with the brief to protect them from their at-risk status. It shocked hundreds of thousands of people and opened up to public scrutiny the shameful secrets that lay buried for so long just beneath the surface of a deeply repressive Catholic society, in particular the period from the 1940s to the 1970s. It challenged popular myths such as the one that more boys than girls were resident in the Industrial Schools and that these schools were places where all young people could learn a trade.

The series caused a national outcry and resulted in dozens of people recounting their experiences in newspapers and on radio and television on a daily basis. Such was the outcry that a Commission to Inquire into Child Abuse was established and the Irish Prime Minister issued a public apology on behalf of the government. This was a wholly new approach to children at-risk and it is difficult to believe that it would have occurred without the involvement of the media.

Suffer the Little Children. The Inside Story of Ireland's Industrial Schools (Raftery & O'Sullivan, 1999) is a further development to this story. Not only does the book recount the stories of individual children who experienced abuse at the hands of "experts," it shows how the State and individuals within the Religious Orders destroyed the lives of countless numbers of these children and, indeed, their families. The book notes that allegations of sexual abuse were made against up to 150 Brothers with eleven charged at the time of publication. Sadly, it also shows how the deeply religious Catholic society of the time allowed this to happen in front of its eyes. Unsurprisingly, the book made it onto the Irish bestsellers list. But children and youth in residential care remained at risk well into the 1990s.

THE MEDICAL EXPERTS BETRAY THEIR TRUST

We have already seen in an earlier chapter that the world of medicine permeates the risk debate. Perhaps the most excessive abuse of such expert power was seen in what has been termed the tragic abuse of medicine during the Second World War (Musto, 1981) This included the legal sterilisation of 350,000 psychiatric patients without their consent, the gassing of 70,000 German psychiatric patients with the active support of a team of psychiatrists and the flourishing of brain research on live psychiatric patients (Muller-Hill, 1991, p. 461).

The year 1999 saw another medical scandal that began to unfold whereby some Irish hospitals were keeping, for research purposes, the organs of infants who had died, but hospital administrations had failed to inform parents. This affected hundreds of families and, again, a Commission had to be established. Yet another recent child protection and welfare scandal, this time related to medical vaccines for children, was dissected in the Irish media with varying levels of sensationalism. As much as 4,250 out-of-date polio vaccines were administered across five health board areas with three other health boards yet to report back to the Department of Health and Children (Irish Times, 9.3.01).

Again, the public is confused about the mixed messages it is receiving from the various expert stakeholders. Even these experts are unsure as to what they should do. A recent advertising campaign by the Irish Blood Transfusion Service informs us that one in four Irish people will require a blood transfusion some time in our lives, yet it is considering whether or not it should place a ban on 15,000 donors giving blood as they may be at risk of carrying variant CJD as this population lived, for various time periods, in the UK and are considered at risk due to the different agricultural practices used.

NEWTOWN HOUSE: WORKING IN AN EMERGING PROFESSION ON THE LEDGE OF THE RISK SOCIETY

The ultimate risk incidence from the point of view of the State is surely the death of a child or youth whilst in its care. We have ensured this when such a high-profile scandal in the Irish residential child care sector involved the death of a 15-year-old girl called Kim O'Donovan. Kim had been placed in the care of a centre called Newtown House in County Wicklow on the east coast.[6] This centre also experienced a scandal involving the alleged sexual and physical abuse of a Traveller child by a male staff member so has gained a degree of notoriety.

The children resident in Newtown House were described as "very disturbed" and many of their other placements had broken down. The staff were largely untrained for the work demands being made on them and they were expected to run what was, in effect, a secure unit in a house entirely unsuitable for that purpose. In terms of support services, the psychological services to name but one were subject to delays of up to six months.

After spending two years in Newtown House, Kim absconded from care and was found dead four weeks later from a heroin overdose in the company of an older male. The judge involved in the case, Peter Kelly, called for an official inquiry to be established and a separate report published by the Social Services Inspectorate (2001) was damning of conditions in the centre and aspects of staff/client interaction. The Social Services Inspectorate's report (2001) notes that Newtown House was originally meant to be used as a specialised group home for younger children but changed purpose in 1996 to provide secure provision. The Inspectorate acknowledges in relation to the children that "at times their behaviour can present risks to both themselves and others" (2001, p. 4). This is clearly the case as one service user had his leg broken when a staff member attempted a physical restraint and seventeen incidents of assaults against staff were documented between July, 1999, and April, 2000 (SSI, 2001, p. 15).

The SSI investigation discovered that none of the senior managers held a relevant child care qualification, and three members of the management team resigned from their posts over a seven-month period. At the time of the inspection there were only nine permanent care staff, although there was provision for 16. There was a 48 percent annual staff turnover, no formal supervision in place "due to pressures of work," and there was no written policy on how clients should be prepared for leaving the unit.

On a more positive note, the centre did have a school on site with two permanent teachers. School was reported as being "a positive experience for most of the young people" (SSI, 2001, p. 34). As with the Youth Encounter Projects, a negotiated curriculum is in use where "the schoolwork is assigned at a level the teaching staff know is within their (the students) ability" (SSI, 2001, p. 34). Finally, the inspection team note that "for some young people, this was their first positive experience of school and for others it helped them to develop their potential" (SSI, 2001, p. 34).

Despite the good work being accomplished in very trying conditions, the Irish media reporting of Newtown House follows similar patterns to the aforementioned child and youth care scandals. An article in the *Irish Times* (19.9.01), for example, reported on the case of a 14-year-old male client, called Billy, who had been sexually abused by a relative who was visited by his social worker after eight months and received no counselling for his abuse.[7] When Billy absconded from Newtown House it was reported that "no social worker went looking for him." Whether this is actually true or not, the public was not informed. Eventually, Billy's parents instituted court proceedings against Newtown House citing poor quality of care. A later report in the same newspaper acknowledged that staff were "operating in an environment of scarcity" and that this scarcity "rather than the actions of untrained staff ... should be the main focus of concern" (Irish Times, 27.02.01). In this environment, children had to wait up to six months to see a specialist therapist.

In relation to court proceedings, child and youth care practitioners from Newtown House argued that they provided for Kim when their centre was established with a different brief for a different client group and "taken the risk of doing that which no one else in society would do" (Irish Times, 9.3.01). The defence Barrister for the East Coast Area Health Board, Paddy MacEntee, informed the High Court that child care workers "were scapegoated any time something goes wrong" and, further, that the judge involved should not "embark on a blame exercise" (Irish Times, 9.3.01). It was also argued that child care workers had to work in an environment where "people working with disturbed children had to make life or death decisions knowing if they did not get it right, they were liable to end up being unsympathetically examined at the High Court" (Irish Times, 9.3.01). Thus, a culture of blame is apparent and there is a lack of investigative rigor in examining both sides of the case. What makes things more difficult for child and youth care practitioners is that they are often told not to speak with the media by their managers. Thus, reporting is often skewed, incomplete, and lacks objectivity.

LET THE COURTS SPEAK

In the late 1990s, in particular, one aforementioned Dublin-based Judge called Peter Kelly arrived at the end of his patience and attempted to publicise the case of what are often termed in the Irish media as "out of control" children. Kelly observed that he was faced daily with children who had no safe place to go and insisted that the Irish State provide *appropriate* residential care places for them. Unfortunately, such *appropriate* places were often extremely difficult to locate and staffing them with qualified personnel remains wholly problematic. Justice Kelly described the juvenile justice system as "a shambles and chaotic" after being forced to send a disturbed and neglected child into a psychiatric hospital, due to lack of alternative accommodation.

In a directive issued in 1999, Judge Kelly proposed that the State provide appropriate residential child care services to children who are in need of special care and/or attention. The directive specified that the Irish Department of Health and Children must provide the High Court with a development plan for each health board in relation to their provision of Special Care Units (Secure Units) and High Support Units (specialist residential care provision in conjunction with other arrangements).

One of the central difficulties in this debate appears to be that the public is confused with regard to the different types of residential care available and it is worth briefly explaining them here. Short-term units are assessment or intake centres. Children are taken in for a six-week to six-month assessment period, and a suitable placement is sought either in foster care or in residential care. A medium term unit should provide for children for a period up to two years whilst family based work is engaged in with a view to returning the child to the child's home of origin after the designated period in residential care. Long-term care is any-thing more than two years, which is considered by most professional as-sociations such as the Resident Managers' Association and the Irish Association of Care Workers to be a less than desirable situation for the child or young person.

Unfortunately, the experience of many residential child care units is that, despite operating with a clear purpose in mind, the immediate needs of young people and the various referring agencies, such as the courts, result in units having to provide a variety of services within one unit for which they were not established. The example often cited from managers of such units is being forced to take in an emergency place-ment in a medium term unit, which is not good practice but is all too of-ten the reality due to resource constraints and a sense of public outrage heightened by the media. Indeed, the Resident Managers' Association noted in 1996 that "Misplacing young people in care can be abusive to residents already in care and it can also be abusive to the young people themselves" (Moynihan, 1996, p. 29).

The profile of children and youth in residential child care frequently includes multiple loss, rejection, deprivation neglect and abuse (McElwee, 2006; O'Higgins, 1996). It should also be remembered that all residen-tial child care has a core feature; it consists of children and young people being looked after away from home by people who are not their parents. This brings many responsibilities and issues with it. Child and youth care practitioners are aware that there are a number of areas a service user coming into residential care will have to deal with including:

- The trauma and separation from their family of origin.
- The sense of bereavement and loss for that family.
- Feelings of guilt and rejection.
- Feelings of having no control over a life which has suddenly been turned upside down.
- Blaming the care workers and agency for their plight and reacting accordingly.
- Feelings of complete loyalty to family of origin regardless of abuse/ neglect suffered.
- Being extremely frightened about the future both for themselves and their families (Impact, 1998, 1).

So what has happened to our child protection service design given the amount of scandals and shortcomings uncovered? Ferguson (1997) claims that, "The striking feature of the childcare system over the past decade has been the dominance of child abuse and protection to its design and operation" (p. 3) and he notes that there is a relatively static pool of professionals involved in the referral of suspected cases of abuse and neglect and that categorising children as high risk ensured a greater level of investigation by social workers. This has the effect of child care being (re)framed more as child protection. Inter-disciplinary planning now marks the social services response to child protection and welfare that, over the course of the 1980s and 1990s, became rather narrow in focus. Family adversity became less important than child abuse *per se* as the focus of abuse and neglect shifted over the past two decades. Despite all of this, over 10 percent of children in care in 2001 still had no assigned social worker working with them (SSI, 2003).

UNDERSTANDING AND NEGOTIATING RISK

It is clear that the nature of care professionals' work with vulnerable children and adolescents can cause particular problems when it comes to the identification and intervention in *potential* and *real* cases of child abuse and neglect. We now live in an era of intense bureaucratisation in child protection. At the same time, as a number of studies both in the UK and Ireland have illustrated, the decisions made by child protection professionals in referring or, indeed, not referring children and adolescents to social services have significant and long-term effects on their lives and the lives of their service users (Beckford, 1985; Buckley et al., 1997; Dartington, 1995; Lindsey, 1994; Utting, 1997; Waterhouse, 2000).

Interestingly, human services personnel now regularly articulate that they feel at the mercy of what they perceive as a largely uncaring public but one very quick to judge when things are perceived to have gone wrong. And, in the midst of all this, the system continues to fail children, youth and their families (see Dunphy, 2006). I am consistently informed by both social care practitioners and social workers that the 1991 Child Care Act has resulted in their work loads increasing considerably, particularly in the area of child sexual abuse and neglect cases. The work has also become more *complex* as procedural and legal issues assume centre stage.

The McColgan Case: Failure of the Experts (Again)

This point was brought to fore in the McColgan case in the North Western Health Board area where four of the six McColgan children were abused by their father Joseph from the late 1970s to the early 1990s. This was a horrendous case of systematic abuse.

When this case surfaced publicly, the questions that concerned child care professionals were (a) whether or not the health board staff had an advanced understanding of child sexual abuse, and (b) could the child protection staff have done more for the children? Sexual abuse was discussed at an Annual Conference of the Irish Association of Social Workers here in Ireland in 1983 so there was, at least, an evolving understanding.

A clear message is that the McColgan children despaired of the professionals (adults) who entered and exited their lives and still the officially documented abuse continued. One of the chapters entitled, "Trapped in a System," elaborates on this point. It documents the family's total of 392 contacts with the North-Western Health Board between 1977-1993. Sophia continually searches for a reason the abuse continued despite the intervention of various professionals. The very last line in the book speaks volumes. "There was a lot of flurry and after that, nothing," said Sophia. "A big zero." Child protection practice still has some serous lessons to learn and, of course, this was all played out in the media. All of this has resulted in what Ferguson (1996, p. 7) has described as an "opening-out" of the routines of the expert system and science of child protection.

If personnel continually choose to either (a) not enter onto programmes of training and education or (b) leave human services for another field, the results for children and youth will be disastrous. An ever depleting pool of staff will be seen in each group home and agency. Inexperience will become the norm. This is neither good for children and youth nor for the field as a profession.

It seems to me that an understanding of risk is now crucial to comprehending child and youth care interventions and, indeed, non-interventions. Firstly, we must ensure that we adequately provide for families and children and youth designated as at-risk by various human services professionals–this is particularly the case when we intervene and remove children and youth from their families. It is continually argued that human, economic, and structural resources can only be put in place if risk surveillance and supervision is scientifically assessed. Of course, the problem in risk assessment is knowing with some degree of accuracy which cases are more or less deserving of our immediate attention. Getting this right is much easier said than done.

It has been argued that there has been a change in both direction and emphasis in child protection and welfare in the latter part of the 1980s as a response to living and working in the risk society (Daniel & Ivatts, 1998; Ferguson, 1998; McElwee, 2001a). In the UK, official inquiries over the past three decades have attempted to single out individual child protection workers rather than to concentrate on institutions and this has had a profound effect on staff morale. This is also increasingly the case in Ireland. Perhaps it is easier to stay "invisible" or "under the radar" and "just work away in a system full of flaws" than to raise one's head and draw attention to issues of practice which are less than appropriate; thus each child and youth care centre is a laboratory in itself. The dangers in this are many.

An example of a global laboratory is given by Thorpe who cites the work of Bauman (1989) on "moral invisibility" where workers in Nazi Germany viewed themselves merely as functionaries and the end result of their (deadly) work was invisible to them. They could not be accorded responsibility, therefore, for the Holocaust as it was always someone else down the line that was really to blame. Thorpe suggests, "... this offers us an important clue as to how moral invisibility and moral distance has been created and is being sustained in child protection" (1997, p. 76).

Communicating Hazards to Non-Experts and Non-Scientists

A great deal of reporting about hazards and their associated risks appear in the guise of media news and features stories concerning accidents, illnesses, natural disasters and scientific breakthroughs. Dioxin, Opren, Saccharin, Asbestos, Tartrazine, Cyclamate, DES, Three Mile Island, Bhopal and Chernobyl are all names synonymous with the risk culture of today. A conflict between the business of news and what social scientists have termed "risk communication" is apparent.

To communicate information about hazards and risks in a way calculated to foster rational decision making requires detailed and precise (if, at all, possible) data about immediate and long-term consequences. One needs to weigh the costs and benefits of a hazard and its alternatives for the individual and for society and to discuss the issues–moral and economic–that inhere in hazardous processes and events. In the 1990s, risks were so diverse that it was extremely difficult to compile a composite list of threats or the set of possible control strategies. There was an almost daily discovery of new threats with massive and widespread publicity which contributed in the creation of a global neurosis which was characterised by mistrust of technology and obsessive preoccupation with risk. One might ask, how can we even attempt to measure risk when Beck (1992, p. 49) suggests we live in Western societies *dominated* by a concern with risk, danger, and safety?

Sensationalising Children at Risk in the Media

Reports in the media of children being the subjects of horrendous abuse are carried on a daily basis. The tragic commentary to which I have already alluded, or what Ferguson calls, "a radicalised consciousness of risk" (1997, p. 15) is perpetuated in many sections of the Irish media, particularly in what is called over here the "gutter press." My experience is that the general tendency of Irish media [is] to cover only the most sensational cases and this is continually articulated at annual conferences of the Irish Association of Care Workers, the Resident Manager's Association, the Irish Association of Social Care Educators and during in-service educational programmes for at-risk children and youth. Thus, the media can have a powerful effect on people entering into and deciding to stay in a particular profession.

Child care and special education for at-risk children and youth in the context of Youth Encounter Projects or Neighbourhood Youth Projects hardly merited a mention in Irish mainstream media until recently. Indeed, one could pick the 1993 Kilkenny Incest case as a benchmark, in that it launched a very public investigation into "expert" practice in child protection and welfare. An editorial in the Irish Social Worker (1993, p. 3) commented that the Kilkenny Incest Case was a good example of the power of public pressure and the willingness of the media to report such issues. By the time of the 1997 annual conference of child and youth care practitioners, a leading RTE documentary reporter, Eamon Lawlor, could comment to the delegates that media attention had become "risk driven and scandal oriented." One result of this is that there remains a preoccupation with case management and not with casework and, as Culpitt (1999, p. 39) argues, the core tasks of the case manager are risk profiling whilst the therapeutic nature of the caseworker/client relationship are those of "competition, quality and customer demand."

Suicide: Ultimate Risk Profiling

Researchers in the Department of Economics at National University of Ireland, Galway identified three potential economic costs associated with suicide: direct, indirect, and human. Direct costs, such as monetary outlays associated with suicide and its aftermath, were estimated to have cost almost €1.8 million in 2001, when 519 people died as a result of suicide. Indirect costs, such as the value of lost output or production arising from suicide, were estimated to cost more than 250 million. Human costs, which refer to the value that individuals place on their lives beyond their capacity to work, were estimated to cost 653 million. In total then, the costs are estimated at €900 million (cited in O'Brien, 2005). Most Irish policy on suicide stems from a 1998 report by the National Task Force on Suicide and, according to the Government, €17.5m was been spent on prevention programmes since then (Hegarty, 2004).

For the past number of years, the official suicide figures have been steadily increasing to the point where suicide is regularly stated "to be at epidemic proportions" and there are now over four hundred deaths annually in Ireland recorded as suicide. Certainly there has been a great deal of research completed on risk indices for suicide amongst different demographic categories such as gender and age. And yet, the highest category for suicide is male youth aged 15 to 25. We know that young people attempting suicide, who persistently express suicidal ideas, particularly where there is evidence of planning and strong intent to die, are at an increased risk of re-attempting suicide (Aggleton et al., 2000). Despite this, how are so many youth not picked up successfully by interventions such as psychology, psychiatry, and medicine?

There is conflicting evidence on the effect of the media's treatment of (fictional and non-fictional) suicide or suicide rates in the overall population. However, various experts do feel that a media effect exists, particularly in individual cases, and that the young are especially susceptible (Hawton, 1995). The much publicised tragic case of the grunge rocker in the US, Kurt Cobain, has filled literally thousands of inches of column space throughout the world (including, of course, Ireland) with several so-called copycat suicides by distraught teens.

What role do the media have in drawing attention to suicide and how best should suicide cases be reported where sensitivity can co-exist with the facts of any particular case? Research completed in the US has found an increase in suicide by readers or viewers of media when the number of stories about individual suicides increases, a particular death is reported at length or in many stories, the story of an individual death by suicide is placed on the front page or at the beginning of a broadcast, and when the headlines about specific suicide deaths are dramatic (Gould, 2001; Hassan, 1995; Phillips et al., 1992). It is argued that certain ways of describing suicide in the news contributes to "suicide contagion" or "copycat" suicides (Schmidtke & Häfner, 1988). Research also suggests that inadvertently romanticizing suicide or idealizing those who take their own lives by portraying suicide as a heroic or romantic act may encourage others to identify with the victim (Fekete & Schmidtke,

1995), and clinicians believe the danger is even greater if there is a detailed description of the method. Research indicates that detailed descriptions or pictures of the location or site of a suicide encourage imitation (Sonneck et al., 1994). Indeed, yet another recent study has argued that young people get a majority of their information on suicide from the media (Beautrais et al., 2004).[8] Thus, the media is a hugely influential source. When a youth in care commits suicide, the media reporting is uncompromising.

Although scandals and examples of alleged incompetent practice appear now in the newspapers with depressing regularity, it should be remembered that their reporting in the British and Irish media reflects *new* public concerns. It remains unclear how prevalent such practices were in the past, and Lowrance (1984) goes so far as to suggest that we have the luxury of going around "searching for possible trouble" (p. 5).[9] It seems that too many cases are dragged into the child protection spotlight at the expense of those children and families that may really require interventions.

The writing was on the wall for two decades. The 1980s and 1990s saw unfolding stages in the risk debate summed up by Howitt (1992) as:

- Concern about under-involvement: leaving children to suffer abuse through a reluctance to intervene.
- Concern about over-involvement: essentially finding abuse where none exists.
- Concern about the quality of care: just how free of abuse are facilities such as homes for children taken into care?

The result of this is that human service experts are put under immense pressure as the public believes that experts can, somehow, *prevent* child abuse. Reder et al. (1993) argue that blame is often accorded to perceived "bad practice" without viewing the facts in an objective and dispassionate framework, and McGrath (1993) has noted that care professionals can easily panic in such situations and that professional support is important. There is a direct connection here with the confused discourse on resiliency where we note that there is no certainty around whom will successfully adapt and thrive and whom will fail to prosper as there is no certainty around to prevent child abuse on every occasion, in every location with all sorts of actors (lay and professional) involved.

CONCENTRATING ON HIGH-RISK CHILDREN AND YOUTH

Unfortunately, problems of "scandalising" child and youth care do not rest solely with residential care staff. It is clear that by the early 1990s, Irish child and youth care workers from community and project settings were beginning to feel the strain of living and working under a public lens of risk consciousness. A recent newspaper article on careers commences thus, "If you're looking for fame, recognition and a bit of glitz in your working life, you may as well stop reading now. Social work will provide none of these" (Irish Times, 25.1.2006).

Over a decade earlier, the Irish Social Worker magazine published a feature which stated, "Social workers in the field of child protection will continue to struggle with the *hazards* that this work unleashes" (1993, p. 4, my emphasis). More recently, the European Social Worker (2005) noted "this perception of low self confidence" and those "moments of truth" which pervade social work (p. 1). These are but two examples from dozens where risk, in a negative rather than positive context, was synonymous with child protection and welfare throughout the 1990s. At the same time, attention was increasingly directed at high-risk children and adolescents and a child protection service concentrated on an even smaller number of cases at the heavy end of the spectrum of risk.

Currently, Irish Health Service Executive spending remains limited on prevention work. At the same time, professionals are being increasingly targeted, which adds to a general feeling of crisis and despair, leading one media commentator to ask how had such complete mistrust taken hold in what used to be one of the most conservative and deferential societies in Europe (O'Toole, 1997). We are a long way from accepting that organisational cultures, rather than simply the individual mindset of workers, have the most impact in shaping what form interventions for children and youth at risk might take.

As with their colleagues in the UK, Irish social workers and child and youth care practitioners take great care in removing children from the home. This approach is partly informed by the UK experience with the Beckford Report (1985) which commented. "... society expects that a child at risk from abuse by its parents will be protected by Social Services personnel exercising parental powers effectively and authoritatively on behalf of society" (p. 297).[10] However, at times, the professionals get it horribly wrong.

This is evident at the time of completing this book in an example where social workers on behalf of the Health Service Executive in the eastern part of Ireland took a family of four children with autism into residential care despite the fact that the parents had been described in one Health Service Executive report as "loving and doing their best in the circumstances." The father of the children called publicly for a "root and branch" review of health services for children with disabilities and a national outcry followed, the parents took the Health Service Executive to court, and they won the case, having their children returned to them. It emerged during this case that it can cost as much as E500,000 to place an adult in an institution but that therapies and education were available for children with autism at a cost of around 60,000 a year for three to four years (O'Hara in Irish Times, 14.3.2005).[11]

Once again, the individual social workers and line management did not get an opportunity to tell their story in the media so the entire social work discipline was called into question by media commentators. The case received blanket coverage in all forms of the media.

The language of risk and uncertainty is also notable in the work of the Irish Journalist, Fintan O'Toole (1997), who remarks that Ireland "has become somehow unreal" (p. 173). In an earlier book (1990) he argues that "in the shifting divided and contradictory reality" (p. 8) real life became as "surreal as avant-garde art" in the 1980s" (p. 13). He notes that the 1980s "was a time of slow crisis, of creeping catastrophe, of petty apocalypse" (p. 9). O'Toole locates "the extraordinary popular scepticism" with leaders to wealth and suggests that "the grand narrative of a society moving from the pre-modern to the modern to the post-modern breaks down in Ireland" (p. 131).

A GLOBAL RISK DEBATE IN CHILD PROTECTION AND WELFARE EMERGES

As the catch-phrase for the TV show, *The X Files*, used to go, "We are not alone." The global risk debate has been discussed by Ferguson (1995) and placed in the context of Irish child protection and welfare. In an important article titled, *Sitting on a Time Bomb: Child Protection, Inquiries and the Risk Society,* he notes the politicisation of child protection and welfare and acknowledges a "new risk profile" where professionals are now publicly challenged and taken to task for what may be perceived as "professional failure." This politicisation has also been noted in the work of Douglas (1994) who observes that risk is always both a political and moral issue "... at all places at all times the universe is moralised and politicised. Disasters that befoul the air and soil and poison the water are generally turned to political account. Someone already unpopular is going to get blamed for it. As we see from the theoretical work of Beck, Lash, and Giddens and the fate of at-risk children who have attended the Irish Youth Encounter Projects, this is easier said than done.

Ferguson (1995) locates his debate in the context of the sanctity accorded to the Irish family (the nuclear version protected in the Constitution of 1937) and the historical reluctance in this country to remove children from the home. Ferguson's sympathy lies with those who are aware of the limitations on their work practices despite the fact they may want to do the right thing. "It concerns the important sense in which we know *too* much about risk" (p. 8) as the expert systems are now in overdrive. Ferguson calls the recent risk debate in child protection and welfare "explosive." Because we can now afford to be reflexive (in the sociological sense), we can radicalise our knowledge base and become experts ourselves. Ferguson rightly asks that we give credence to what cannot be done for children at-risk due to limitations of human and financial resources and unintended consequences and inevitable knowledge gaps. We should actively question or, "radically engage" as Ferguson terms it, in adapting to the risk society in child protection and welfare. He concludes by stating:

> The more we take account of the new parameters of child protection in the risk society, the less likely it will be that inquiries will be necessary because the quality of professional judgements will be such that, as far as is humanly possible, good intentions can go right. (Ferguson, 1995, p. 10)

Later, Ferguson (1997, p. 6), notes that social work has become more investigative and intrusive since the 1970s. Mapping out the transition from physical abuse and neglect to emotional and sexual abuse within Social Services Departments, he supports Giddens's thesis for a more dynamic view of late modernity which "does justice to the *opportunities* as well as the *dangers* inherent in the modern child protection system."

FEAR OF A PROCEDURAL AND LEGALISTIC MORAL CLIMATE IN THE RISK SOCIETY

Social services are increasingly protecting themselves through process regulation. Buckley et al. (1997) ask rhetorically, "Are the developments of formalised guidelines for the management of child abuse and neglect cases and greater inter-agency and inter-professional collaboration the most appropriate way to advance the protection of children?" (p. 205). Similarly, Ferguson (1997) states. "… the crux of the issue concerns the need to get the right kind of response to the "right" families and avoid inappropriate proceduralised investigative interventions to those who require different kind of "welfare" response" (p. 9).

Parton et al. (1997) suggests that an emphasis on proceduralism (simply following orders or ensuring forms are filled in with little thought to context) is now the experience of the Western world. One of the concerns shared by practically all academics and practitioners in Ireland is the fear that child and youth care work will become overwhelmed and driven by procedure rather than competent practice and this may also be attributed to the risk society. Simply put, practitioners are afraid to place themselves in a position where a potential allegation may be made about them. The work environment has become both more complex and proceduralised.

This apparent tension between the legalised, formalised and bureaucratised political climate of child protection and welfare (risk society consciousness) informs daily practice. Thus, child and youth care and social workers continually complain about formal supervision being inadequate and limited. So what is going on? Ferguson (1997) argues that the child protection system represents a classic form of advanced modern institutionalised risk system and cautions us, "Future challenges, or problems arise, however, in how colonising the future opens up new settings of risk which, in turn, must become institutionally organised– as the progression of the inquiries demonstrates" (p. 11).

Certainly a valuable point that Ferguson alludes to is that those who point out discrepancies in the system tend to be "scapegoated" as "professionals live as well as work in the risk society." In Giddens' frame of reference–we all ride the juggernaut. Such a point was also made by Slovic and Fischhoff (1977) where they asserted that scientists and policy makers who point out the gambles involved in societal decisions are often resented for the anxiety they provoke. Ferguson emphasises the centrality of processes of reflexivity in the creation of self-identity and asks us to "break away from limited definitions of protection." This, in itself, would be worthwhile. Let us look more closely at the situation in the U.K.

CHILD PROTECTION AND THE RISK DEBATE IN THE UK

The situation with regard to living and working in the risk society is little different in the UK to the one we experience we Ireland. Research completed by Bridge (1991), Brown (1991), Warner (1992), Clyde

(1993), Levy and Kahan (1991), Parton et al. (1997), Utting (1997), Waterhouse (2000) all attest to the fact that approaches to child protection and welfare have come under intense critical and public scrutiny.

Social workers debate the merits of including competence in their work practice and evaluation and the road has been littered with casualties. O'Hagan makes the point that incompetent social workers have featured strongly in the media during the 1980s and 1990s. He cites cases involving the elderly, mentally ill, adolescents and social workers neglecting protection models generally (1996, pp. 2-3) which fundamentally influenced the controversial Central Council on Education and Training for Social Work (CCETSW) revised Paper 30. Social workers have realised the risk society influences their training and work practice as the CCETSW Paper 30 states social workers must, "be strategic thinkers, able to weigh up the advantages and disadvantages of proposals, and to anticipate the possible consequences of decisions or actions." The inquiry report into the much publicised and tragic death of Jasmine Beckford could not have been more critical of the social services:

> … Jasmine's fate illustrates all too clearly the disastrous consequences of the misguided attitude of the social workers having treated Morris Beckford and Beverley Lorrington as the clients first and foremost. (London Borough of Brent, 1985)[12]

In *Child Protection: Risk and the Moral Order* (1997, p. 245), the authors conclude that, "Statements about risk have become the key moral statements of society and lie at the heart of child protection work." In the book, they map out what has occurred in social work practice over the past two decades (a move from the "battered baby" to a focus on "child abuse"). We are now experiencing notions of risk being given a much greater significance than was the case historically (shifting location) and yet social policy has missed the fact that a wider social and political analysis could very usefully inform practice.

Parton et al. claim that child protection and welfare services in the UK are overwhelmed by the sheer number of alleged reports and referrals of child abuse coming in. Research from the USA is cited where it is thought that as many as 50% of reported cases of alleged abuse are unsubstantiated (Parton et al., 1997, p. 2). The authors argue that it would be more helpful for social policy makers to view a number of representative cases of child abuse and neglect and respond to these findings, than to review only the highly publicised scandals in the UK such as the watershed Cleveland case, the Orkneys and the Beckford case. Crucially, they argue that "Debates about risk must thus lie at the hearts of attempts to reframe and redirect future policy" (Parton et al., 1997, p. 16. They cite the findings of the Audit Commission (1994) as evidence for their position that resources are wasted and misdirected.

Drawing from the earlier work of Parton (1996), the authors claim that we have moved beyond the medico-social model and that concerns in child protection and welfare may be understood as reflecting increased anxieties and uncertainties on the one hand and as a way for staff of coping with their new-found situation of societal scrutiny. An important point raised by Colton et al. (1995) is that social workers are very aware of available resources in determining their assessment of children in need as has been noticed in the Irish context.

Parton et al. (1997) note the central irony of child protection and welfare in the 1980s and 1990s. "More than ever, practitioners have to walk a fine balance and the costs of getting that wrong could lead to considerable public, political and media opprobrium" (p. 219). Luhmann (1993) quips that "The fear that things could go wrong is therefore growing rapidly and with it the risk apportioned to decision-making" (p. xii). Experts, themselves, have started to argue publicly about the significance of signs and symptoms and that the high profile cases of the 1980s and 1990s have taught us to question our social construction of child abuse. The authors are critical of the Dartington Report's failure to decide whether their research overview was on children in need or on child abuse. They quite rightly comment that the type of language one chooses to use (or, indeed, not use) will have important ramifications for the way questions are phrased and responded to by interviewees and interpreted by researchers. The term "child abuse" is both negotiated and socially constituted and must be understood in terms of how it impacts on society in a macro framework and organisations in a micro framework. Ferguson (1993, p. 3) has also commented on this international trend where professionals were perceived to have either under reacted or over reacted in their work and were in a no win situation in terms of the media scrutiny which is, itself, scandal oriented.[13]

CONCLUSION

Irish identity is changing and the fall off in both male and female numbers of religious orders has meant a profound shift in the terrain of volunteerism and professionalism. The premier Association for residential child care managers (Resident Managers' Association) which was founded by the religious in the 1930s now has only one active priest member who remains in practice in Dublin. The Catholic Church increasingly has to compete with a variety of external influences, especially from the mass media (O'Grady, 2001).

Earlier in the chapter, I presented a vignette from child and youth care practice. What does it mean, then, in the context of the overall discussion? Perhaps unsurprisingly given the media (over)emphasis on scandals involving the courts, child sexual abuse, physical abuse, neglect and residential child care, children and youth attending the Youth Encounter Projects have been left off this new politicised at-risk agenda. Indeed, I completed an archive search in the *Irish Times* newspaper over a five-year period between 1995 and 2000 and discovered that the Youth Encounters Project was only mentioned once and, even then, appeared under a much more general article on a potential court case concerning disruptive pupils and access to education (Irish Times, 19.2.1998).

There is little doubt but that front line child and youth care workers and social workers increasingly see themselves as operating within a high-risk rather than a high-opportunity society (Dunphy, 2006; McElwee, 2006). The situation in Ireland and the UK is akin to the situation elsewhere where "The overwhelming feature of the age is not physical–the threat of annihilation–but social: the fundamental and scandalous way in which the institutions, almost without exception, fail it" (Beck, 1995, p. 69).

It is proving more and more difficult to attract volunteers into child and youth care and child protection and, indeed, an argument rages as to the place of volunteers in these disciplines with some arguing for their continuance and others believing such work should be the preserve of professionals. It is interesting, for example, that the Samaritans organisation reports that the female to male volunteer ratio is now 2:1 (McElwee, 2006).

There is hope in the risk terrain. The Limerick project has somehow managed to, on the one hand, provide for some of the most at-risk children and young people whilst at the same time operate within Beck's complex risk society. How could this be the case and what are the Youth Encounter Projects? The next chapter attempts to provide some answers to these questions.

NOTES

1. The non-statutory sector includes voluntary service providers of which there are thirteen private companies operating residential child care and several high profile organisations such as Barnardos and Focus Ireland.

2. This surely suggests that some are there against their will (Ferguson, 1993, p. 4).

3. This is particularly evident in a trilogy of television documentaries aired for RTE, the Irish State television station, titled *States of Fear* (1999) that explored the provision of residential services for vulnerable Irish children during the 1940-1980s period. A number of religious and lay care providers were exposed as allegedly being cruel, hurtful and abusive of children in their care with the State showing various levels of disinterest.

4. The Irish Christian Brothers in Canada changed its name in the early 1990s, dropping "Irish" out of the title as senior figures were concerned that the Canadian public would associate the order too closely with their Irish counterparts (Phelan, 1999).

5. The later Task Force Report (1981, p. 52) stated that "the underlying concept of such projects is that they should provide an alternative educational option to boys and girls aged between ten and fifteen years who fail to conform to the normal school regime." The primary focus of the Youth Encounter Projects was to avoid having children being removed from their homes and placed in residential care. By 1980, there were fifty students attending these projects.

6. This centre was formally called Trudder House.

7. The Irish Times is the newspaper of record in Ireland.

8. Please see (Irish) National Suicide Research Foundation for discussions.

9. This apparent fondness for searching for trouble was communicated to me by some of the parents of the children and youth I interviewed for this study. They claimed that journalists only arrived at their housing estates with notebooks in hand when something negative such as a stabbing, a drug seizure, an episode of joy-riding, a murder, or a suicide had taken place and, "never to write stories about any of the good stuff we are involved in."

10. Indeed, the much quoted Report on Kimberley Carlile notes: "Society, rightly in our opinion, is not prepared to tolerate too heavy-handed disruptions to family life, and expects careful judgement to be exercised in our deciding on the appropriate action to be taken in any particular case. This more flexible approach offers some security to families. But, given that human judgement is fallible, society must tolerate occasional failure. Staff who follow up suspicions of child abuse are not creating these risks. They are inheriting the risks, and are accepting them on our behalf" (London Borough of Greenwich, 1987, p. 136).

11. Official figures suggest that one in 166 children goes on to develop an autistic spectrum disorder, a 10-fold increase since the figures were first recorded in the mid-1990s.

12. Jasmine Beckford died aged four and a half in July 1984 at the home of her step-father and her mother in North-West London. She was emaciated and chronically undernourished but had died as a result of cerebal contusions and subdural haemorrhage. She had previously been the subject of a Care Order in 1981 due to severe injuries noted at hospital. Judge Pigot described her social worker as showing "naivete almost beyond belief."

13. Studies completed in the United States have noted that the media tend to report on specific instances of hazards that produce or are accompanied by specific harms.

REFERENCES

Aggleton, P., Hurry, J., Warwick, I. (Eds.). (2000). *Young people and mental health.* John Wiley and Sons Ltd.

Barratt, J. K. (1998). *The report of the 1997 inquiry into the "Trotter affair": Report by J. K. Barratt to the Council of the London Borough of Hackney.* London: London Borough of Hackney.

Bauman, Z. (1989). *Modernity and the Holocaust.* Cambridge: Polity.

Beautrais, A. L., John Horwood, L., & Fergusson, D. M. (2004). Knowledge and attitudes about suicide in 25-year-olds, *38*(4), 260-5.

Beck, U. (1992). *Risk society. Towards a new modernity.* London: Sage.

Beck, U. (1995). *Ecological politics in an age of risk.* Polity: Cambridge.

Beck, U. (1997). Politics of risk society. In J. Franklin (Ed.), *The politics of risk society* (pp. 343-366). Cambridge: Polity Press.

Beck, U. (1997). *The reinvention of politics: Rethinking modernity in the global social order.* Cambridge: Polity.

Beck, U. (1997). Capitalism without work. *Dissent, 44*(1), 51-6.

Beckford Report. (1985). *A child in trust: The report of the panel of inquiry into the circumstances surrounding the death of Jasmine Beckford.* London Borough of Brent.

Bridge Childcare Consultancy Service. (1991). *Sukina: An evaluation report of the circumstances of her death.* London: Bridge.

Brown, J. D. (1991). Staying fit and staying well: Physical fitness as a moderator of life stress. *Journal of Personality and Social Psychology, 60,* 555-561.

Buckley, H., Skehill, C., & O'Sullivan, E. (1997). *Child protection practices in Ireland: A case study.* Dublin: SEHB/Oak Tree Press.

Causon, P. (1997). Who will guard the guards? Some questions about the models of inspection for residential settings with relevance to the protection of children from abuse by staff. *Early Child Development and Care, 133,* 57-71.

Charles, G. (August, 2001). Accountability, failure and success. *CYC Online,* Issue 31. www.eve-net.org/cyc-online/cycol-0801-charles.html.

Clyde, L. (1993). *Report of the inquiry into the removal of children from Orkney in February 1991.* House of Commons, Session 1992/93, Paper 195. London: HMSO.

Colton, M., Drury, C., & Williams, M. (1995). *Children in need: Family support under the Children Act (1989).* Aldershot: Avebury.

Culpitt, I. (1999). *Social policy and risk.* London: Sage.

Daniel, P., & Ivatts, J. (1998). *Children and social policy.* London: MacMillan.

Daniluk, J., Leader, A., & Taylor, P. (1985). The psychological sequelae of infertility. In J. Gold (Ed.), *The psychiatric implications of menstruation.* Washington: American Psychiatric Press Inc.

Dartington Social Research Unit. (1995). *Child protection: Messages From research.* London: HMSO.

Department of Health and Children. (2001). *National children's strategy.* Dublin: DOHC.

Dept. of Health and Children. (2003). Dublin: DOHC.

Dingwall, R., Eekelar, J., & Murray, T. (1995). *The protection of children: State intervention and family life.* London: Avebury.

Douglas, M. (1994). *Risk and blame: Essays in cultural theory.* London: Routledge.

Dunphy, S. (2006). *Wednesday's child.* Dublin: Gill and McMillan.

European Social Worker. (2005). *1*(2), 1-9. Retrieved from http://www.ifsw.org/cm_ data/ESW_2005.pdf

Fekete, S., & Schmidtke, A. (1995) The impact of mass media reports on suicide and attitudes toward self-destruction: Previous studies and some new data from Hungary and Germany. In B. L. Mishara (Ed.), *The impact of suicide* (pp. 142-155). New York: Springer.

Ferguson, H. (1993, Autumn). The manifest and latent implications of the report of the Kilkenny incest investigation for social work, *The Irish Social Worker, 11*(4), 4-5.

Ferguson, H. (1995). Sitting on a time bomb: Child protection, inquiries and the risk society. *Irish Social Work, 13*(1), 8-10.

Ferguson, H. (1997). Understanding man and masculinities. *Men and Intimacy: Proceedings of a Conference hosted by St. Catherine's Community Services Centre, Carlow and Accord.*

Ferguson, H. (1997). Child welfare and child protection in practice. Are we getting the balance right? *The Child Care Act 1991–Promoting the Welfare of Children/Making it Work in Practice. Conference Proceedings.* Midland Health Board/Western Health Board.

Fewster, G. (2002). Touch. Threads Digests of CYC–Net Discussions. *The International Child and Youth Care Network.* Available at cycnet.org.

Fischhoff, B., Slovic, P., & Lichtenstein, S. (1977). Knowing with certainty: The appropriateness of exterme confidence. *Journal of Experimental Psychology: Human Perception and Performance, 3,* 522-564.

Friedson, E. (1990). *Professionalism, caring and nursing.* Paper prepared for the Park Ridge Center, Park Ridge, Illinois. Available http://itsa.ucsf.edu/eliotf/Professionalism,_ Caring,_a.html

Garfat, T. (1988), The magic of children and youth: A participatory exercise. *Child and Youth Care Quarterly, 17*(2), 70-85.

Garfat, T. (1998). On the fear of contact, the need for touch, and creating youth care contexts where touching is okay. *Journal of Child and Youth Care, 12*(3), 3-10.

Garfat, T., & McElwee, N. (2001). The changing role of family in child and youth care practice. *Journal of Child and Youth Care Work, 16,* 236-248.

Garfat, T., & McElwee, N. (2004). *Effective interventions with families.* Cape Town: Pretext.

Giddens, A. (1994). Living in a post-industrial society. In U. Beck, A. Giddens, & S. Lash (Eds.), *Reflexive modernisation* (pp. 56-109). Cambridge: Polity.

Gould, M. S. (2001). Suicide and the media. In H. Hendin, & J. J. Mann (Eds.), *The clinical science of suicide prevention* (pp. 200-224). New York: Annals of the New York Academy of Sciences.

Hassan, R. (1995). Effects of newspaper stories on the incidence of suicide in Australia: A research note. *Australian and New Zealand Journal of Psychiatry, 29,* 480-483.

Hawton, K. (1995). Media influences on suicidal behavior in young people. *Crisis, 16*(3), 100-1.

Hegarty, S. (2004, October 23). Looking for answers. *Irish Times.*

Howitt, D. (1992). *Child abuse errors*. Hemel Hempstead: Harvester-Wheatsheaf.

Impact. (1998). *Submission to the expert review group on behalf of care workers*. Dublin: National Care Workers Vocational Group.

Inglis, T. (1987). *Moral monopoly: The Catholic church in Irish society*. Dublin: Gill and McMillan.

Irish Social Worker. (1993). *Editorial. 11*(4), 3.

Irish Social Worker. (1993). *Feature. IASW response to the Kilkenny inquiry report, 11*(4), 6-7.

Joint Committee on Social Care Professionals. (2003). *Report of Joint Committee on social care professionals*: Author.

Kemshall, H., Parton, P., Walsh, M., & Waterson, J. (1997). Concepts of risk in relation to organisational structure and functioning within the personal social services and probation. *Social Policy and Administration, 31*(3), 213-32.

Kendrick, A. (1997). Safeguarding children living away from home: A literature review. In R. Kent (Ed.), *Children's Safeguards Review for the Scottish Office* (pp. 143-275). Edinburgh: The Stationery Office.

Kennedy, K., & Gallagher, C. (1997). Social pedagogy in Europe. *Irish Social Worker, 15*(1), 6-8.

Kennedy Report. (1970). *Report of the Committee of reformatory and industrial schools system*. Dublin: Stationery Office.

Kirkwood, A. (1993). *The Leicestershire enquiry 1992*. Leicester: Leicestershire County Council.

Kreuger, M. (2002). Touch. Threads Digests of CYC–Net Discussions. *The International Child and Youth Care Network*.

Langan, M. (1996). Introduction. In N. Parton (Ed.), *Child protection and family support: Tensions, contradictions and possibilities*. London: Routledge.

Lash, S. (1994). Reflexivity and its doubles: Structure, aesthetics, community. In U. Beck, A. Giddens, & S. Lash (Eds.), *Reflexive modernisation* (pp. 110-173). Cambridge: Polity.

Levy, A., & Kahan, B. (1991). The Pindown experience and the protection of children. Stafford: Staffordshire County Council.

Lindsey, E. A. (1994). *Health within illness: Experiences of the chronically ill/disabled*. Unpublished doctoral dissertation. University of Victoria: Victoria.

London Borough of Brent (1985). *A child in trust (Jasmine Beckford Inquiry Report)*. London: Author.

London Borough of Greenwich. (1987). *A child in mind: Protection of children in a responsible society: Report of the commission of inquiry into the circumstances surrounding the death of Kimberley Carlile*. London: Author.

London Borough of Lambeth. (1987). *Whose child? The report of the panel appointed to inquire into the death of Tyra Henry*. London: Author.

London Borough of Wandsworth. (1990). *Report of the panel of inquiry into the death of Stephanie Fox*. London: Author.

Lowrance, W. (1984). Improved science, heightened societal aspirations and the agenda for risk decision-making. In L. Zuckerman (Ed.), *Risk in society*. John Libbey and Co. Ltd.

Luhmann, N. (1993). *Risk: A sociological theory*. New York: Aldine de Gruyter.

Maier, H. W. (2001, Sept). New days are coming. CYC Online, Issue 32. www. cyc-net.org/cyc-online/cycol-0901-majer.html.

McElwee, N. (1998). The search for the holy grail: Social care in Ireland. *Irish Journal of Applied Social Studies, 1*(1), 79-105.

McElwee, N. (2000). *To travel hopefully: Views from the managers of residential child care units in Ireland.* Galway: Social Scientific Publishing.

McElwee, N. (2001). Legislative and service initiatives: A personal perspective. In K. Lalor (Ed.), *The end of innocence: Child sexual abuse in Ireland.* Dublin: Oak Tree Press.

McElwee, C. N. (2001a). *Aspects of risk. At risk and resiliency in the context of the Youth Encounter Project system in Ireland.* Unpublished Doctoral Thesis. Waterford: Waterford Institute of Technology.

McElwee, C. N. (2001). *Removing the label of at-risk and moving towards an understanding of high-promise children and youth in a resiliency context: Lessons from a five-year study.* Paper to the International Forum for Child Welfare Conference on The Children's Agenda: Familiar Issues, Emerging Concerns. Limerick, Ireland. August 31.

McElwee, N. (2005), *Not just a city problem: Darkness on the edge of town.* Paper to the South Kerry Life Education Mobile Conference, Killarney, Co. Kerry. October 7.

McElwee, N. (2006). Suicide. *Irish Journal of Applied Social Studies, 7*(2), 1-27.

McElwee, N., Jackson, A., McKenna, S., & Cameron, B. (2003). *Where have all the good men gone: Exploring males in social care in Ireland.* Athlone: Centre for Child and Youth Care Learning.

McGrath, K. (1993, Autumn). The effects on those at the heart of the Kilkenny inquiry. *Irish Social Worker, 11*(4), 10-11.

Mitchell, D. (1999, August 6). Response to child abuse. *The Irish Times.*

Moynihan, P. (1996, March). *The importance of a clear strategy for residential care.* Focus Ireland Conference Papers. Dublin: Focus Ireland.

Muller-Hill, B. (1991). Psychiatry in the Nazi era. In S. Bloch & P. Chadoff (Eds.), *Psychiatric ethics* (2nd ed.). Oxford, UK: Oxford University Press.

Musto, D. (1981). A historical perspective. In S. Bloch & P. Chadoff (Eds.), *Psychiatric ethics* (2nd ed.) (pp. 13-30). Oxford, UK: Oxford University Press.

National Children's Strategy. (2001). Dublin: Stationary Office.

O'Brien, C. (2005, October 12). Economic cost of suicide is 900m. *Irish Times.*

O'Grady, M. (2001). *An introduction to behavioural science.* Dublin: Gill and McMillan.

O'Hagan, K. (Ed.). (1996). *Competence in social work practice: A practical guide for professonials.* London: Jessica Kingsley.

O'Hara, P. (2005). Quoted in *Irish Times*, March 14.

O'Higgins, K. (1996). *Disruption, displacement, discontunity.* UK: Avebury.

O'Toole, F. (1990). *A Mass for Jesse James: A journey through 1980's Ireland.* Dublin: Raven Arts Press.

O'Toole, F. (1997). *The Ex-isle of Erin: Images of a global Ireland.* Dublin: New Island Books.

Parton, N. (1985). *The politics of child abuse.* London: McMillan.

Parton, N. (1996). Social work, risk, and the "blaming" system. In N. Parton (Ed.), *Social theory, social change and social work* (pp. 98-114). London: Routledge.

Parton, N., Thorpe, D., & Wattam, C. (1997). *Child protection: Risk and the moral order.* London: MacMillan Press Ltd.

Phelan, J. (1999). Child and youth care in Canada. Seminar to Social Care Faculty at Waterford Institute of Technology.

Phillips, D. P., Lesyna, K., & Paight, D. J. (1992). Suicide and the media. In R. W. Maris, A. L. Berman, J. T. Maltsberger et al. (Eds.), *Assessment and prediction of suicide* (pp. 499-519). New York: The Guilford Press.

Rafferty, M., & O'Sullivan, E. (1999). *Suffer little children: The inside story of Ireland's industrial schools.* Dublin: New Island.

Reder, P., Duncan, S., & Gray, M. (1993). *Beyond blame–Child abuse tragedies revisited.* London: Routledge.

Rose, N. (1996). The death of the social? Refiguring the territory of government, *Economy and Society, 25*(3), 327-56.

Schmidtke, A., & Häfner, H. (1988). The Werther effect after television films: New evidence for an old hypothesis. *Psychological Medicine 18,* 665-676.

Share, P., & McElwee, N. (Eds.). (2005). *Applied social care: An introduction for Irish students.* Dublin: Gill and McMillan.

Slovic, P., & Fischhoff, B. (1977). On the psychology of experimental surprises. *Journal of Experimental Psychology: Human Perception and Performance, 3,* 544-551.

Social Services Inspectorate. (2001). *Newtown House high support unit. Inspection Report.* Dublin: Social Services Inspectorate.

Social Services Inspectorate. (2003). *Annual report.* Dublin: Government Publications.

Sonneck, G., Etzersdorfer, E., & Nagel-Kuess, S. (1994). Imitative suicide on the Viennese subway. *Social Science and Medicine, 38,* 453-457.

Task Force Report. (1981). *On child care services.* Dublin: Stationary Office.

Thorpe, D. (1997, January). Regulating late modern childrearing in Ireland. *The Economic and Social Review, 28*(1), 63-84.

Utting, W. (1997). *People like us: The report of the review of the safeguards for children living away from home,* London: The Stationery Office.

Warner N. (1992). *Choosing with care: The report of the Committee of Inquiry into the selection, development and management of staff in children's homes.* Department of Health, London: HMSO.

Waterhouse, R. (2000). *Lost in care: Report of the tribunal of inquiry into the abuse of children in care in the former county council areas of Gwynedd and Clwyd since 1974.* London: The Stationary Office.

Williams, D., & Lalor, K. (2000). Obstacles to the professionalisation of residential care in Ireland. *Irish Journal of Applied Social Studies, 2*(3), 73-90.

doi:10.1300/J024v29n01_06

Chapter 7

"Learn What You Like and Like What You Learn": The Youth Encounter Projects and St. Augustine's Special School, Limerick City

SUMMARY. Mark Twain once famously quipped, "I never let schooling get in the way of my education." Paul Simon, the American folk singer, begins one of his songs "When I think back on all the crap I learned at high school, it's a wonder I can hardly think at all." These men could just have easily been discussing schooling in Ireland, for this is the way many Limerick children and youth felt about formal school life prior to their involvement with St. Augustine's Youth Encounter Project. But it is prior to their involvement.

This chapter provides a demographic profile of the pupils of that project and explores aspects of the day-to-day life of the project as a child and youth care intervention by examining some of the influences of risk replacement or resiliency projects that have influenced provision of services. This Limerick YEP attempts to alter the approach

---

[Haworth co-indexing entry note]: "'Learn What You Like and Like What You Learn': The Youth Encounter Projects and St. Augustine's Special School, Limerick City." McElwee, Niall. Co-published simultaneously in *Child & Youth Services* (The Haworth Press, Inc.) Vol. 29, No. 1/2, 2007, pp. 165-199; and: *At-Risk Children & Youth: Resiliency Explored* (Niall McElwee) The Haworth Press, Inc., 2007, pp. 165-199. Single or multiple copies of this article are available for a fee from The Haworth Document Delivery Service [1-800-HAWORTH, 9:00 a.m. - 5:00 p.m. (EST). E-mail address: docdelivery@ haworthpress.com].

doi:10.1300/J024v29n01_07

from one that is risk, deficit, and psychopathology-oriented to one that is protection, strength, and asset focussed. A question posed is, "Has the early intervention enrichment programme assisted the pupils to reintegrate successfully within the community?" By reintegrate I mean the ability to attend a regular school, hold a job, live again with their family and such things. This chapter also explores the establishment of the Youth Encounter Projects in Ireland in the context of an important but largely overlooked study completed by Egan and Hegarty over two decades ago (1984). No official review has been published since.

doi:10.1300/J024v29n01_07 *[Article copies available for a fee from The Haworth Document Delivery Service: 1-800-HAWORTH. E-mail address: <docdelivery@haworthpress.com> Website: <http://www.HaworthPress.com>* © *2007 by The Haworth Press, Inc. All rights reserved.]*

KEYWORDS. Special education, Limerick Youth Encounter Project, risk, resiliency, youth work, youth development

A college professor had his sociology class go into the Baltimore slums to get case histories of 200 young boys. They were asked to write an evaluation of each boy's future. In every case the students wrote, "He hasn't got a chance." Twenty-five years later, another sociology professor came across the earlier study. He had his students follow up on the project to see what had happened to the 200 boys. With the exception of 20 who had moved away or died, the students learned that 176 of the remaining 180 had achieved more than ordinary success as lawyers, doctors, and businessmen. The professor was astounded and decided to pursue the matter further. Fortunately, all the men were in the area and he was able to ask each one, "How do you account for your success?" In each case, the reply came with feeling, "There was a teacher." (Butterworth, 1993, pp. 3-4)

Schools are acknowledged as being able to promote pupils' competencies and prevent the development of unhealthy social and health behaviours as they enjoy unequal access to pupils, parents, and teachers, clinical psychologists, social agencies and the health care system (Anthony, 1987; Garfat & McElwee, 2004; McElwee, 2001; Rhodes & Brown, 1991; Rutter, 1980).

It is well recognised that an important foundation supporting economic development is education. In 1967, a comprehensive system of free secondary level education and transport in rural areas was introduced. The numbers of pupils who sit their Leaving Certificate examinations has increased exponentially from only 12,000 in 1965 to 65,000 at the end of the 1990s (Commission on the Points System, 1999) which represents a completion rate of about 81 per cent of the relevant age cohort (O'Grady, 2001). What of the other 19 percent?

Youth Encounter Projects lie at the heart of the educational at-risk terrain in Ireland. The Department of Education and Science understands the Youth Encounter Projects to use negotiated career, counselling and academic remediation (where mild disabilities are negotiated) to break the "cycle of poverty" of disadvantaged or at-risk children and assists in the realisation of potential. The projects recognise that parents' experiences of the rejection of school are reinforced through their children's schooling today and that the "cycle of disadvantage" can be broken by focusing primarily on structural explanations, while not ignoring ameliorative actions (Government of Ireland, 1997).

One widely quoted North American study estimated that for every $1 invested in an intervention programme, it produces a net return of $7 in terms of income tax yield (Schweinhart, Barnes & Weikhart, 1993). "Success" or "failure" in the formal educational system depends on a number of factors often outside the control of individual pupils, and schools are significantly constrained by "questions of ideology, governance, and resource allocation" (Gilligan, 1998). Teaching disadvantaged young people to simply conform to dominant society's norms, therefore, is often unhelpful, because such programmes fail to adequately embrace issues of cultural diversity. We are finding, more and more, that there are considerable differences in the familial socialising of children from certain geographical areas as their demographics radically shift. For example, some 70,000 people migrated to Ireland in the 12 months to April 2005, the highest annual immigration figure on record and the number of non-nationals living in the State is estimated to be 350,000, accounting for 8-9 percent of the population of 4.13 million currently living here, according to CSO estimates. Seventeen percent of these immigrants come from Poland and 9% from Lithuania to take but two examples of countries of origin (McElwee, 2006). This is having an effect on child and youth care practice as front line workers try to make sense of a changing environment in terms of family dynamics.

Indeed, family dynamics have been identified by several commentators as important (see Madge, 1986). Consistency, self-discipline, home supervision, personal ability, helpful, understanding parents or care-givers, and positive peer influences are frequently absent in the lives of disadvantaged children and youth. This is a crucial point in the emerging discourse on at-risk and resiliency in Ireland. Resiliency is not just about getting a class of at-risk or vulnerable children to merely pass examinations. Rather, it is about celebrating diversity and nurturing the individuality of a pupil whilst passing on coping skills and facilitating self-mastery. And, it should be remembered that the children and youth coming to projects like St. Augustine's are coming from very challenging backgrounds. I present a brief case study of one of my interviewees to illustrate this point below.

CASE STUDY ONE: JAMES

James is the eldest of six children. The family live in a Corporation Estate in Moyross.[1] At his time of involvement in the Limerick YEP his parents were alive and living together. Both his mother and father left school at primary level and both were unemployed. With regard to the cultural climate of the home there were some daily newspapers, only a few books, a colour television, a radio, and a record player. His problem behaviour came to attention of the authorities at the age of twelve. He was referred to the Limerick YEP by a social worker for non-attendance at school. James had court appearances for malicious damage prior to coming to the YEP and was addicted to solvents. There was also evidence of alcohol abuse. His father was known to be violent. His family was well known to the social services. On leaving the YEP, James could read. He has spent time in prison.

RISK-FOCUSED PREVENTION

In the introduction to this book, it was noted that risk may be under-stood from the perspective of exposure (vulnerability) or from the perspective that concentrates on positive adaptive behaviour (resiliency). Risk-focused prevention attempts to reduce, eliminate, or mitigate the effects of factors that put people at-risk as identified in epidemiological and etiological studies. The Youth Encounter Projects provide children and adolescents with opportunities, or what is termed in child and youth care discourse as "teachable moments," for them to acquire a broad range of competencies that would facilitate a full complement of connections to self, others, and the community. Factors such as school goals, expectations, discipline, and reward systems can significantly influence a child (Garfat & McElwee, 2004). Change in both the child and the environment may be established when the focus is on systemic, ecological, organisational reorientation that involves full participation by all the actors involved. Over and over, the research points to interventions that promote social competence, problem solving skills, mastery, autonomy, and a sense of purpose for the future as predictors of successful resiliency.

MEETING THE RESILIENCY PERSPECTIVE

As we have seen in an earlier chapter, international research indicates that assets are inversely related to risk behaviours and that these are additive with each increment of assets accompanied by a reduction in the number of risk behaviours (Garmezy & Neuchterlien, 1972; Gore & Eckenrode, 1994; McElwee & Monaghan, 2005; Ungar, 2004). The Youth Encounter Projects, as child and youth care intervention programmes, focus on *resiliency* rather than *risk* as they attempt to assist in the individual's response to risk factors. A number of the identified processes below of resiliency are implemented by the Youth Encounter programmes, with these perspectives in mind:

- The process is long-term and developmental. It is difficult to measure resiliency in the short-term as children need time to overcome certain obstacles in their lives.
- The process views children with strengths rather than with deficits or risks. Resiliency looks to the ways in which children make sense of their lives and builds on the child's perceived worldview.
- The process nurtures protective processes so that children can succeed by changing systems, structures, and beliefs within schools and communities (Winfield, 1994).

Garmezy (1983) argues that children who attend such schools tend to develop individual resiliency attributes such as positive peer interactions, a high degree of social responsiveness and sensitivity, intelligence, empathy, a sense of humour and problem-solving skills.

THE RESILIENCY PERSPECTIVE: INVOLVING THE WIDER ECOLOGY

Early intervention may be described as actions by agencies other than the family to facilitate the development of young children and to improve their life chances at an early age before they come into contact with formal education. Nonetheless, the Youth Encounter Projects build on the notion of parental involvement which, until the 1980s, was almost non-existent in the Irish context (Fitzgerald, 1995; Garfat & McElwee, 2004). A working partnership between the home environment and the school is constructed where possible. The Director of St. Augustine's is quick to comment that, in his experience, "All children want to be in school, part of the set-up really. It is only their adverse circumstances that create obstacles in this." With regard to the teacher/parent relationship, all concerned want the best for the pupils and all parties learn from one another. Parental engagement imparts to children "a positive sense of self, physical health, access to positive models, and trust in others as resources" (Consortium on the School-Based Promotion of Social Competence, 1996, p. 273).

This change in emphasis towards ecological inclusion has found expression in the Report of the Special Education Review Panel (1993) which proposed seven principles to facilitate development of educational services. These include:

- all children … have a right to an appropriate education;
- the needs of the individual child should be the paramount consideration when decisions are being made concerning the provision of special education for that child;
- the parents of a child with special educational needs are entitled and should be enabled to play an active part in the decision-making process;
- a continuum of services should be provided … ranging from full-time education in ordinary classes, with additional support as may be necessary, to full-time education in special schools;
- … appropriate education for all children with special educational needs should be provided in ordinary schools;
- only in the most exceptional circumstances should it be necessary for a child to live away from home in order to avail of an appropriate education;

- the State should provide adequate resources to ensure that children with special educational needs can have an education appropriate to those needs. (pp. 207-208)

An Alternative Approach in Education:
The Historical Background to the Youth Encounter Projects

> Safe Haven: A place that is perceived (in this case by youth and their families) as safe from physical, emotional, intellectual, and cultural harm.

The first Youth Encounter Project opened in the home town of *Angela's Ashes* author Frank McCourt, Limerick City, in October, 1977, followed by Cork in 1978 and two schools in Dublin in 1978 and 1979. Unfortunately, the school on Sean McDermott Street in Dublin proved to have many problems right from the beginning and eventually closed, with the school in Limerick very nearly closing just two years after opening.[2]

The Youth Encounter Project's specific brief is to deal with "disadvantage within disadvantage" where disadvantage is perceived to have a broad base in home life, community life, and pupil behaviour. As noted earlier, research indicates that the school and community environments of at-risk children have significant impacts on the shaping of their worldview. This is now understood to be particularly the case for males (Peterson, 1988; McElwee & Parslow, 2003). The Youth Encounter Projects were to embrace a socio-ecological perspective because it was acknowledged that the quality of home life for the majority of the pupils was well below the norm of their national school counterparts.

The central premise behind the Youth Encounter Projects was that they would be a non-residential, community-based resource and a system of guidance and care as well as a more traditional centre of learning. They would embrace elements of formal education, would provide vocational training and have a strong leaning towards recreation and social activities and a negotiated curriculum. The schools would have a four-tiered approach utilising life skills education (communication, problem solving and decision-making); basic skills (reading, writing, speaking, and maths); counselling (personal and group) and participation in outdoor pursuits (summer programmes). These special schools were to "throw as much light as possible" on disadvantage, delinquency and the relationships between formal and informal education.[3]

The Youth Encounter Projects, then, were established as special *national* schools for children at-risk utilising a negotiated curriculum (with)in the formal State school context.[4] The curriculum is adapted to meet the student's perceived and individualised needs. To facilitate this, woodwork, arts and crafts, cookery, and recreational studies are provided in addition to a summer programme culminating in a residential camp. A curriculum profile at the project is provided in Table 1.

The term "informal" is widely used to describe aspects of the Youth Encounter Projects such as the negotiated curriculum, the summer camp, and the summer programme more generally. They are also described as a form of compensatory education, which can have many hidden connotations. It seems fair to suggest that the complementary emphasis on the environment outside the school, and, more generally, the primary importance of personal relationships, are all characteristics of the Youth Encounter Projects, which entitle the system to be called "informal" by comparison to the national primary school system as a whole and which make them a child and youth care intervention.[5] Specific programmes, content, and curriculum are important, but the mere perception that school, itself, can be a positive experience may be protective for the child or young person at-risk.

Community Care

It is worth briefly commenting on community care in the context of the Youth Encounter Projects and the ecological approach (Bronfenbrenner, 1979). Community care is recognised as a sound strategy in the delivery of health and welfare services. Such care may be provided by informal, quasi-formal, or formal helpers or a combination of all three.

TABLE 1. St. Augustine's Limerick YEP School Year Curriculum Programme (2005 Data)

Programme Elements	
Junior Certificate Schools Programme	Swimming
Information Technology	Woodwork
Staff Meeting	Gardening
Domestic Programmes	School Maintenance
Social Programmes	Physical Recreational Activity
Summer Programme	Outdoor Bound Activities (Sailing/Canoeing/Surfing)

Community care was established in Ireland for families experiencing distress after the publication of the McKinsey Report on the Management of the health services and provided an administrative framework for the emphasis on community care that had been evident in official reports throughout the 1960s. Community care should be readily accessible, preventative in orientation, and personalised. The importance of community care in the educational context is noted by a number of commentators (Gilligan, 1998; McElwee, 1996; Wehlage et al., 1989).

Sourcing Pupils for the Youth Encounter Projects

Children attending the Youth Encounter Projects may be sourced from a number of areas such as primary schools, secondary schools, health boards, education welfare officers, the children's court, juvenile liaison officers, the national assessment units, parents, relatives and the pupils themselves. I return to this later in this chapter.

Costing the Youth Encounter Projects

The Youth Encounter Projects were seen by Government Departments as expensive (see Table 2). There was, originally, to be a pupil-teacher ratio of 1:7 whilst there is currently a principal and four teachers making the ratio 1:6. Funding for the projects comes from the Department of Education and Science in the context of delinquency and disadvantage as opposed to handicap in the more conventional sense (Egan & Hegarty, 1984).[6]

The Egan and Hegarty Report: Profiling the Children of the YEPs

There has been little critical research published on the Youth Encounter Projects and yet the Mid-Western Health Board (1991), the Report of the Special Education Review Committee (1993), McElwee

TABLE 2. Breakdown of the Limerick YEP Funding (2004 Data)

Category	Amount
Directors Salary	€64,000
Full time teachers	€40,000 (average)
Part time teachers	€34 (per hour)
Bean a Ti (Gaelic for "Woman of the House")	€28,000

(1995), McKenna (1996) and Bates (1996) commented positively on its overall contribution to development for vulnerable children at-risk. Egan and Hegarty, from St. Patrick's College in Drumcondra, Dublin, evaluated the Youth Encounter Projects in the early 1980s. This ground-breaking but largely neglected study utilised four categories to describe the current status of past pupils of the Youth Encounter Projects;

1. settled and unsheltered (if a past pupil was working, looking for work, or keeping a home without any evident signs of trouble);
2. settled for the time being but still in a sheltered environment (applicable to ex-pupils who left the projects but went to another, similar one such as a Neighbourhood Youth Project);
3. unsettled (but still better off than when they originally came to the projects);
4. at-risk and in trouble to varying degrees (Egan & Hegarty, 1984, p. 168).

Over a seven-year period, between 33% and 50% of the children attending the Youth Encounter Projects had a significant degree of learning deficit and, on average, the entrants are 3-5 years below the population norm in reading proficiency. There is an established regression towards concrete thinking amongst the pupils. Overall, Egan and Hegarty discovered that 50% of the entrants to the Youth Encounter Projects completed the programme that was designed for them with another 30% completing most of the programme. About 20% only stayed in the project for six months and never settled down. Fifty percent of the pupils were considered no longer at-risk after their involvement with the project, 25% could still be categorised as at risk, and 25% required some form of secure care (locked youth detention) after leaving their project.

Egan and Hegarty (1984) discovered that one parent was absent from the family home in 40% of the children admitted to the Youth Encounter Projects, 75% of the parents were unemployed, in 55% of the homes violence was common, and 33% of parents and older siblings of the pupils in the projects were "commonly known to the Gardai for serious crimes." The authors broke their analysis down into three categories which included parental relationships, quality of home living, and sibling influence.

One of the more salient conclusions of Egan and Hegarty (1984) was that the Youth Encounter Projects, as they were constituted at the time, had little or no chance of making an impact on the formal school system. The projects concentrated on attracting applicants with near zero school attendance, children exposed to family violence, and delinquents. By

1984, over 100 students had passed through the Limerick programme spending an average of 12 to 24 months there. By 2004, over 300 students had passed through the programme.

St. Augustine's Special School

St. Augustine's Special School was the first Youth Encounter Project established in Ireland in 1977 and is located in inner-city Limerick. Originally, it resided in the Limerick Youth Services building and the present use of the building was facilitated to the school by the Augustinian Order in 1981.[7] The school was described as having the most disadvantaged pupil population of the YEP projects, yet it scored well in a number of areas (Egan & Hegarty, 1984).

Nonetheless, out of 227 pupils who attended the Limerick Youth Encounter Project over a 19-year period (1977-1996), none of the pupils passed the formal School Leaving Certificate examination.[8] Indeed, if we take a random look at one of the file categories in the school, that of "pupils in 1993," we note that 12 did not even reach sixth class. This is a cause for serious structural concern in terms of social policy formulation, educational strategy, and personal concern in terms of the expectations children attending St. Augustine's Special School and their parents may have had.

The poor performance on those formal education variables in the subject group at the point of admission into the project shows us how disadvantaged the pupils were. None of the pupils were regular school attendees, all were classed as "often absent," five of the boys and three of the girls had been expelled from the formal school system, none of the pupils had attained the norm expected reading age, none of the pupils had attained the norm expected maths age, and only two of the thirteen males were described as "gifted creatively."

Family Histories of the Interviewees

The family histories of the pupils at the project are also crucial for understanding the pupils. Out of the seventeen interviewees in my study, four of their parents were deceased at the point of first contact, all thirteen males and all four females lived in Corporation Estates, four of the males and three of the females had criminal activity in their family constellations, three of the males and one of the females had chronic illness in the family, and six of the males had psychiatric illness in their immediate families. All of these contribute to their overall risk status.

Geographical Profile of the Pupils of St. Augustine's

The students attending the school invariably come from the large housing estates of Limerick, which constantly feature in the Irish media for their high frequencies of serious assaults, drug dealing and murders. For every girl attending the project there are four boys and there is a waiting list of prospective pupils.

Egan and Hegarty (1984) found that the Limerick and Cork Youth Encounter Projects should really be considered *regional* Youth Encounter Projects as none of their pupils came from the immediate locality of these schools. Also, the schools are located in business areas in the centre of cities, which was not the case with their Dublin counterparts.

Social Exclusion and Urban Authority Housing

In 1992, the Irish Government published an important Housing (miscellaneous provisions) Act, which built on the Housing Act Ireland 1890, the Housing Financial and Miscellaneous Provision Act 1932, the 1960 Housing Act and the 1988 Housing Act. Between 1931-1940, a total of 822 houses were built in Limerick City. Between 1961-1971 the Corporation provided some 1,811 dwellings mainly located at the south of the city. The 1991 census of population stated that there was a population of 55,554 in Limerick City. Limerick and its suburbs have a current population of 75,356. Its population declined between 1981 and 1991 while the population of the suburbs increased. Some 40% of the registered unemployment in the mid-western region is in the Limerick city area (MWHB, 1996). Numerous factors militate against the positive development of these high-density Corporation housing areas in Limerick[9]:

- Deficient housing.
- High unemployment rates.
- Low incomes.
- Excessive dependence on social welfare.
- High percentage of families suffering from stress-related matters.
- Problems with juvenile crime, truancy, and vandalism.
- Indications of drug/substance and alcohol abuse (Hickey, 1995, p. 25)

There is a considerable amount of literature on social exclusion and urban local authority housing (McCafferty, 1999). The most plausible location of an Irish "underclass" is in public sector rented households in major urban centres (Nolan & Whelan, 1999, p. 112).[10] Almost 25% of the population in the aforementioned Corporation estates left school before the age of fifteen as compared with 12% for the wider city area (MWHB, 1996, p. 14). Indeed, for some it is a cultural norm and has been institutionalised through two generations or more.

The pupils of St. Augustine's typically come from families where long-term unemployment, financial problems, alcohol and substance abuse, suicide, tragic deaths, single parenting (70% first time births to lone parents) multiple partners, and early pregnancy are the norm. Added to these are violence, criminal activity, inadequate parenting, little effective communication between families and school authorities and a lack of formal education.[11] Thus, in terms of agreed understandings of social *disadvantage*, the pupils have to be acknowledged as seriously disadvantaged. Of all the areas in Limerick, Southill Estate features most negatively in the Irish media and is recognised by the interviewees in this study as being "risky" (i.e., joy-riding, stabbings, shootings, murders) . Let us explore the demographics of this estate in more detail.

Southill Estate: Community Climate and Resources

Southill Estate was constructed from 1966-1972 and the corollary of providing housing on an emergency basis is that priority is attributed to purveyance of houses per square mile. Southill is situated on the southern periphery approximately two kilometres from Limerick City centre and incorporates the following areas: Keyes Park (167 dwellings), Kincora Park (133 dwellings), O'Malley Park (530 dwellings), and the notorious Carew Park (251 dwellings).[12] O'Connell (1993) suggests that many of those housed in peripheral urban estates have been re-housed from overcrowded and insanitary inner neighbourhoods. Indeed, between 1990 and 1993 there were 560 official re-lettings in a part of the estate that contains only 418 houses (Limerick Corporation, 1995).

By September, 1977, the population of Southill was approximately 5,365. Of those 44% were children under the age of fourteen while 80% of all married couples were in the 20-33 age grouping thus indicating that the majority of people who first moved into the area were young couples seeking their first residence (Counihan, 1973).[13] By 1995 the population was 5,297 (11% of the city's total population). There were 1,149 families living in 1,131 houses in 1994 with this figure revised to 1150 in 1999 (McCafferty, 1999). In 1995 unemployment stood at 2,395 people between the ages of 18-65, a rate of 80% of eligible workers.

The spiral of social disadvantage is self-perpetuating, a point which was detailed over thirty years ago which recognised minority groups as particularly disadvantaged in terms of where they live, attempting to secure jobs, inadequate education and discrimination. In terms of an overall picture of poverty and social exclusion, households with more than four children (21% of families in Southill East), households with young female heads, single adult households with children (33% of families in Southill East), and households headed by an unemployed person (71% under the age of 30 in Southill East) have been acknowledged as risk indices and dominate Southill (McCafferty, 1999). As high a figure as 71% of those under the age of 35 had never been employed, which is 2.5 times the Limerick City rate (Gordon, 2000).

The second major catchment area for the pupils of St. Augustine's is Moyross.

Moyross Estate: Community Climate and Resources

A major development was undertaken by Limerick Corporation in 1973 with the commencement of the Moyross Development on the northside of the city. In all, some 870 dwellings were provided during the period 1971-1978 (LCDPR, 1986). Thirty-seven per cent of the population were under the age of twelve with 20% of the population single-parent households. Moyross has approximately 1,200 households with a population of six thousand people. A number of schemes have been put in place to counteract the social exclusion experienced in Moyross such as in-school support programmes, home-school liaison co-ordinators, remedial and concessionary posts, educational support projects, resource teachers and teacher counsellors, an early start pre-school programme, a schools' psychological service, intervention and prevention programmes for traveller children, special classes/units, suspension or expulsion, the Youth Encounter Project, youthreach, school attendance officers, and parenting courses.

CONNECTING CONTINUUMS

The preceding discussion on social disadvantage and at-risk clearly illustrates the fact that the parents and children must be seen in terms of a connected continuum, whereby each is dependent and related to the other. Restricted opportunity for such families has led to an increased focus on the present rather than the future. This fact has been of crucial importance in the thinking behind developing educational programmes in disadvantaged and at risk areas of Limerick with the Moyross Intervention Education Pilot Project prioritising;

- the empowerment of parents towards partners in the educational process;
- the adaptation of the curriculum instructional timetable to help satisfy subject demands;
- the extension of the school day by one hour to allow for the provision of intensive parent-teacher-child interactional learning.

Like Southill, it is acknowledged that the area has an increasing number of lone-parent families with poor social and environmental facilities (McClure, 1995). The programme managers make the point that parental involvement is quite sophisticated with enrichment classes, in-school learning, parental input into educational planning, and "parental project management" all listed as key tasks in the partnership programme. It is thus acknowledged that changes occur through a developmental process that necessitates considerable nurturing, a willingness to share power, and a commitment by parents to take on new responsibilities.

The School Files and Constructing At-Risk Profiles

Over a period September to March, for example, a total of 72 children were referred to the project: 21 females and 51 males. The addresses confirm the fact that the pupils overwhelmingly come from Moyross (18), Southill (22) and Weston (12). Of the referrals, 10 were made by mothers of pupils, 4 by fathers of pupils and 5 were made by the pupils themselves.

Having obtained a general sense of where the pupils are from in Limerick and who referred them into the project, let us now take a closer look at the interviewees. In Table 3 we note that the main professional grouping to refer pupils to the project in addition to parents or separate students who were not referred by parents in this instance are, in fact, social workers (7). Gardai and School Attendance Officers also play a strong role in referring children to the school (3) with parents (2), local teachers (2) and the Neighbourhood Youth Project (2) sharing equal referral numbers. The youth service only referred 1 pupil. This is in keeping with the recent findings on youth at-risk of Forkan (2001).

The type, content and reasons of referrals coming in to the project are varied. Out of the study cohort, one male came in after being in care, another male came in after returning from England and was not in any formal school, a further male came in after being assessed by a special school (mental handicap/intellectual impairment), and a fourth male was homeless at the time of initial referral.

TABLE 3. Sources of Referrals for Interviewees of the Limerick Youth Encounter Project (n = 17) ⁃

Referral Agencies	Number of Pupils
School Attendance/Gardai	3
Welfare Officer (YEP)	N/A
Welfare Officer (Other)	N/A
Social Worker (MWHB)	7
Parents	2
Local Teachers	2
Neighbourhood Youth Project	2
Youth Service	1
Clinical Assessment Centre	N/A
Self-Referral	N/A
Ex-Student	N/A

We get a sense of the profile of children coming into the Limerick project from the following two examples chosen at random from the case files which include letters of referral from two separate sources and a response letter from the project. Again, I have changed some of the details by "cutting" and "pasting" from several reports for illustrative purposes.

Referral Letter: Example One

Dear Dr. O'Shea,

We, as staff, are very concerned about Andrew Bailey. This is his third year with us and we feel that we are unable to meet his needs. He is becoming more difficult to manage, is aggressive and, at times, cruel to children. We fear that he may injure somebody soon. Parents have complained about their children's hair being pulled, being kicked and struck.

Andrew consistently used bad language to pupils and teachers. On one occasion, he hit a teacher. I can no longer permit this to happen as pupils and teachers have rights too. Can anything be done to help him? ... We would very much like to see some therapeutic programme prescribed for Andrew as we feel much of his aggression, apparent cruelty and erratic behaviour is a cry for help.

At this stage, I feel that we cannot continue to maintain him as he is, and we hope that you can be of assistance. We will appreciate any advice or support you can give as we would genuinely like to help Andrew.

Yours sincerely,

Sr. Bernadette Xavier Walsh

Referral Letter: Example Two

Re: Liam O'Flynn
Date of Birth: 14.3.1983
Date of Report: 12.2.1995

Liam attended the school for a period of some weeks. In general, I found Liam to be very apathetic and disinterested in his work. He actually did any work I gave him but he would need encouragement to complete the task. His concentration is poor. He usually just sat quietly at his desk daydreaming when not actively engaged in a task, i.e., writing or reading. Liam often seemed very tired, yawning a lot, moving and responding slowly to any demands.

Liam's levels of academic functioning are very low. On the Drumcondra Maths Tests, scored for the beginning of second class, he scored well below average in all sections–computation R.S. 7/S.S. 80. Concepts 14/81 and Problems 7/75. Total 28/74 which would put him on the 4th percentile rank.

In English on the Schonnel, he scored a reading age of 7.3 years, on the Holborn 6.09 and a comprehension age of 7.6. On the Jackson, he showed no knowledge of phonics and evidence of b/d confusion. On the Drumcondra English Attainments again scored for the beginning of 2nd class, he scored slightly below average in vocabulary (12/109), average in word analysis (13/99) and well below average in comprehension (5/70).

I found that Liam responded poorly to tokens such as stars on his work. He tended to be more giddy in front of his peers than when on his own in the class.

Signed: Susan McCloud
Educational Psychologist

The individual behaviour of each potential pupil is also a source of concern for the staff at the project. At times, the project decides not to take in a pupil as the school cannot meet all the perceived needs of all children. This confirms the fact that the staff are aware of the limitations of the project as we can see from one example of a response sent back to a referrer as provided below (names have been changes to protect identity and the year of the letter has also been changed to ensue confidentiality).

Response Letter: Example One

20.4.1991
Re: Conor O'Brien

Dear Dr. Smith,
At our recent Referrals Committee meeting, it was decided that Conor O'Brien would not have his needs met at St. Augustine's. On the information submitted to us, it would seem that Conor requires considerable professional skills which are not available on our staff.

Yours sincerely,

John Hanna (Director)

Finally, I provide an extract from a psychiatric evaluation of one of the pupils.

Psychiatric Evaluation: Example One

Name: Geraldine Hickey
Address: 1 Oakey Terrace, Moyross, Limerick
D.O.B. 12.12.1982
Age: 13 years, one month

Geraldine Hickey was admitted for psychiatric evaluation to this facility. She presented as stubborn, disobedient and aggressive. On further enquiry, parents stated that she was violent in the home context. She was negativistic–refused to do normal daily routines, oppositional–would do exactly opposite of what she was asked to do, explosive–both verbally and physically if her demands were not met, manipulative, and attention seeking.

At school, Geraldine's behaviour was disruptive. She would become verbally abusive and uncooperative. She was disinterested in learning and progress in school was retarded. There was no evidence in the history suggestive of over activity, emotional or biological disturbance, or psychosis.

Personal History

Geraldine was born following a near full-term pregnancy. Delivery was assisted by forceps. Baby was kept in an incubator for seven days as there was delay in cry. Her motor milestones were found to be delayed with slightly arrested development of mental milestones. Achievements at normal school were delayed.

Physical Illness

Geraldine spent several short stays in hospital due to accidents in the home. On one occasion, aged three, she fell down the stairs and broke an ankle and a shoulder blade. On another occasion, she split her lip after hitting her head off the front door. She also received stitches in an arm wound after putting her hand through a glass panel in the bathroom door.

Mental State Examination

At the first session, Geraldine came across as a child with limited intelligence and poor speech and language development. On subsequent assessment, her problematic behaviour was evident.

Physical Examination

This revealed poor muscular co-ordination and a minimal weakness in upper and lower limbs. She was investigated to outrule chromosomal anomalies due to the fact that her parents were older than the norm when she was born. The routine bloods investigations and EEG were within normal limits.

"HAVE WE COME HERE FOR FORGIVENESS?"

The school's location presents some difficulties in security provision for the Director and staff of the school. Vagrants tend to shelter in the laneway and there are frequent reports of criminal activity in the area, which has included fighting, drug dealing, and stealing alcohol from a nearby public house. Indeed, Egan and Hegarty (1984) comment on the fact that problems of accommodation, programme design, and the actualisation of the student population created tremendous difficulties at times. Entrance to the school has always required the unlocking of a large steel gate and use of an intercom system. Every time the school gate and door are opened and admission is facilitated, they close immediately in a sense shutting the project out from the world and the world from the project.[14]

The lack of an outdoor playing area, particularly for the younger children, raises further problems for staff and students (Egan & Hegarty, 1984). The children and youth are concerned at the limited cramped space afforded to them by the Department of Education and Science.[15] Perhaps one of the reasons the summer programme is so anticipated by the children is because it brings with it the promise of wide open spaces, green fields, mountains, lakes and the seaside where the pupils can "wander lonely as a cloud" or remove themselves "far from the madding crowds."

STAFFING AT THE YOUTH ENCOUNTER PROJECTS: THE RESILIENCY PERSPECTIVE

The Director of the Project notes that staff of St. Augustine's need certain qualities to survive and prosper in a child and youth care intervention such as this one. Indeed, the qualities of staff are key in a child and youth care intervention. Since the establishment of the project, there has been very limited staff turnover and with the Director's recent retirement, another long standing teacher was successful in becoming Director. This ensures a climate of consistency for the current pupils, ex-pupils, graduates and their families.

Staffing of the Youth Encounter Projects consists of the Director, four schoolteachers, a community worker and a Bean an Ti (Gaelic for "woman of the house"). In addition, there are two special needs assistants, a part-time secretary, a part-time woodwork teacher, and a maintenance person. There is also a strong voluntary contribution from parents, ex-pupils, and friends of the school all dedicated to the principles of resiliency. Originally, a welfare officer was seconded from the Department of Justice but has since been withdrawn after some years. The Youth Encounter Projects provide the service of a full-time community worker whose responsibility it is to strengthen the project within the community and home environment of the students by liaising between the school and home.

The experience of the staff is that professional development, school policies, and school cultures that promote learning and achievement for both student and teacher work best in replacing risk with resiliency. Resilience in coping with the transition at early ages is likely to be associated with having a good match between the child's entry characteristics and the teacher's expectations for classroom behaviour (Taylor, 1991).

The perceived responsibilities of the Director and staff have changed over the years as one might expect. These largely reflect the changes in the Irish education system. There is a degree of variation between the 1984 designated responsibilities and the 2004 designations but several categories have remained constant. The responsibilities of the Bean an Ti have remained fairly constant over the 1984-2004 period. She no longer has a role in home counselling and has a diminished role in counselling overall and her responsibility for the summer programme has decreased dramatically due to funding issues. The Bean an Ti still retains a limited role in teaching and has increased her role in aftercare for the pupils.

Significant changes have taken place between the 1984 and 2004 dates (see Tables 4, 5, and 6). Teaching staff have become less involved in court related work, home counselling, in dealing with referrals, clubs activities, placements, aftercare, community groups, and admissions. They have increased to primary responsibility their summer programme activities.

The Director has more responsibility for court work and significantly less time for actual teaching which he sees as disappointing and is concerned at this loss of direct teaching contact with the pupils. The Director has become less engaged with arranging and supervising the work placement.

TABLE 4. Perceived Responsibility of the Teachers 1984 and 2004

Area	1984	2004
Court related work	X	n/a
Home counselling	XX	X
Referrals to other institutions	X	n/a
Non-attenders	XX	X
Teaching	XXX	XXX
School supervision	XXX	XXX
Counselling	XX	XX
Clubs	XX	n/a
Work placement	XX	n/a
Aftercare	XX	X
Other community groups	XX	X
Admissions	XX	X
Summer programme	XX	XXX (some staff)

XXX   Primary responsibility
XX   Secondary responsibility
X   Some responsibility

TABLE 5. Perceived Responsibility of the Bean an Ti 1984 and 2004

Area	1984	2004
Court related work	n/a	n/a
Home counselling	X	n/a
Referrals to other institutions	n/a	n/a
Non-attenders	XX	n/a
Teaching	XXX	X
School supervision	XX	X
Counselling	XX	X
Clubs	n/a	n/a
Work placement	n/a	n/a
Aftercare	n/a	X
Other community groups	n/a	n/a
Admissions	n/a	n/a
Summer programme	XXX	X

XXX   Primary responsibility
XX   Secondary responsibility
X   Some responsibility

TABLE 6. Perceived Responsibility of the Director 1984 and 2004

Area	1984	2004
Court related work	X	XX
Home counselling	XX	XX
Referrals to other institutions	XXX	XX
Non-attenders	XX	X
Teaching	XXX	X
School supervision	XXX	XXX
Counselling	XXX	XX
Clubs	X	n/a
Work placement	XX	X
Aftercare	XX	XX
Other community groups	XXX	XXX
Admissions	XXX	XXX
Summer programme	X	X

XXX   Primary responsibility
XX   Secondary responsibility
X   Some responsibility

The Negotiated Curriculum:
"Learn What You Like, and Like What You Learn"

Classes begin at 10:00 am with the girls and boys divided into mixed classes depending on their ability and age. There is a constant emphasis on attempting to mirror the pupils' needs with the school programme. The school motto is "Learn what you like, and like what you learn." The Junior Cert Schools Programme fits the needs of each individual child. This is not to say that everything in the school is negotiated. There are some school rules as seen below:

1. Physical violence to staff or pupils will warrant immediate suspension, followed by consultation with parents, which may lead to indefinite suspension.
2. No solvents, alcohol, tablets of any kind allowed on the premises.
3. No pupil to attend school under the influence of any solvents, alcohol, or tablets.
4. If a pupil breaks (1) or (2) pupil will be brought home, parents informed, and the pupil will be suspended.
5. School furniture and equipment to be treated carefully–any serious breach–the parents will be informed and the pupil suspended.
6. Any pupil sleeping "rough" (i.e., out of the house) will not be allowed to attend school until he returns home.
7. Pupils leaving the premises (repeatedly) without staff permission during school hours–their parents will be informed and the pupils be suspended if the case warrants it.
8. If a pupil is constantly involved in minor breaches of discipline, the following procedures will be followed:

   a. Pupil will meet with staff to try and solve the problem.
   b. Parents will be called if (a) fails.
   c. If (a) and (b) fails, the pupil will be suspended and parents informed.

9. If pupils are constantly refusing to take directions from staff and be uncooperative, the procedure in number 5 will be adopted.

In practice, my experience is that the above rules are interpreted as elastic and organic by all concerned, but there is a common understanding of zero tolerance. The fact that they are there, however, means that they can be invoked if a member of staff feels particularly upset at a pupil.

Freidus (1992) has noted a number of curricular features of programme design and delivery that impact strongly on children and these include:

- Curriculum practice which is clearly grounded in a theoretical framework.
- Curriculum goals which are clearly articulated.
- Activities and materials which are consistent with theory and goals.
- Teachers who understand and share the theory and goals of the chosen approach and who have been carefully trained to develop and/or implement appropriate classroom practice.
- Teachers who are knowledgeable about children, about content, about pedagogy ... the learner, what is to be learned, how to promote this learning.
- Teachers who believe in the curriculum they are implementing and work together, collaborating, supporting and reinforcing one another's practice.

The curriculum has been adapted from the formal Irish national curriculum bearing such criteria in mind. The type of education provided could be termed "culturally friendly" in the positive sense of the term. For example, the pupils might learn to read a bus timetable that proves particularly useful, as their normal mode of transport is the bus service (car ownership being alien to many of their households). Nature, history, geography and contemporary social issues are taught indirectly to the children through verbal interaction, painting, and woodwork (McKenna, 1996) again drawing parallels with the Rutland Street Project's informal pupil-centred approach.

The production of cribs and crib pieces for Christmas and Halloween masks and costumes is undertaken with great enthusiasm with students involved in the general upkeep of the premises. This includes sweeping and washing the floors, emptying rubbish bins, and doing the laundry. The school offers swimming, sailing (the project was recently given a sailing boat by the Limerick Harbour Board), soccer and mini-hockey and is fortunate in that it owns a mini-bus that is essential for the school children to be mobile both during formal school term and the summer holidays. The sports on offer carry the agenda of team building and responsibility. Confidence is fostered through setting realisable goals that the pupils may attain.

The school has access to a small plot of land in a rural area in County Limerick for the children's use. Caring for the land and the vegetables and mingling with pets and animals comprises part of the sessions for the pupils. The thinking behind this is that the children get to see a process from start to finish as they are with the teachers when the seeds are bought, plant the seeds, nurture and harvest them and, finally, eat them. This organic sense of continuity is something that the children rarely experience in their lives, and the experience appears to be enriching for the majority.

The approach and process to education here is seen as far more important than merely receiving an educational Certificate. The students are not merely permitted to "take" from the school all the time. A sense of civic responsibility is imbued in the children by weekly visits out to a day and residential centre for children with an intellectual impairment where the children take the residents on swimming outings. They are responsible for the safety and enjoyment of their charges and this is undertaken with a profound sense of seriousness. Every Thursday night, the community worker collects the pupils and travels out to a residential centre where the pupils of St. Augustine's put on a disco for residents and day pupils. This is clearly a case of real community empowerment where the people help each other to develop. Some of the pupils also assist in the Special Olympics for people with a mental handicap. This can have a profound effect on the ex-pupils years after they leave the school.

The staff of the school believes that the balance between academic education and the creative therapeutic programmes are of primary importance as they encourage the children to come to school and offer a programme that is relevant to them, whilst incorporating their needs. The negotiated curriculum on offer at St. Augustine's, then, is of major importance in maintaining the children's attention and interest as the pupils have substantial room to choose subjects that they feel are relevant to them both collectively and as individuals.

THE IMPORTANCE OF FOOD AS A SOCIALISING AGENT AT THE PROJECT

One of the more positive aspects of the Youth Encounter Projects is the emphasis on food, as was Bruno Bettleheim's Orthogenic school, where food is understood as being the "great socialiser." The project provides both breakfast and lunch for the pupils. School commences at 9.30 am Monday to Friday with breakfast and ends at 3.00 pm each day. Due to the social and economic circumstances prevailing at home, some of the children lack adequate diets and do not eat regularly. An important side benefit of eating with the pupils is the fact that an opportunity arises to provide a form of instruction that lies between the formal and informal health guidance.[16]

Nutritional needs are sometimes unheard of in some of the homes of children attending the project. Indeed, I had the sobering experience during one of the summer camps I attended of bringing a number of children out to a restaurant in west Cork. This was not the normal practice due to resource inadequacies within the school, but the Director was particularly pleased with the collective efforts put in by the pupils that day during canoeing practice and wanted to treat the children. One of the girls informed me that this was the first time she had ever been inside a restaurant. Despite the fact she was permitted to choose whatever she wanted from the menu, she still chose a coke, chips and a burger. I could only surmise that this was an acceptable meal to her but, more importantly, it was familiar and safe. She had great difficulty reading a basic menu and I had to negotiate this with her.

Another of the interviewees, Robert, informed me that the only time he ever had a Christmas dinner was at St. Augustine's. Unfortunately, this is not just unique to this study. Gormley et al. (1989) also comment on the types of food considered as desirable by certain Irish "inner-city" children, such as chips, burgers, sausages, tea and toast. The fact that Robert had decent dinners in St. Augustine's did not leave his memory. When I interviewed him in prison in 1999 and 2000, he again discussed the importance of food to many of the pupils.

Part of the school curriculum in St. Augustine's (and the National Council for Educational Awards Examination Syllabus and Schools Completion Programme) involves the children, on a rotating basis, preparing meals with the Bean an Ti. There is no doubt that the kitchen programme has been successful using a number of criteria. Children often say that the kitchen is their favourite room in the school, and Egan and Hegarty (1984) suggested that as many as 80% of the pupils learned more respect for food while they were in the school.

In the Limerick project, the pupils cook lunch and assist in the serving of the meals. Pocket money is then given to the students who assist with cleaning and the other necessary chores and in recognition of their culinary expertise. At 11:00 am a light snack is provided for the children. Again, the psychology borrows from Bettleheim's "food is the great socialiser" thesis and Maslow's hierarchy of needs concept. If the basic need for food is not met, the children will not be physically able to concentrate on schoolwork. The pupils are very much involved in the daily running of the school. This gives them a sense of responsibility and achievement. For at least part of the day, the pupils are needed and important to someone else. Some of the children come from environments where the only time-keeping that has to be followed in the home is getting up on time to make it to the labour exchange, social welfare offices, and to various Garda (police) station visits.

Finally, a summer programme operates at the project. Let us briefly explore this programme and examine some of the influences behind it. The school offers a youth programme during the summer that also includes children not attending St. Augustine's but deemed to be at-risk by referees. Originally these programmes were intended to be run by the community worker and the welfare officer but, in practice, all staff have been involved. An open house policy is used during the summer whereby children and adolescents are allowed to utilise the facilities for a number of hours daily in the context of "learning through leisure." They can play pool, basketball, table tennis, and board games and obtain light refreshments.[17] In effect, the summer programme is a combination of the welfare and community programmes without the school programme. Such an approach has the support of a number of international studies such as Jenkins and Smith's (1990) American study and Borge's (1996) Norwegian study of influences on children's development where it was noted that organised leisure activities may assist in preventing behaviour problems in children and youth.

Anecdotal evidence based on my experiences being with the children and young people was reinforced in the later formal interview data and suggests that the annual summer camp is the most eagerly awaited event of the school year by the pupils. Those pupils who behave during term time are "rewarded" with the summer programme camp. Nonetheless, when the pupils do arrive at the summer camp, the child and youth care orientation of the project is obvious.

THE OTHER 23 HOURS

The brief residential summer camp experience is understood as an effective child and youth care intervention as it makes use of the "richness of the milieu" (Durkin, 1993; Gudgeon, 1986). The camp experience allows the pupils to view one another through a different lens. As the primary aim of the camp is simply around having fun, the pupils really want to be there. This facilitates greater entry into a therapeutic relationship (Treischman, Whittaker & Brendtro, 1969). Low risk, but high gain, activities are encouraged such as learning to wash down a canoe whilst moored, learning to tie specific knots for night hikes, getting together a first aid pack for use during sporting activities such as abseiling. "Teachable moments" are then used by the staff and volunteers to discuss organisation, leadership qualities, peer interaction, safety and health issues, appropriate assertiveness and the like. The self-esteem of pupils rises as they can see tasks being accomplished where adults provide unconditional positive regard. The pupils can and do ask for assistance without shame or fears that they will either be rejected or laughed at and through carefully selecting tasks suited to individual levels of competence, task accomplishment and self-mastery results. Thus, the summer camp provides a meaningful but realistic environment for at least some of the features of a resiliency perspective to be explored.

RECREATIONAL RISK: REPLACING AT-RISK WITH HIGH-PROMISE

Recreational risk replacement therapy is a major component of the St. Augustine programme. Competency-oriented, relevant, empowering, and democratic recreational risk can have a major impact on at-risk youth, particularly when this involves a residential child care experience. Durkin (1993) argues that it is summer camps, in particular, that provide a social system suited to the care and treatment of at-risk youth by providing a fun camp environment that does not break the continuity of life in the school community. Crucially, summer camp is constructed around the 24-hour needs of children and youth as opposed to the more traditional nine-to-five needs of many adults. Durkin suggests that summer camp allows for immediate feedback and encouragement of prosocial behaviour amongst the participants who are removed from their inner-city neighbourhoods with all the associated influences. In terms of the resiliency debate, self-mastery and self-esteem are encouraged by requiring participants to experience both self- and team-oriented tasks such as choosing a site area to put up tents, cooking for the group, choosing games, and engaging in role play in games and the like.

Writing about the situation in the United States, Dustin (1982) and Mitchell (1983) have suggested that the desirability of recreational risk is high for those individuals with lower mastery of other more formal social settings such as work and home life. The experience of summer programmes at Jefferson school in the United States was that an emphasis on enrichment as opposed to remedial classes proved beneficial.

This thesis has been supported by my various studies completed on adolescents at-risk in various locations in Ireland (McElwee, 2001), by Hogan's (1997) study of outdoor pursuits with delinquent youth, Laste's (1997) study of children who witness family violence (1997), and Bates' study of young offenders in open settings (1996).

Hunter (1987) notes that outdoor pursuits create an environment for adolescents to rethink and rebuild their negative attitudes. In order to accomplish the task of completing an orienteering course or abseil down a cliff face, adolescents have to learn to work together so they are indirectly learning the social skills society expects from people more generally.

Studies carried out by Cason and Gillis (1994) suggest that the longer the adventure programme lasts, the more significant the improvement is on self-esteem and self-confidence because of an emphasis on pro-social behaviour.

THE WAY FORWARD: RESILIENCY IN THE FACE OF ADVERSITY

Certainly my experience has been that the earlier a "disadvantaged" or at-risk child is reached, the more effective a school-based programme may be (Gibbons, 1990; MacDonald & Roberts, 1995; Savage, 1994). This has been evident since the 1960s in mainstream international socio-educational research (Deutsch, 1964; Lynch, 1999). Despite revisions, the current Irish national curriculum remains challenging to both the life opportunities and life expectations of children designated as "disadvantaged" (Report of the Special Education Review Committee, 1993).

According to Sagor (1996) and Wang, Haertel, and Walberg (1995), schools can provide support to students, particularly those at risk, through resilience-building experiences that focus on five themes:

1. Competency (feeling successful)
2. Belonging (feeling valued)
3. Usefulness (feeling needed)
4. Potency (feeling empowered)
5. Optimism (feeling encouraged and hopeful)

Experiences that relate to these five factors are likely to enhance students' motivation and self-esteem and, consequently, their achievement (Edwards, 1997).

CONCLUSION

This chapter has presented a descriptor of St. Augustine's Youth Encounter Project by tracing its historical roots and contemporary way of being with youth. It is disappointing that the Youth Encounter Projects have functioned without formal, regular networking between them. This may be largely due to the individual preferences staff members entertain towards more mainstream academic subjects in some schools and the creative subjects in others and the overall importance they place on particular recreational programmes such as the summer programme. It was suggested, for example, that the Limerick school held a low-key approach to the academic programme and that this served to remove conflict between the pupils and teachers.[18]

The Youth Encounter Projects aim to develop scholastic, vocational, and personal capabilities and strengths in the pupils whilst recognising that a more positive ideology towards school and school work must be fostered both with the children attending the projects and their families and communities. The value of both the classroom and the school "as symbolic and practical sanctuary for the vulnerable child" (Gilligan, 1996) must be emphasised. In Egan and Hegarty's 1984 review, 50% of the pupils completed the programmes assigned to them with 30% leaving for various reasons prior to programme completion. Twenty-five percent of the pupils of the Youth Encounter Projects remained at-risk, in sheltered environments, or in some kind of institution with a further 35% requiring care in a more secure environment. In the final analysis, the Youth Encounter Projects have met sone of their primary aims, at least, that of overcoming truancy amongst their pupil base.

The Youth Encounter Projects are invaluable because they adopt an ecological approach to working through relationships based on use of self, which are individualised to the needs of each pupil. Self-mastery, social competence and belief in the future are fostered in the pupils by staff and volunteers that believe in the therapeutic child and youth care relationship. But how do the pupils perceive their own lives? How do they make sense of the Youth Encounter Project system and, crucially, how do they understand risk in the context of life in Limerick? Let us explore this.

NOTES

1. A Corporation Estate is dedicated housing that is built, operated, and owned by a local council or corporation and that is typically provided at nominal rent to the needy.

2. The Limerick YEP had to have a change of patron from the Limerick Youth Services to the Augustinian religious community to ensure its survival.

3. Many in the field of child protection and welfare would advocate the acceptance of behavioural maladjustment as a category of psychological disability as with physical, mental or sensory disabilities.

4. National schools because of the age range and educational backgrounds of the children.

5. McManus (1995) has suggested that schools can offer a safe environment in which children can explore insecurities, distrust and anger if they have a resiliency outlook.

6. An area of contention in the past was the fact that the schools had to discuss all areas of expenditure with the administrative officer, a member of the steering committee.

7. The Director and Board of Management are currently negotiating with the Department of Education for monies for either the renovation of the school or its relocation to more suitable premises.

8. The Leaving Certificate is the examination taken at the end of secondary school in Ireland. Traditionally, a student had to obtain five passes to achieve the Leaving Certificate.

9. Southill is one such large-scale local authority housing area where unemployment is estimated at 80%. At the start of the 1990s, the level of unemployment in Moyross was estimated at 70% (MWHB, 1991), but by the middle of the decade this figure had increased by ten percent to 80%.

10. There are many difficulties with employing the term underclass not least the fact that many people do not actually constitute a class in the classic sociological tradition and because some people move in and out of the underclass for brief periods. Categories are disputed.

11. The housing estates in which the children typically reside have been portrayed as a conglomerate of hopelessly dysfunctional families condemned to spawn a new generation of dysfunctional youth that, in turn, will reproduce dysfunctional families.

12. The area also houses a number of Industrial Estates with Galvone, located adjacent to Childers road, being the largest. At one time this employed approximately 800 people.

13. The total population of Southill has decreased over this period.

14. One of the ex-pupils informed me that he had heard of Frank McCourt's book, *Angela's Ashes* and the emphasis on living in dirty lanes. He noted the irony of the school suffering from being hidden away down a dirty lane in 1999.

15. The U.S. Department of Education (1997, p. 45) has noted that ... educational disparities are not simply the result of risk factors that cause emotional or physical harm, or that alienate children from school. Many students at risk of developing low skill levels are emotionally and physically healthy, and they enjoy a relative amount of academic success in warm caring (*yet substandard*) schools (my emphasis). This seems to be the case in St. Augustine's and, more generally, in the Youth Encounter Projects.

16. The Bean an Ti (Woman of the House) plays a particularly strong role in the Limerick Youth Encounter Project as a whole and early on was assigned a primary responsibility.

17. The State is not obliged to ensure that children receive any physical education.

18. Nonetheless, Egan and Hegarty (1984, p. 94) claim that the Youth Encounter Projects can be termed genuinely *informal* because they do concentrate on personal relationships, the teachers have a degree of flexibility to cancel classes and try something else if things are not going well and there is an emphasis on the environment outside the school. Sixteen years later, this is commonly understood as the resiliency approach.

REFERENCES

Anthony, E. J. (1987). Risk, vulnerability and resilience: An overview. In E. J. Anthony & B. J. Cohler. (Eds.), *The invulnerable child* (pp. 3-48). New York: The Guilford Press.

Bates, B. (1996). *Aspects of childhood deviancy: A study of young offenders in open settings*. Unpublished doctoral dissertation. Dublin: University College Dublin.

Boldt, S. (1997). *Hear my voice: A longitudinal study of the post-school experiences of early school leavers in Ireland*. Marino Institute of Education: Dublin.

Borge, A. (1996). Developmental pathways of behaviour problems in the young child: Factors associated with continuity and change. *Scandinavian Journal of Psychology, 37*, 195-204.

Butterworth, E. (1993). Love: The one creative force. In I. Canfield & M. A. Hansen (Eds.), *Chicken soup for the soul* (pp. 3-4). Deerfield Beach, FL: Health Communications.

Cason D., & Gillis, H. L. (1994). A meta-analysis of outdoor adventure programming with adolescents. *Journal of Experiential Education, 17*(1), 40-47.

Commission on the Points System. (1999). *Final report and recommendations*, Dublin: Stationary Office.

Consortium on the School-Based Promotion of Social Competence. (1991). Preparing students for the twenty-first century: Contributions of the prevention and social competence promotion fields. *Teachers College Record, 93*, 297-305. *Resilience in Children and Adolescents: Process, Mechanisms and Interventions*. USA: Cambridge University Press.

Counihan, B. (1978). *Five years a growing: A case study on community Development in a new urban community 1973-1978*. National Federation of Social Service Councils.

Deutsch, M. (1964). The disadvantaged child and the learning process. In A. Passow (Ed.), *Education in depressed areas*. New York: Bureau of Publications, Teachers College, Columbia University.

Durkin, R. (1993). Structuring for competence, relevance and the empowerment of children and those who care for them: A case study of the Sage Hill programme. *Journal of Child and Youth Care, 8*(3), 63-75.

Dustin, D. (1982). *Life wish*. Paper presented at the National Recreation and Park Association Congress (Louisville, Kentucky, October 26, 1982).

Edwards, C. H. (1997). *Classroom discipline & management* (2nd ed.). Upper Saddle River, NJ: Merrill.

Egan, O., & Hegarty, M. (1984). *An evaluation of the Youth Encounter Project*. Dublin: Educational Research Centre, St. Patrick's College.

Fitzgerald, D. (1995, November 14). Teaching and parenting. *The Irish Times*.

Forkan, C. (2001). *Needs, concerns and social exclusion: The millennium and beyond*. Waterford: Centre for Social Care Research, Waterford Institute of Technology.

Freidus, H. (1993). Recurring themes and current issues. *Curriculum Resource Handbook*. New York: Kraus International Publications.

Garfat, T., & McElwee, N. (2004). *Effective interventions with families: The Eircan perspective*. Cape Town: Pretext.

Garmezy, N. (1983). Stressors of childhood. In N. Garmezy & M. Rutter (Eds.), *Stress, coping and development in children* (pp. 43-48). New York: McGraw Hill.

Garmezy, N., & Neuchterlien, K. (1972). Invulnerable children: The facts and fiction of competence and disadvantage. *American Journal of Orthopsychiatry, 42*, 328-329.

Gibbons, J. (1990). *Family support and prevention: Studies in local areas.* London: HMSO.

Gilligan, R. (1996). The role of teachers and schools in protecting children at risk of abuse or neglect. *Oideas* (Journal of the Irish Department of Education), *44*, 26-45.

Gilligan, R. (1998). The importance of schools and teachers in child welfare. *Child and Family Social Work, 3*, 13-25.

Gordon, L. (1989). *Heroes of their own lives: The politics and history of family violence. Boston 1880-1960.* London: Virago.

Gordon, L. (2000). *Southill. An area with hope after all?* Unpublished diploma dissertation. Waterford: Centre for Social Care Research, Waterford Institute of Technology.

Gore, S., & Eckenrode, J. (1994). Context and process in research on risk and resilience. In R. Haggerty, L. Sherrod, N. Garmezy, & M. Rutter. (Eds.), *Stress, risk and resilience in children and adolescents: Process, mechanisms and interventions* (pp. 19-63). Cambridge University Press.

Gormley, T. R., Walshe, T., & Comrican, K. (1989). *Assessment of school meals and of growth food intake and food likes/dislikes of primary school children in inner city Dublin schools.* Dublin. Combat Poverty Agency Research Report. Series No. 1.

Government of Ireland. (1997). *Sharing in progress: National anti-poverty strategy.* Dublin: Stationary Office.

Gudgeon, C. (1986). Pack up your troubles: A childcare worker approach to summer camp. *Journal of Child Care, 2*(5), 101-104.

Haugh, K. (1996). *Partners in education newsletter.* Limerick: St. Kieran's, Southill.

Havighurst, R. (1965). *The bulletin of the National Association of Secondary School Principals, XLIX*, 110-127.

Hickey, S. (1995). *A sociological analysis of an urban community in crisis.* Unpublished diploma dissertation. Waterford: Centre for Social Care Research, Waterford Institute of Technology.

Hogan, A. (1997). *Outdoor recreational pursuits.* Unpublished diploma dissertation. Waterford: Centre for Social Care Research, Waterford Institute of Technology.

Hunter, I. (1987). The impact of an outdoor rehabilitation programme for adjudicated juveniles. *Therapeutic Recreation, 21*(3), 30-43.

Jenkins, J., & Smith, M. (1990). Factors protecting children living in disharmonious homes: Maternal reports. *Journal of the American Academy of Child and Adolescent Psychiatry, 29*, 60-69.

Laste (1997). Unpublished Dissertation. Waterford: Waterford Institute of Technology. *Limerick Corporation Development Plan Review.* Limerick Corporation.

Lynch, K. (1989). *The hidden curriculum: Reproduction in education. A reappraisal.* Lewes: Falmer Press.

MacDonald, G., & Roberts, H. (1995). *What works in the early years? Effective intervention for children and their families in health, social welfare, education and child protection.* Essex: Barnardo's.

Madge, N. (1983). *Families at risk.* London: Heinemann Educational Books.

McCafferty, D. (1999). Poor people or poor place? Urban deprivation in Southill East, Limerick City. In G. Pringle, J. Walsh, & M. Hennesy (Eds.), *Poor people, poor places. A geography of poverty and deprivation in Ireland* (pp. 203-224). Dublin: Oak Tree Press.

McClure, B. (1995). *Barnardo's family support project Moyross, Limerick.* Limerick: Policy Statement.

McElwee, N. (2001). Child sexual abuse: Legislative, policy and service initiatives. In K. Lalor (Ed.), *The end of innocence. Child sexual abuse in the Republic of Ireland.* Dublin: Oak Tree Press.

McElwee, N. (2006). *Strand 1 application.* Athlone: Centre for Child & Youth Care Learning.

McElwee, N., & Monaghan, G. (2005). *Darkness on the edge of town: An exploratory study of heroin misuse in Athlone and Portlaoise.* Athlone: Athlone Institute of Technology.

McElwee, N., & Parslow, D. (2003). The importance of male role models in Irish residential child care. *Irish Journal of Applied Social Studies, 4*(2), 47-58.

McKenna, S. (1996). Walking the roads. The children of St. Augustine's. Unpublished diploma dissertation. Waterford: Centre for Social Care Research, Waterford Institute of Technology.

Mid-Western Health Board. (1991). *Child care practice policy statement.* Limerick: MWHB.

Mid-Western Health Board. (1996). *Review of Child Care and Family Support Services 1995.* Limerick: MWHB.

Mitchell, D. (1999). Response to child abuse. *The Irish Times*, August 6.

O'Grady, M. (2001). *An introduction to behavioural science.* Dublin: Gill & McMillan.

Peterson, A. C. (1988). Adolescent development. *Annual Review of Psychology, 39*, 583-607.

Pikes, T., Burrell, B., & Holliday, C. (1998). Using academic strategies to build resilience. *Reaching Today's Youth, 2*(3), 44-47.

Report of the Special Education Review Panel. (1993). Dublin: Government Publications.

Rhodes, W. A., & Brown, W. K. (1991). *Why some children succeed despite the odds.* New York: Praeger.

Rutter, M. (1980). *Changing youth in a changing society.* Cambridge, MA: Harvard University Press.

Sagor, R. (1996). Building resiliency in students. *Educational Leadership, 54*(1), 38-41.

Savage, M. (1994, April). Can early indicators of neglecting families be observed? A comparative study of neglecting and non-neglecting families. *Journal of Multi-Disciplinary Child Care Practice in Northern Ireland, 1*(1), 27-35.

Schweinhart, L. J., Barnes, H. V., & Weikhart, D. P. (1993). *Significant benefits: The High Scope/Perry preschool study through age 27.* Ypsilanti, Michigan: High Scope Press.

Taylor, A. R. (1991). Social competence and the early school transition: Risk and protective factors for African-American children. *Education and Urban Society, 24*(1), 15-26.

Trieschman, A., Whittaker, J., & Brendtro, L. (1969). *The other 23 hours: Child care work with emotionally disturbed children in a therapeutic milieu.* New York: Aldine de Gruyter.

Ungar, M. (2004). *Nurturing hidden resilience in troubled youth.* Toronto: University of Toronto Press.

U.S. Department of Commerce. (1997). *America's children at risk report.* CENBR/ 97-2. Washington: DC.

Wang, M. C., Haertel, G. O., & Walherg, H. J. (1995). *Educational resilience: An emergent construct* (Clearinghouse No. UD 030 726). Philadelphia, PA: National Education Center on Education in the Inner Cities.

Wehlage, G. G., Rutter, R. A., Smith., G. A., Lesko, N., & Fernandez, R. R. (1989). *Reducing the risk: Schools as communities of support.* New York: Falmer Press.

Winfield, L. F. (1994). *Developing resiliency in urban youth.* NCREL Monograph. http://www.ncrel.org/sdrs/areas/issues/educators/leadrsho/leOwin.htm.

doi:10.1300/J024v29n01_07

Chapter 8

Listening to At-Risk Youth

SUMMARY. In this chapter I describe the micro "risk society" of Limerick City and St. Augustine's Youth Encounter Project in terms of the social and cultural background of the interviewees, their perceived family and community identity, and their wider socialisation influences. The project is situated down one of the notorious Limerick lanes made famous in a deftly realized and beautifully written story of a boy coming of age during the 1930s and 1940s in Catholic Ireland, *Angela's Ashes,* and has been a safe haven for children and youth since 1977. In this chapter I present direct quotations from my young interviewees organised around the risk concept in their own dialect and inflections.

Past and present students of St. Augustine's are viewed in the context of family, school, and community whilst considering three broad questions: What are the important risk factors associated with each setting? What factors at the individual level are associated with resilient outcomes? What mechanisms at the social ecological level promote resilience in individuals? doi:10.1300/J024v29n01_08 *[Article copies available for a fee from The Haworth Document Delivery Service: 1-800-HAWORTH. E-mail address: <docdelivery@haworthpress.com> Website: <http://www.HaworthPress.com> © 2007 by The Haworth Press, Inc. All rights reserved.]*

KEYWORDS. Safety, self acceptance, belonging, youth work, youth development, child and youth care

---

[Haworth co-indexing entry note]: "Listening to At-Risk Youth." McElwee, Niall. Co-published simultaneously in *Child & Youth Services* (The Haworth Press, Inc.) Vol. 29, No. 1/2, 2007, pp. 201-247; and: *At-Risk Children & Youth: Resiliency Explored* (Niall McElwee) The Haworth Press, Inc., 2007, pp. 201-247. Single or multiple copies of this article are available for a fee from The Haworth Document Delivery Service [1-800-HAWORTH, 9:00 a.m. - 5:00 p.m. (EST). E-mail address: docdelivery@haworthpress.com].

A lot of people, especially this one psychoanalyst guy they have here, keep asking me if I'm going to apply myself when I go back to school next September. It's such a stupid question, in my opinion. I mean, how do you know what you're going to do till you do it? The answer is you don't. I think I am, but how do I know? I swear it's a stupid question.

–Holden Caulfield, *The Catcher in the Rye*

The chapter is written in an interpretative, relational child and youth care perspective and it is worth exploring in a little more detail what I mean by "relational" in this context. Relational research, for me, is qualitatively different from some other perspectives in how one might approach "doing" research. For example, I talk about research partners rather than research subjects, the youth helped generate the questions on which this chapter is based, the youth had a hand in deciding how the chapter might be presented. There is, then, a cultivated relationship between me and the youth over a five-year period and, indeed, has since been maintained with some of them. The chapter has also given me cause to reflect quite a bit on what actually happens in child and youth care interventions.

Schön (1983, 1996) introduced the idea of the "reflective practitioner" by which he meant a practitioner who consciously thinks about what she is doing both as she does it and after she has. Schon elaborated about "reflection-in-action" and "reflection-on-action" and suggested that it was the ability to reflect both in, and on, action that characterised the effective practitioner. There has been a recent focus on meaning-making in child and youth care discourse that invites a researcher into the territory of reflection (see Garfat & McElwee, 2004; Krueger, 2004; McElwee & Monaghan, 2005). Garfat (2005) goes on to suggest that "The field of child and youth care needs reflective child and youth care practitioners both to improve immediate practice and to enhance the possibilities for future practice" (p. 2).

CASE STUDY ONE: PATRICK

Patrick is the second eldest of seven children. The family live in a Corporation estate in Southill. At the time of his involvement in the Limerick YEP his parents lived together at intervals. Both his parents left school at primary level and both were unemployed. Management of the family budget was deemed to be poor. With regard to the cultural climate of his home there were no newspapers, only a few books, a black and white portable television, no radio, and he had few personal belongings. His problem behaviour came to the attention of the authorities at the age of twelve. Pat was referred to the YEP by a Juvenile Liaison Officer for "truanting from school with no parental support." He had previous court appearances for larceny and had been placed on probation. Patrick had been taking solvents and drinking heavily and was listed as "being in physical and moral danger due to his living arrangements" and he regularly suffered from burns. Both his mother and father were hostile to authority. Patrick was listed as having a poor attitude to school discipline, interest in school, application to school tasks and relationships with teachers. On leaving the YEP Patrick still could not read properly. He has spent time in prison.

FRAMEWORKS AND CONTENT

In relation to youth offending and early school leaving, we in Ireland have been obsessed with the identification and quantification of risk factors and with establishing mechanisms to deal with them for a generation. Indeed, this forms the basis for most of our efforts to alleviate disadvantage and, in turn, youth offending. But does it miss the point? (Stokes, 2004, p. 22)

The results below are divided into three content-led sections generated utilising frameworks analysis (see Richie and Spenser, 1984) discussed in an earlier chapter: (a) personal risk/risk factors; (b) risk to friends and peers; and (c) risk in a familial context. I have done this because this is exactly what the youth asked me to do in one of our initial group interviews. Four thematic sub-sections, safety, self-acceptance, belonging, and finding opportunity were further developed from a phenomenological child and youth care perspective. I present my results thematically with selected representative quotations utilised to illustrate broad consensual themes and I have kept the actual language and rhythm of the children and youth in an effort to make the text as genuine to their experiences as possible.

CATEGORIES A1 (PERSONAL RISK/INDIVIDUAL FACTORS) B1 (RISK TO FRIENDS AND PEERS)

The School as Resiliency Environment: Safety, Self-Acceptance, Belonging, Finding Opportunity

> Dave is the fifth child in a family of ten siblings ranging in age from four to twenty-seven. The family lived in a Corporation estate in Moyross where there were two living rooms and four bedrooms. At the time of his involvement in the YEP both his parents were alive and living together. Both parents left school at primary level. Dave's father has an unskilled permanent job. Management of the family budget was "fair." In the home there were weekly newspapers, a few books, a colour television and Dave has some personal belongings. He came to the attention of the authorities at age thirteen for persistent truancy but he had no court appearances for criminal behaviour. There was no evidence of drug or alcohol abuse. Dave was reliable, responsive to direction, emotionally competent, and showed good concentration, helpfulness, and independence in the YEP. His social interaction was positive. He returned to the school to act in a voluntary capacity for a time and has not served a prison sentence. He is now the father of two children.

The school environment has been identified as a social institution second only to the family in its developmental influences on children and young people. Unsurprisingly, the area of school (i.e., the project itself) and how it was seen to impact on the interviewees was a major source of interest. Seventeen sub-themes across categories Personal Risk/Individual Factors and Risk to friends and Peers in relation to school were recorded. The project was understood to have a number of quite diverse roles for the pupils ranging from being a source of peer support to a physically and emotionally safe environment. In essence, the project fulfilled four central roles for the ex-pupils including physical and emotional safety; self-acceptance; emotional, cognitive, and physical belonging, and; a place to find opportunity. These four areas have been identified as being crucial in re-integrating youth at-risk in child and youth care literature.

Primary Role as Diversion: Safety, Finding Opportunity

All of the interviewees commented that they found life in their previous national schools very difficult for a number of diverse reasons. Joe recounts that the project became somewhere he could find a sense of self-acceptance. "When I was on the dole when I was just finished school and during school term, I hated it because I had nowhere to go. So, basically, what I used do is to pass away the time. I used to come in here during the summer holidays and work for a few hours." Some of the children were being bullied in their schools prior to their admission into the project and were fearful of being isolated out for attention or of not being listened to because of past negative experiences. Amanda remembered, "Because they picked on you in other schools and down here is nice. They are nice and they give you the chance here, learning and everything. Out there, they think I know nothing but [here] they sit down and they listen to you and they don't force you to do anything."

Other interviewees felt shamed by mainstream teachers who, they felt, isolated them and "picked on them." Being expelled from one of the formal schools prior to taking up a place at the project was not unusual. Fred explains, "That is what I think like. I got expelled. I got expelled from three schools now and then I got into that school and that quietened me down."

Source of Peer Support:
Safety, Self-Acceptance, Belonging, Finding Opportunity

The project also acts as a focus of peer support as Jane suggests: "Because they tell other kids how great it is and then their mothers send them up." Many of the pupils are acquainted with each other from their respective housing areas and there is a very strong sense of loyalty to the project. Several interviewees commented that they could act naturally and "be themselves" in front of their peers in the project and ask the type of questions that they would ordinarily be too shamed to ask in their old schools. Whilst attending the project, pupils are facilitated with acquiring specific skills such as first aid and orienteering to name but two and are continually shown the more positive aspects of team participation and team building. Shane realised that his fear of appearing stupid in front of peers in his old school held him back, but the project had a different approach. "I don't know, some of the lads, me personally anyway when I was growing up, I needed for a while, I needed one-to-one attention and you can't get that in a normal school. You are not going to put up your hand and say you don't know something when you don't because your friends are around you or people, they don't have to be your friends, people in general, so you are not going to say it, it is too embarrassing.'

Removing Children from At-Risk Environments: Safety

All of the interviewees were well aware that the project removed them from at-risk environments at least for the hours that they attended either school or some of the games and outings outside formal school hours. A sense of physical risk is apparent in the following quotation. "Well if they don't, they will end up on the streets every day and up for a mugging. I have seen kids from between as young as two years of age up to twelve and all they are doing is hanging out on the streets. Some of them actually cause damage to houses. If they were in this school then they wouldn't give any damage to it." Ironically, Eamon admitted, "And then I went into Augustine's and I was hanging around with all the same people that I was fighting against." Eamon is able to demonstrate that a change in environment can make a significant difference in how an individual will behave towards his peers.

Shane was aware that he lacked direction prior to coming to the project. "Um, well coming in here obviously like, because I left school and I came in here and this kind of started me on the right road because I wasn't sure what I wanted to do. And then I came in here and after here then like, I had a lot more understanding about work and the way you are supposed to behave and do you know like? I thought that I could do my own thing, but obviously the world doesn't work like this. You know, when you come here, you learn that."

Maintaining Outcast Status

Perhaps the only manifestly negative feelings around the project itself was that it could serve to remind the pupils that they were, in fact, in a special school set up for them because they were unlike other children in mainstream schools. This was particularly felt due to the location of the school, which is in an alleyway frequented by what the interviewees described as "winos" and "mentos."

Entry to the Project: Safety

The pupils enter the project because they are considered to be at-risk either by a family member or by a professional. Larry noted that it was his mother's attitude that resulted in his entry to the project. "...My mother kind of figured out I was doing it like, she figured out herself. That was why she got me into the school and got me off to work, because I was expelled from other schools like. She kept me off the roads." The pupils are aware themselves that one can go to the project if one drops out of the formal school system, as explained by Brian. "It is a place they go, they can leave school early." Some of the pupils were extremely disruptive in a formal school environment and were forced to leave and seek education elsewhere. "Well, I can yeah, well one school I gave a teacher a leg of a chair. I just bashed something through the window and the other school I was just misbehaving."

Shane noted that he was physically at-risk in terms of his general health and well being which affected his integration into a normal school environment. "What happened is I took a year out of school. I got yellow jaundice and some sort of liver thing and I had to take a year out of school. When I went back to school then, I couldn't fit in because I didn't know the people, you know. I kind of lost contact with them and I thought then that I was way behind everybody else and, you see, when I went back to school I was put back into the class that I left. So I didn't know the people around me and I just wasn't comfortable and I used to "mitch" from school then, pretend I was going to school and not be there, because I wasn't happy there."

Relationship with the Project:
Safety, Self-Acceptance, Belonging, Finding Opportunity

The relationship with the project for both the male and female interviewees can be described as excellent. Not one interviewee made a negative comment about either the staff or the curriculum. When asked about the staff the sense of positivity is apparent in the following three comments. Justin stated simply, "They are grand the way they are. They can't really do much more for you." Brian noted that the project itself "Is not doing anything wrong," and Fred observed, "And they send you out to farms then and brings you a whole load of places, you know? It is a good school like, no point in saying it is not like, because it is."

The majority of ex-pupils still return to the project to meet up with staff as Amanda explains. "I still go in to see John Hanna every now and again. Life is the same for the other kids in there now. The school does everything. There's not much to do in Limerick. In the school, your mind is always occupied, like. They do everything in the school. They tell you about how to do loads of different things." Eamon further stated, "They should do what they are doing, teaching them what to do, cause it is a decent school like, keep on doing what they are doing."

Fred describes how the project is seen to work for the ex-pupils because it is more informal in its approach to instruction and integration.

"There is a laugh in there and kids running and it is alright, you know? It is all right when you want to be, do you get me, and the Headmaster, JH, he is all right. He is all right to talk to. All the people in there would know him from their own area or someone from up town or something like that."

The interviewees do recognise some of the shortcomings of the project, but these are structural rather than directed at staff, with Brian noting, "I would give them a bigger school, you know, just keep them going the way they are, but just give them a bigger school." Joe noted that the project was under-staffed. "But I think, I don't think that St. Augustine's can do anything better unless they got more teachers. That would help them all."

The interviewees further recognised that the project could help to overcome some of the perceived shortcomings in their family environments because of the positive school attitude, a point seen by Justin. "Because a normal school doesn't have patience to sit down with a child, he is just put in a corner and wasted. There's no push from parents, they don't come if their kids go to school. Parents don't give them a push. I got more inside St. Augustine's than in a normal school. They make time for you. They open you up to a lot of opportunities that you wouldn't get. I would recommend the School but it depends on the sort of child. It should be a child who doesn't get on. I always praise the school. I loved going to St. Augustine's."

Some of the pupils indicated a preference for the more traditionally academic subjects such as English or maths, whilst other pupils favoured the excursions to the countryside. The fact that the school has changed the thinking and behaviour of some of the interviewees is also recognised, with Fred acknowledging, "It has changed me a small bit, like. When I was kind of wild before, when I was with them, I kind of quietened down a small bit, you know when I went to school and all that. It is all right. They helped you as well. There is people that did help you, like you know, it is a good school, you get a lot of help in there ..."

Jane maintains such respect for the project that she has proactively sought out a place for one of her relations. "But it was grand like, the kids loved us, so, my nephew is in there now. My nephew is only seven and he is trying to get in there already. You are going to go to St. Augustine's are you and my sister asked me to reserve that. And he is very clever like, he can take care of himself until about fifth class, then go."

Length of Time Spent with the Project: Belonging

A number of the interviewees (in fact, all of the four females) indicated that they would like to have remained in the project for a longer period than was permitted by state funding, with Fred elucidating on the positive aspects of the project.

> Oh, I tried one school and they wouldn't leave me in there, and they said there wasn't that much space, and they said to call back in a few months time there would be space or something like that. Then I think my mother went into JH. JH then came out and said would you like to join up in the school or something like that and someone came with JH and said would you like to try it out? So I went in to try it out anyway and so when I was in there one or two days I got a thing for a bus, you know a bus pass? I got the bus pass and all that and then I went in there for one or two weeks and I started lightly and all the pool tables were in there and there were a lot of things like woodwork and art and all that kind of thing. You could cook there and I liked all that kind of thing, so I stayed there. I was in there about four or five years. I thought it was nice there. We used to be painting the walls inside and outside the school as well, so I thought it was all right in there, I would love to go back there.

Indeed, Joe was keen that he would not upset any of the teachers for fear that he might not be asked back to participate on the project during recreational activities. "I would imagine, yeah, eh, like in St. Augustine's School, I wouldn't like to get into a row with any of the people, because I know them so long, I wouldn't like to have to leave the school."

Summer Camp: Self-Acceptance, Belonging, Finding Opportunity

The annual summer camp held in County Cork was identified as a major source of fun and an opportunity to leave Limerick City behind and explore other ways of doing things. This was clearly seen as the highlight of the year for many of the interviewees. The impact of the summer camp may be judged by the fact that three of the boys stated that they wanted to be sports instructors and cited the summer camps as being influential in this regard. Fred looks back fondly on his time spent on camp.

> Oh, it was good like, it is about five year ago now, do you get me, since I was, about five year ago since I was down there like, so the last time I thought it was good like. I would love to go there again, that kind of a way, do you get me. I would like to go to a good few

things, cause you do canoeing and all that and I like canoeing and all that, done swimming down there and all that kind of stuff as well.

Shane also commented that the role of the project staff was crucial during the summer months when most schools were on holidays as the pupils had a significant amount of time on their hands.

I don't know if the school can do much for you, if you are living in the environment or if you are around it, like when you are outside the school. It really has nothing to do with the school, do you know, but I suppose, they, they work to some programmes to keep the lads doing something and that is brilliant, because the summer is a long time to be out of school and that is excellent like what they are doing. But at night when they are at home, I don't think there is anything they can do.

Truancy: Self-Acceptance, Belonging

A major finding was that the area of truancy featured less significantly in the interview data than I expected, as the project was established partly with remedying truancy in mind. A number of the interviewees did bring up the fact that they had either been removed from school or elected to remove themselves. Perhaps one reason that truancy was not a major source of conversation during the interviewees was that attendance rates at the project were described by the director of the project as "excellent."

CATEGORIES A2 (PERSONAL RISK/INDIVIDUAL FACTORS) B1 (RISK TO FRIENDS AND PEERS) C2 (RISK IN FAMILY)

Thoughts Around Childhood and Risk

Tommy comes from Limerick City. He is the second child in a family of four siblings. Both his parents left school at the primary level. Tommy's father died suddenly, his mother works as an industrial cleaner. In the home there were some daily and weekly newspapers, a few books, a colour television and a radio. He was an affable lad but did not attend formal primary school, because he, "Simply did not like the place." He was not in trouble with the authorities and had no previous court appearances. He was referred to the YEP for truancy. Tommy's mother was anxious for him to attend the project. He showed leadership potential early on and this was both cultivated and encouraged. Tommy had an interest in music and sport and had no real difficulty with reading. He has had a long involvement with the project and the children look to him as a positive role model. He has not been to prison.

Risk Taking Associated with Childhood and Youth: Belonging, Finding Opportunity

All of the interviewees associated risk taking with childhood and youth. Basically, they saw this period as one where they could experiment, albeit with varying consequences, as admitted in the following quote by Eamon referring back to his time in the project. "I was only a young fella and there was no talking to me, I just wanted to have a laugh." One of the other male interviewees was aware that such behaviour could only be excused for a time. "When you get older you cop onto yourself, you know when you are fifteen, fourteen, you do all mad things like, like breaking windows, but when you start getting older you cop-on and you say to yourself, why did I do that when I was small like, do you get me, I mean I would have been like this, do you get me and all that kind of stuff." This view is supported by Shane who noted that "... I don't know when you are younger maybe, say if you go back a few years ago, if you saw someone doing something risky and you thought it wasn't too bad, you might join in yourself because it seems like fun. You have nothing to do, you are bored or whatever, but now when you grow up, everyone thinks for themselves, so you can't stop somebody doing something they want to do."

Excusing Criminal Behaviour: Finding Opportunity

Several of the male interviewees were clearly of the opinion that their past criminal behaviour could be excused by the fact that they were only "messing" and "were too young to know any better." Nonetheless, some of the behaviour involved violent acts against other people, joyriding, and house burglary. Eamon admitted that he had been "Going around robbing, when I was a young fella like. And you know beating up people, you know the usual like, going around with gangs and that like, so my Mother got me into St. Augustine's and I quietened down and I am out of prison so far like and I am not locked up." He was unable (or unwilling) to explain his behaviour. "I was just like that anyway, man." This is a cause of concern.

CATEGORIES A3 (PERSONAL RISK/INDIVIDUAL FACTORS) B3 (RISK TO FRIENDS AND PEERS) C1 (RISK IN FAMILY)

> Mary comes ninth in a family of fourteen siblings. A number of her siblings have an intellectual impairment. Her family lives in a Corporation house in the inner city where there are three bedrooms and two living rooms. Both her parents left school at primary level and both are unemployed. In the home there are no newspapers, no books, no radio, and a black and white television. Mary had no personal possessions when she came to the YEP. Management of the family budget was poor. Mary was referred to the YEP by the District Health Nurse. At the time of her initial involvement with the project there was no evidence of her using drugs or alcohol. She was self-conscious and withdrawn. Mary has returned to education in her adult years and hopes to sit formal examinations. She has not been to prison.

Crime. Crime was a significant feature across all the interview data, with each interviewee making reference to criminal behaviour in some format. Several of the interviewees were more open about crime than others and some admitted they had engaged in criminal behaviour in their childhood (i.e. up to the age of eighteen). Interestingly, none of the interviewees stated that they were involved in criminal activity at the time of the last formal interviews.

Opportunistic Crime: Belonging, Finding Opportunity

As mentioned, several of the interviewees stated that they engaged in crime (in their earlier years) more as a source of fun than for any tangible benefits. Shane, for example, stated that he often engaged in crime simply because he was with his peers as opposed to it being premeditated. "Oh, all stupid things. If there was an ornament in the porch, I would run in and pick it up or one of the boys would run in, ornaments then sell them for a $10 and get a few cans and things like that, like." Although Brian had a criminal record, he could barely remember what he was arrested for exactly: "Well, when I was a young fella years ago, I got arrested." He seemed unable to rationalise his actions or the consequences, but after prompting remembered he might have been "Walking through private property" and Joe also recounted his behaviour in a casual manner. "Em, well let's see, we used to skin cars and we were robbing clothes and shops and carrying weapons."

On the other hand, Shane was very clear about his choice not to get involved in crime, even if it was opportunistic. He explained he would not rob a car,

> Because first of all it is somebody else's and I have just had my own taken and I know the feeling, like, I have never been into that. I couldn't do that, honestly. I couldn't do something like that, I couldn't take something belong to somebody else and watch what they are going through because of it, you know, I am just not that type of person.

Of course, in this choice he had to run the risk of upsetting his peers and being alienated.

Learned Familial Behaviour: Belonging

There is no doubt that for the majority of the youth, criminal involvement was the norm rather than the exception within their families. One of the interviewees was regularly given his uncle's motorcycle to ride even though the bike had no valid insurance or tax. Both were aware of this fact. Brian noted he had been driving the bike and that, "Yeah, it is not mine." On the other hand, Shane deliberately chose not to follow the same path as his brothers into crime, expressing a moral reasoning.

Risk Acceptance–Belonging, Finding Opportunity

For many of the interviewees, crime provides that much needed buzz so common in the international literature on risk and resilience. Even Shane, who generally avoided criminal activity, recounted with great enthusiasm where he played with his friends in a building site area under demolishment despite the fact that it was patrolled by private security and the Gardai. "Well, what we used to do which was absolutely crazy. I think I told you this before, we used to play it in ranks down there on the back road, when they were blowing it up and we found it brilliant." Seeking out thrills by chasing after trucks was also a favourite of the children. "Right, first thing I used to do is hanging off the back of lorries."

CATEGORIES A4 (PERSONAL RISK/INDIVIDUAL FACTORS) B4 (RISK TO FRIENDS AND PEERS) C2 (RISK IN FAMILY)

Neil comes fourteenth in a family of nineteen children. The family live in a Corporation estate in Moyross where there are two bedrooms for the entire family. At the time of his initial involvement in the Limerick YEP his parents were alive and living together. Both his parents left school at primary level and, although his father was skilled, he was unemployed. His mother was also unemployed. Management of the family budget was listed as poor. In the home there were no newspapers, no books, a black and white television, and a record player. Neil had no personal belongings. His problem behaviour came to the attention of the authorities at the age of twelve. There was no evidence of drug or alcohol abuse when he came to the project. In terms of general ability his understanding, fluency and vocabulary are listed as poor. His accuracy and comprehension of reading are poor, as are his accuracy and fluency of writing. He has great difficulty in computation and problem solving. Neil's general knowledge is poor, interest in music, ability at sport, interest in outdoor pursuits and environmental studies also poor. Neil could read when he left the YEP. He has spent time in prison.

Having a Child

Having a child is understood collectively by the participants as grounding an individual, as providing a reason to live, and as a source of social status. When asked the question, "What kinds of things do you think have made a difference to the way your life has gone so far? One of the answers was, simply, "Having a child." The males also acknowledged that having a child changes one life, albeit to differing degrees. Three of the four females had children at the time of final interview, as had four of the males.

A Child Provides an Individual with Status–Self Acceptance, Belonging

All of the interviewees that had become parents themselves said having a child gave a person a certain degree of status within one's own community and that this status could not be taken away by anyone else. This was connected to the prevailing sense of local identity. Indeed, one of the female interviewees noted that the child compensated for her poor choice of male partner. "The fella I have is an ugly sick cunt, I hate him." This comment was later supported by her admission that "And no matter what happens to you and your fella it is you that has delivered the child. You are kept going and you are not going around hanging in corridors and it keep you occupied. They keep you going on your feet all day." On the other hand, Eamon was thankful that he got to spend time with his child at the weekends. "Oh, I sees the child every week and she is, do you know Moyross? She lives out there yeah and so every weekend I gets the child for the weekend then."

INSIGNIFICANCE OF A CHILD–FINDING OPPORTUNITY

The interview data suggests that, on the one hand, a small number of the participants attempted to consolidate their male status by becoming a parent and, on the other, a child was seen as something inconsequential as seen in future aspirations. "Hopefully settled down, nice gas, peace of life like, nice gaff, hang around with the boys and a child." Interestingly, the child comes last in this list.

Grounding an Individual: Safety

Several interviewees suggested that if one had a child it would assist in curtailing risk activities as seen in the following quote.

> I think, well, if the, if there is some, if they entice them to get into more trouble, like if you get a girlfriend, they might, they have a good chance of quieting down, they are not as wild, and then when they start going out with the girl, maybe they have kids, they quieten down. If they have got a good job, then I'd say there would be a good chance of them settling down and having kids.

Irresponsibility Around the Father Role

It is unfortunate that two of the males felt that the father's responsibility should stop at providing financial assistance to the mother as evidenced by the following comment. "Gives her money now and then like." Also, there is a worrying trend towards wanting a baby simply because a male feels that he can physically procreate. At the time of the final interviews Justin's partner was expecting a child later in the week, and when asked about his future hopes, the impending child was mentioned almost as an afterthought. "Sports, I have done. Work. Meeting new friends. Seeing different ways. Doing a bit of travelling around on the Asgard. Seeing what is out there. Maybe the child coming along." Eamon stated that he wanted a child, "Because I have one already like and I am not with the girl, so I just want a child like, you know a son or something like, a daughter." Another one of the male interviewees was unsure what fatherhood would mean. "Man, I don't even know how I feel about it to tell you the truth. Not really. All I would be thinking about is money and having a nice house. You do what you have to, man, to get what you want."

CATEGORIES A5 (PERSONAL RISK/INDIVIDUAL FACTORS) B5 (RISK TO FRIENDS AND PEERS) C3 (RISK IN FAMILY)

All of the male interviewees were concerned with risk in a general context–either getting injured or, perhaps, killed. This extended out to various family members. The threat of ending up in prison was very real for some of the interviewees, and male interviewees ended up there for a range of criminal offences from motoring offences to armed robbery. Two ex-pupils were arrested whilst committing an armed robbery only a few hundred yards from Limerick prison. Unsurprisingly, alcohol and drug misuse came up regularly in conversations with both males and females. Fatherhood and motherhood were listed as being potentially important for the interviewees. A number of the ex-pupils were fearful of being isolated from their peer groups and engaged in certain risk behaviours so that they could maintain their peer affiliations. Finally, in terms of behavioural disapproval and parental punishment, the interviewees expressed fear around physical punishment.

Death and Safety

The threat of a violent death hangs over many of the pupils of the project. A comment from one of the female interviewees illustrates this point. "I'd be afraid in case you die and stuff like that. But you have to face it. You always have to face your fear." Although not part of the sample group for this research, four ex-pupils died in tragic circumstances over a twelve-month period. In one family alone, two brothers committed suicide, one of the ex-pupils was stabbed and died later in hospital of his injuries. The male interviewees were also fearful of death with Fred admitting that, "The most frightening thing is dying. That would be the most frightening thing" and Amanda stated that "Drowning or anything like that" was her greatest fear.

Prison–Belonging, Finding Opportunity

Prison featured significantly in the interview data (approximately 33% of the male ex-pupils over a twenty year period have served prison sentences). Of the thirteen male interviewees, four had served time in prison between 1995 and 2000. Prison is seen as having no redeeming qualities by all of the interviewees. When I asked Robert if he thought the experience of being in prison was in any way useful, he answered,

> No. To be honest with you, man. Since I came in here I just don't have no more conscience. You get used to it because he would have done it to me. Around town if they told someone that you didn't do anything about it (meaning retaliating) it just isn't on. The guys would try to do the same thing to you. They think they are big.

It is also obvious that some of the interviewees feel that they are further discriminated against in having to serve prison sentences in the first instance. Fred admitted that,

> … you don't get off lightly like that. You get the same treatment that anyone else would, that is like me getting caught robbing a car like. You would get twelve months, that is like someone from Corbally or somewhere like that, they would get the same thing as me like, twelve months as well like, so nothing would be different between them.

Concerns Regarding Consequence

As noted earlier, this study indicates that the parents of the pupils tend to use physical and concrete punishment styles as opposed to negotiating possibilities and alternatives to unacceptable behaviour. Jane stated that the beatings she received also extended to her mother. "When my father pummels my mother up, he would beat me senseless." Paul also recounts how his drug taking behaviour was dealt with severely by his father. "Well, back then I was young like, so my mother like, my father like would have digged the mouth off me basically like for taking drugs." When one of the female interviewees became pregnant and informed her mother, the reaction is telling. "She hit me. I thought that she would kill me, cause she did with the rest of them...." Perhaps one of the worrying aspects of this quote is that there is no surprise voiced with the reaction from her mother. Yvonne reported that she was fearful of her father. "No, eh, nervous if I didn't know a fella, well I used to be frightened of my Father, like."

CATEGORIES A6 (PERSONAL RISK/INDIVIDUAL FACTORS) B6 (RISK TO FRIENDS AND PEERS)

Risk Avoidance/Acceptance

Alongside school, risk avoidance versus risk acceptance is an area of particular note in the at-risk and resilience literature. This is an important area as the findings here disconfirm the widely held view that youth at-risk often do not think about risk.

Risk Is a Personal Thing:
Safety, Self-Acceptance, Belonging, Finding Opportunity

This study illustrates that the interviewees, in the main, do actively consider risk and how engaging in risky behaviour might affect them. Fred's first reply around risk was that, "Just like, that is like risky, that is risky now isn't it. Or me trying to swing from tree to tree, that is risky as well like, how are you going to make all them kind of things like?" However, when pressed about risk he answered, "No, I never think of something like that, I thinks about mad things again, I don't think about war and all that." For Fred, risk was associated mainly with criminal activity. "Risky, anything I mean like, do you get me, like crashing a car and going through a windscreen or something."

Robert, who was in prison at the time of final interviews, held a very definite view of risk. "Risk to me, man, is going into a credit union and some fucker pulls a gun on me. That's a risk. That's a risk. Opening a door at three or four in the morning. They're risks to me. They're all dying to get it. I'm just looking out for myself. Myself and that's it...." When asked about risk in the sociological context of authors such as Giddens and Beck, Robert replied,

Not at all. Not at all, man. That's not risk to me. Risk to me is walking down the road at twelve o'clock at night or being caught robbing or crashing a car into a river. Mad things like that. I wouldn't be thinking about things like that (meaning global risk). I don't know how to explain it. It's weird like. Fifteen years ago, all you would be worried about in Limerick is keeping up with the big boys like. Just trying to be them. Like with Susan (child care worker with S.T.A. project), if she met me now she would say, "Jesus, you've changed."

This intense understanding of risk was also shared by one of the female interviewees.

Well, I think risk means death. It's trying to stay alive, stay out of prison and out of trouble and stuff. That's risk, you're doing something your not supposed to do but you try to get away with it. Or you're fighting with someone and you're risking your life there on the line fighting with him cause he could shoot you or kill you. That's what risk means to me.

Justin noted that he liked engaging in what were obviously high-risk behaviours. "I like jumping from heights. I'd go parachuting or bungee jumping. I'd put my head to dangerous things." One of the female interviewees was aware that risk could be linked back directly to her own behaviour. "Going upstairs with a fella and getting pregnant is definitely risky. Going with a bloke that another girl is going out with is risky, because she could kill you."

An interesting area of data was around whether the interviewees enjoyed engaging in risk behaviours by themselves or with their peers. The answers were mixed. For Justin, peer presence was not a major factor in his risk-taking behaviours and he would act "Both on my own and with friends. My friends are all game, you'd naturally do it with them, but if I was on my own, I'd still do it. There's a bit of a risk line inside me." Both Brian and John indicated that they would prefer peers to be present. Some of the risk behaviours were risky to innocent bystanders as illustrated by Eamon who expressed no moral difficulty with "Going around robbing ... and you know beating up people, you know the usual like, going around with gangs and that like."

Again, there is some duality in this as Amanda is aware that there is always some degree of risk present on the roads. "Because you don't own the roads and next thing when two people start fighting and next minute there is one stabbed and you are just walking the other way like, just for no particularly reason like, just blue is the main reason like, blue and both stab each other then, that is the main reason for that." Jane noted that she would engage in risky behaviour with peers. "Friends. I couldn't do it. I'd be too shitty afraid. A bottle of cider...."

Fighting: Belonging

For all of the male interviewees, fighting with children and teenagers from housing areas located near their own homes of residence was considered to be part of everyday life, although not all chose to become directly involved. Pat recounted,

> Beatings, walking up the road and there are two separate gangs and one of them has a row with another one and next minute holy shit erupts, starts and like we are all fighting and like whichever gang is the strongest, say my gang is the strongest, half their gang run away and we would have the other half and you would kill the other half then if you know what I mean.

A sense of passive tolerance of violence was also the case with some of the females. An area that could easily cause a physical row between girls occurred if one girl was perceived to have "chatted up" another girl's partner. "Yeah, moving from fella to fella to fella, you will get done quicker than you get a slap."

Avoiding Weapons: Safety

One of the more revealing areas of research for this study has been around my attempts to understand the precarious balance between risk avoidance and risk taking behaviours amongst the interviewees. For example, some of the males state that they actively sought out street fights for the buzz but tended, as much as possible, to avoid particular scenarios considered to be too dangerous. One such situation most often mentioned in the interviews is when weapons such as knives, guns, axes and baseball bats are involved.

> ... when you are living in a place like Moyross man, it's different boy, you can't mind your own business. Once you are known, you could get your door blown in at four o'clock in the morning and confronted by two guys in balaclavas and get shot to fuck, or get stabbed. You have to survive. It's the truth, that's what it's like.

The manner in which children and young people in this study categorise acceptable and unacceptable violent injury is, I feel, unique. Robert admits that, "I never got shot at. I got stabbed by a knife in a couple of places when I was fourteen. I was on a track (meaning railway track) and this guy was annoying me and I told him to fuck off, but he kept coming over to me. He had something in his jacket, so I bust a Budweiser bottle off his head." Robert wilfully inflicts serious injury on another young person in this scenario, but there is a clear sense that the other youth "deserved" this as Robert claims to have acted only after the initial stab injuries were sustained by him. Nonetheless, he broke a bottle over another boy's head causing him serious harm. The perceived sense of normality in this incident would, no doubt, shock many an unenlightened reader, but I was told this in a totally matter-of-fact tone.

Robbing: Finding Opportunity

Robbery and stealing featured regularly in the interview data from both the males and female interviewees. None of the interviewees voiced any surprise at the fact that several of their peers were involved in criminal activities. For John, "Robbing cars" was a regular activity. Eamon's response to questioning around robbing was casual acceptance. "Oh, yeah, robbing, robbing, I used to do a lot of drugs back then ..." The fact that some of the interviewees might get caught robbing did not deter them. "Like taking something that is not belonging to you and someone came in a caught you and gave you a few belts or something like that." The long-term effect of being involved in such behaviour may best be summed up in a quote from Robert.

> I was as I was a mad fella. I was a cheeky cunt. I was mad. But they all knew it because I was robbing cars when I was twelve. I robbed cars inside and outside Moyross. There was nothing to be doing only drinking and robbing cars. And you would go home and your father would beat the fucking head off you. All that tension in your head like. When you are young you think you can take it. I never had a chance to live like you. Stay on top. I feel like I'm an old fella of thirty and I'm only seventeen. When I get out of here I'm back into it all again. Who's in here? Who's out here? Who is the main man? What's what? Who is with who?

Using Needles: Safety

The most common drugs mentioned during the interviews included "Hash," "Es," and "Speed." Eamon observed that he would regularly "Take drugs like. Just like popping Es and As. Popping As and speeding and when you come down then you want more...." All of the interviewees voiced concern at the injection of drugs and stated that they would avoid this behaviour due to the health implications. Eamon was horrified when asked whether he considered injection of drugs a risky activity and answered, "What? Never in my life. Never." Earlier in his interview he noted, "Yeah, all that like, be careful like sticking needles in your hand then and all that like, stay away from all that kind of thing."

Facing Fears: Self-Acceptance, Finding Opportunity

A number of the interviewees were aware that they had to face up to any fears, whether these were emotional or physical, a point noted by Siobhan who claimed that, "The best thing to do is to face it and pretend that you are not frightened and just go through with it." Shane used a similar strategy.

> Well, the way I used to handle things that frightened me or that I couldn't cope was, I suppose, if I would avoid it as much as I could and if I couldn't avoid it I would got into it head on, like if it was an argument with someone or something more like, I would go into it as much as I could and if I couldn't handle it. I suppose I just wouldn't talk to the person that was putting me on the spot or so to speak I would get away from it as much as I can or else lie my way out of it or get out of it some way. I would just get myself away from the situation.

Avoiding Conflict: Safety

All of the interviewees stated they would avoid conflict if possible, and this category links directly to the category of weapons. Shane had witnessed a good deal of trouble at home and was keen to avoid a similar pattern himself.

> No, I wasn't, honestly, I wasn't, I never kind of got into trouble, I kind of, I don't know, I kind of, you see the two lads at home used

to get into trouble and I used to see what used happen so I have honestly managed to stay away from all that.

Pat noted that the most sensible thing to do when confronted with danger was, "If I was fighting, deck off, I would run away like." He was more specific when talking about the use of weapons in a street fight. "If people come towards me with a baton or something, knives, I would take off."

Fred was more direct and stated that he would "Run" and later in his interview he elaborated "That is true isn't it, there is nothing else I should be saying now is there." Justin said that he would like to "Walk away with no problems," because the safest option was to "Stick to a normal routine, don't wander too far and don't annoy anyone you don't know." Joe was also clear about how he would deal with conflict. "Yeah, everything was I just didn't like it. I always hated it, if I ever saw trouble I would walk away from it." The reaction from one of the female interviewees was similar. "Well, if I were to do it, I would prefer to do it by myself instead of getting more people into trouble."

There was a feeling that sometimes one had to engage in risk behaviours, because there were no other options. A pertinent example of this is Robert who notes that in prison you have to act in a certain way to survive.

> … you'd have to be careful though. Life here is shit. I'll have to spend the next four years of my life banged up here with fellas from Dublin and Cork–criminals and fucking rapists and mad fucking bastards. It would drive you mad and when you get out you would be worse that when you came in. I'll be in until I'm twenty-one. I'll be an old fella.

Later in the same interview, Robert admitted,

> When I get out of here I'm going to get a nice house for the girl and child. I want to get away from the scum here. I'll kill one of those "hairies." This is a shithole, man. This is a bad jail. The screws are bad; they could come in through your cell door and kill you, like. There is people hanging themselves here, people are dying, and they are not doing it because they are mad about his place. That's why I just want to get the fuck out of here … There's no choice in here, no choice.

He noted that he sometimes had to be violent to survive in prison.

> Yeah. Well, we were playing pool. He said, "Your man lost." And I said, "Can I have my table?" And he said, "No. I'll fucking have you." He was making an eejit out of me. You can't walk away, because if you do they will all be at you (referring to the prisoners watching the game of pool). So he pushed me and I busted a pool cue off his face and he jumped back up, so I busted a pool cue off his face. They brought me out and, as they were doing that, I ran back and hit him in his head and he was bleeding and I hit him with a chair. They moved him down to Spike Island and they chucked me into the chokey (referring to the isolation cell). All over a game of pool. You mightn't want to fight, but you have to. If you let one fella at you, they all go at you. That's the way it goes.

Personal Safety

All of the interviewees were concerned with aspects of their personal safety as apparent in the above quotations. Robert expressed fear that when he got out of prison he would have to return to his old housing estate where the gang hierarchy would have changed since his time there.

> No. I'll tell you now, if I had money and a nice car. You don't get any of that stuff living in Moyross so you're out robbing the whole time. You wouldn't be out looking for a job, because there aren't any. It's mad. After a while you see that you just can't get out of it. When I get out, I'm just going to go back into Moyross. Some fella will come along and try to make the name that I had before (meaning challenge his gang position). If I quieten down, they will think he is only a shithead. I will go back to Moyross.

Gangs: Self-Acceptance, Belonging, Finding Opportunity

All but two of the males in this study claimed to be members of "informal" gangs in their respective housing estates in their early teens. They state that they achieved both status and safety through "hanging around with the lads."

> Say if you go with a group of lads and there is a younger and an older generation and, after a while, the older generation start touching on (meaning grow out of delinquent behaviour) and then

you move up and then you are known. You have to be hard. Guys fight against each other and then guys from Ballinanty could come down to your house and go knocking on your door. Blow two holes in you.

It is also obvious that both the teachers at the project and parents were fearful of the pupils joining gangs.

Like our mothers and fathers, they are afraid in case we get into gangs that we shouldn't be getting into, like that do drugs. And in case we start fighting and basics like. Like everyone else's mother and father are afraid because they treat you like they're your daughters or they're your sons–that's the way they treat you, the staff do. They'd be afraid of the same things that your mother and father would be afraid of, like getting drunk, drugs, fighting, locked up.

Knowledge of How to Survive: Safety

Several of the interviewees spoke of the need to have specific knowledge of how to survive their own neighbourhoods and that other teenagers lacked this despite their access to formal schools. Siobhan felt that this was particularly around "looking for trouble from fellas." "I feel safe; you know what I mean because I know a lot of people and I'm more streetwise compared to the people that go to posh schools and stuff, "Cause they go out at night and they're all dressed up and they have mini skirts so far up. They're not as streetwise as us.' This perception of knowledge extends out to other areas also and this is where the project is credited by the ex-pupils.

At St. Augustine's, they learn you more about life; they learn you more about reality. Inside in St. Anne's or any posh schools, they wouldn't tell you, "You better watch out for yourself." St. Augustine's here do a reality test.

They say like there's drugs going around, you know. Here, now, they's streetwise kids. They mightn't be as smart as some streetwise kids or whatever, but they're as smart as they can get going around the roads and making sure that they have their life to live. You hear on the radio now that so and so got stabbed down in some street. Now those people aren't as streetwise as us. I mean we know how to look after ourselves. We know what places to go and what places not to go. But other people don't.

Taking Drugs–Belonging, Finding Opportunity

As mentioned earlier, drug taking was a regular part of life for many of the pupils and their peer groups but was considered to constitute "risky" behaviour. Jane admitted taking drugs and was philosophical about this. "I suppose, that happens all the time." This was despite the fact that the pupils knew this was risky behaviour. "Risky, take drugs like. Just like popping Es and As. Popping As and speeding and when you come down then you want more so you rob money for more, so drugs leads to robbing and everything, like, you know what I mean."

Drinking–Belonging, Finding Opportunity

The consumption of alcohol was a regular aspect of life for the interviewees and their families. When asked about risky activities, Joe answered, "…And the third would be drinking, alcohol." When Amanda was asked to name a risky activity, she named drinking. The average age of first taking alcohol amongst the interviewees was thirteen.

Safe Sex: Safety, Belonging, Finding Opportunity

The interviewees were concerned with the practice of safe sex, and two of the female interviewees did mention that they would use condoms, as not to do so was "risky." Nonetheless, Joe stated that in his experience in the project, the pupils were uneducated on such matters.

> … One reason is that if they had more schools, most schools there is no such thing as sex education, most of them are a few years ahead, you know, don't know the facts of life and then if you want the kids to learn the facts of life then they have a word to their mother and father and their mother and father speak to them, and I think that most parents won't do it, therefore most of them don't have a clue about contraception and the likes.

STDs: Safety

Drawing out the issue of safe sex in more detail, two of the female interviewees expressed concern with acquiring a sexually transmitted disease. They stated that their boyfriends may be having sexual intercourse indiscriminately without the use of "rubbers" (condoms) and they were unaware of how many partners each boyfriend may have. "He is not with me every day of the week like, he is off somewhere else. I hope I never catch anything. I never got one of them."

Smoking–Finding Opportunity

All of the interviewees were well aware of the detrimental effects of smoking. "Em, yeah, after all, eh, not to smoke, it's bad for you," but the majority of them claim they were smoking regularly. Again, the age of starting to smoke was young, with the average being between eleven and twelve years of age. Joe was the oldest of the interviewees to commence smoking and, once again, the role of peers was influential in this regard. "I got into joining a dart team and darts were a cheap game; I started then." This concern with smoking extended to family members. "If I found out they were smoking ..."

Medical/Health Issues

Medical and health issues featured in the interview data with several of the participants being hospitalised during their time in the project. In terms of risk behaviours, one of the females who had a young baby had refused to undertake a health scan and admitted, "I never got a scan, I got nothing."

Threat of Violence on the Roads: Safety

Despite the above quotes on avoiding conflict, the fact that some of the pupils become involved in fights is not always mere coincidence. One of the more disturbing aspects of hanging around the roads is the young ages of the children involved, as noted by Joe.

> Well if they don't, they will end up on the streets every day and up for a mugging. I have seen kids from between as young as two years of age up to twelve and all they are doing is on the streets, some of them actually cause damage to houses. If they were in this school then they wouldn't give any damage to it.

CATEGORIES A7 (PERSONAL RISK/INDIVIDUAL FACTORS) B7 (RISK TO FRIENDS AND PEERS) C3 (RISK IN FAMILY)

Significant Persons

The literature on risk and resiliency continually points to the role of significant persons in assisting children to overcome significant adversity. It is unsurprising, therefore, that the Director of the project, the school staff, and family members featured regularly in the interview data. Again, in terms of adopting a specific child and youth care perspective, we see that safety, self-acceptance, belonging, and finding opportunity all appear in this category.

Parenting, Child Rearing Practices and Risk

As noted in this study, the parental role is crucial in the psychosocial development of children. One American study indicated that working class mothers were more indulgent during infancy in comparison to their middle class counterparts. By the time the child had reached age five, the working class mothers were less openly demonstrative of affection, more rejecting, and more strict about sexual behaviour (Wolff, 1973). Siobhan noted with some humour that, "I'm nearly eighteen now, you'll laugh at this but it was only during the summer. You see, my mother and father are very protective of me and I'm not allowed to stay out."

Expressed Feelings Towards Family Members: Safety, Belonging

All of the research participants, with the exception of one, could be described as "extremely concerned" with the fate of their family members and showed strong attachments to them.[1] The depth of concern was most apparent in the answers given by the ex-pupils as the two fears were that a family member would get injured through a violent act or might die. "Something happening to one of my family," and "A bad beating happening to my family" or "My family getting hurt, or losing my child." Amanda said, "... I'd worry about the baby."

Joe was fearful that something bad could happen to his family by virtue of where they lived.

The worst thing, I think, is getting them something they can do or having people barred at the door. I remember once years ago, my

> Mother was sitting at home with my brother and there was a family living next door to me and both our house and their house were Corporation Houses, so this fella came up and he kicked in the back door and my brother ran out to him and the family next door.

He claims that he made a decision when he was in his early teens that he would endeavour not to cause his mother any trouble.

> Well first of all, my mother was a lone parent when my father died and I was the oldest in the family, so I had to help my mother look after my brother and two sisters. Basically, the only thing I did in school was cause trouble in the morning; I wouldn't go. She had it hard enough, when my father died she had a hard enough time, and I just turned around and she had a hard time and the last thing she needed was Guards calling, so, I was mostly thinking about my mother than anyone else.

Siobhan believed that her dreams could be predictive.

> I don't know but you wouldn't know what would happen in Limerick. I'm very protective of all my family and my friends. When I dreamt my grandfather had a heart attack, he had a heart attack two hours later and I was woke up. I'm afraid in case any of my dreams come true now because most of them do. When I dreamt my grandfather had a heart attack, my mother came running downstairs and she asked me what happened and I told her what happened and about an hour later my uncle knocked on the door and told my mother he had a heart attack. I'm afraid in case any bad things in my dreams come true.

The participants are protective of their family members even when they understand the potential repercussions. "Well, the only thing I do dangerously risky nowadays is if someone hit my family I would set out like, if some harm came to my family like, that would be something risky, because what I would do afterwards, I would lose it like and I would go up and do damage to them as well like, that would be something like, you know."

Yvonne suggested that "The only people I would help out is my family," because they were all close to each other. "Oh, we do yeah, yeah, we are all close" and Jane said, "My mother gives me anything and everything, anything I want that." Siobhan was keen to point out her relationships. "Yeah, you always have to look out for somebody. Like, I look out for my friend and I look out for my mother and father, brother and sister, you know what I mean if anything happens to them."

It was touching to see that the interviewees tried to help out their family members. "My mother, when she is upset, you know, we try our best." All of the interviewees, with the exception of Robert, stated that their parents had done the best they could for them and were doing enough. "The way they are, loving us and protecting us." Joe wanted to acknowledge the role of his mother.

> I just think my Mother, 'cause my Father died when I was eleven, so I was living with my Mother until he died and then my Mother brought us up that we could do better and we weren't clubbing or anything like that. She had a tough life, she was only thirty six, she brought us up as best she could and she couldn't have done a better job.

Robert does not agree and felt that his parents should have provided more financial support to him. "Give me money, like. They should never have slapped the fucking head off me for going up the roads. I was wild, though. A wild man." As is the case with many children, the majority continue to locate their homes of origin and return there even when they can provide for themselves. "I have my own house like and I stays at my mothers the whole time. My mother feeds me now."

Family Expectations for the Pupils: Finding Opportunity

It is clear from the research that the parents of the interviewees in this study are concerned with the immediate physical needs of their children but display a general sense of disregard for "deferred gratification." In fact, this seems to be absent in the majority of the home lives of the children with a limited number of exceptions. Joe recounted that his mother wanted him simply to be content with his life as it is. "Hopefully the way I am now. Hopefully that I will still be working and eh hopefully still be with my girlfriend and hopefully be happy."

The Role of Peers and Risk Avoidance/Risk Behaviours: Safety, Self-Acceptance, Belonging, Finding Opportunity

The majority of participants like to engage in risk behaviours with their peers present as distinct from on their own with Jane admitting,

"No, I wouldn't be able to do it myself, I wouldn't have the bottle like if you know what I mean." Involving peers in risk behaviours are engaged in for a number of reasons including wanting to share the risk with a peer, to act as a look-out during risk activity and to dissipate the blame if any of the participants get caught. The participants are divided when it comes to whether or not they would engage in assisting peers to avoid risks.

> I would never tell my friends not to do something like, because I just wouldn't do it myself. Cause to tell them not to do something they will say, "Ah, go away you shittyhole and this and that," so if they want to do something, just let them do it. You just don't do it, just leave them off. That is the way I look at it.

It is obvious that some of the participants are fearful of being rebuked and falling out of favour with their peers should they express a desire not to engage in risky activities. It is not just that the peers may not listen to advice. "If you walk away like and especially in a young fella you are the one that is shitty. All the boys stay away from you then and so you have to do them like and even though if someone else walked away, I would be calling them shitty as well like, so you know what I mean like, everyone was the same like."

Minimising Risk and Promoting Resiliency:
The Expressed Attitudes of the Pupils to the Teachers:
Safety, Self-Acceptance, Belonging, Finding Opportunity

All of the teachers were mentioned as being approachable by the interviewees and it was recognised that the teachers spent a considerable amount of one-on-one time with the pupils. "Yeah. It's great in here. They teach you, they're fun, they're not like other teachers, you can talk to them if you need to talk to them. I think they're ok the way they are." When asked about specifics of the project, Jane answered, "The same really. They should have Laura back as well. It was brilliant with her."

Attitudes of the Teachers to the Pupils: Safety, Finding Opportunity

The attitude held by teachers is crucial as the interviewees recognise that they can be trying on teacher's nerves. "I can't think of any. Because I'm hyper, I got up teachers' holes for screaming and shouting. The teachers would throw you in the corner for carrying on…." It is the teachers who reward the pupils. "When you are finished your work you can go and play a game a pool or something and the other schools you can't...."

The Director of the Project:
Safety, Self-Acceptance, Belonging, Finding Opportunity

The Director of the school was singled out time and time again in the interviews as a positive role model and was thought of as a father figure by some of the pupils.

> When I came to St. Augustine's first, even up to now, I think that John didn't know much about me. He is more like a father now and I was only telling him recently that when I was living here first, John didn't treat me any different. He treated me like, one of the family. If he had anything he would give it to me and he would explain things to me. If I needed any money or anything like that he would explain it to me, sit down and explain it. I thought John, he was like a fatherly figure to me, so I couldn't say a bad word about him.

Clearly, the research participants understood that there was method to the Director's particular style of delivery with Amanda recalling, "Well yeah, he made a difference, he kept me out of trouble like." When I enquired further how this was achieved she replied, "Nothing really, what he done was the way he talked to you like and that like, well I was only a young person back then like and would just really talk to me and really talk and have a buzz."

The Director's emphasis on nature was not lost on the children, despite the fact they lived in sprawling urban housing estates and rarely got the opportunity to travel to the seaside or forest parks without some form of charitable assistance. The Director of the school would use these opportunities to instruct and discuss with the children such issues as life, death, loss, and bereavement and the importance of respecting the environment. A simple example is the fact that the seaside huts were there for the children year after year and the Director used this to illustrate how vandalism can be annoying and hurtful to them all. The pupils were able to make sense of this in the context of stability and consistency. An example of the reaction of the pupils to the Director's style can be seen in the following quote.

> Even one day when we were going down to camp (in Cork) and we knocked down a rabbit. JH said "Did we knock down that rabbit?"

and he was so upset that he thought he had knocked down the rabbit. And he said "Amanda. Look into my eyes and tell me the honest truth if I knocked down that rabbit." Jesus, we were all totally knackered. "Did I knock down that rabbit?" So I said, "We didn't kill him." Even the year before we came across a dead bird on the way to camp and JH made us all stop and we had a proper funeral for it and everything. We even made a sign and buried it at the side of the road. A dead bird!

The disciplinary approach utilised by the Director of the school won him uniform respect with the children. Patrick spoke fondly of the Director and noted the crucial resiliency role he played for his development.

JH I would say, he made a difference to me anyway, he did anyway, because before I went into the school I was stone mad and pure running mad around the roads like and in the school I quietened down and well stayed out of prison and if I didn't join the school, I would have got prison like, I had to do something.

Perhaps most importantly, the Director was consistent and fair with all the pupils, having no specific "pet." Indeed, according to Joe (the ex-pupil with the longest involvement with the school) the Director raised his voice only once in over ten years. To accomplish this is the very essence of an effective child and youth care practitioner.

CATEGORIES A8 (PERSONAL RISK/INDIVIDUAL FACTORS) B8 (RISK TO FRIENDS AND PEERS) C5 (RISK IN FAMILY)

Sources of worry for the interviewees included many of the things that might concern a general population such as smoking, health issues, and injury to either themselves or their family members. However, one notices that their environments throw up other sources of potential risk such as hanging around the roads, being innocently caught up in a street fight, and their own deaths.

Death of a Parent

Along with the death of oneself, the interviewees were concerned with their families and, particularly, their parents. Justin admitted that, "I don't know, it all depends on what is making me frightened. Maybe feeling threatened with your life, but it never happened to me. If someone died in your family or close friends." Only two of the interviewees were somewhat indifferent concerning the potential death of a parent. "Any of them getting hurt or dying. Although, I'm in two minds about it. If they don't give a fuck about me, I say fuck 'em. They are your flesh and blood. They do like but they are just animals, they care about your money and that's it."

Injury to a Parent

Perhaps the first thing one notices when viewing this category is the random nature of potential injury to parents. "The worst thing I think is getting them something they can do or eh, having people barred at the door ... now basically I wouldn't like to see my family getting blamed for something they didn't do."

Death of a Sibling

Robert articulated the fear that one of his brothers could become involved in a random act of violence. "I'm afraid of a fella calling to me at four o'clock in the morning and ending up being shot in the head. That could happen to you or to your brother...."

Death to One's Own Child

As with the fear of death to oneself, this fear also extended to children. When asked what would Amanda be most concerned about, she replied, "Losing my child" as did Yvonne. "Em, lose my child, OK."

Injury to Sibling

Yvonne was equally concerned that a family member might get injured. "And my family getting hurt or me getting hurt."

Injury and/or Death of Oneself

As with many adolescents, the interviewees expressed fears around their own deaths. "I'd be afraid in case you die and stuff like that." Several of the interviewees expressed the concern that they could be injured in their environments. "Oh, of course I would, I would worry. That is like one fella was walking down the road and he got shot and you could be dead and who would know like, he would be in hospital for months and you are thinking to yourself what is going to happen, is he going to die or is he going to live or anything like that, do you get me." When Siobhan was asked what she would be worried about, she answered. "In case I got hurted or they got hurted or something bad happened to them." This translates itself into the ex-pupils having to be careful as to where they frequent. "Well, keep out of pubs. Coming from Moyross is bad luck. I'd worry about the baby. Lots of people.... I don't usually go out unless I have all my family with me. My aunts and uncles and cousins. In my circumstances, you have to be careful. I could get stabbed. If I fell that a person doesn't like me, then I don't talk to them and think that's their tough luck. But they might think that's cheeky." Justin also expressed fear at a potential beating. "If something had happened to the family or getting a beating, getting a bad beating."

CATEGORIES A9 (PERSONAL RISK/INDIVIDUAL FACTORS) C6 (RISK IN FAMILY)

Work

Formal work did not feature highly in the expressed worldview of the interviewees. Work was found by several of the interviewees through informal contacts. "I went out on the roads and down to Knockryan, down there and there Mike Ryan got me a job and I am working ever since then."[2] Work was generally understood as providing a route out of Limerick and as a means of improving one's life situation as opposed to something one might do as a matter of course. It was also considered the norm that one would not pay taxes to either local or central government and that cash was the most preferable form of payment.

Life Improvement: Finding Opportunity

Several of the interviewees saw formal employment as an opportunity to improve their lives. Money could assist in freedom of movement and in providing an avenue out of Limerick. Work was understood to be "a necessary evil" in some cases and the majority of the interviewees wanted to work only on a part-time basis if at all possible. Eamon admitted that there was significant room for improvement in his attitude towards work. "Em, work harder, work a lot harder like." This might be explained by a comment he made later in his interview as he felt that his labour was of a transient nature. "Well on and off, like we will say, I was working up in Dell and they leave you go, they always do like and...."

A Route Out of Limerick/Enables One to Travel: Finding Opportunity

Formal and informal work was seen by several interviewees as providing a route out of Limerick City. Brian had undertaken a work placement on the ship "the Asgard" and intended to return to the ship and sail over to America. Another one of the female interviewees wanted to run a rural pub in County Limerick. Justin acknowledged that he only wanted to seek part-time employment "Because it's a handy number" and he would not have to pay tax and work within the formal system.

CATEGORIES A10 (PERSONAL RISK/INDIVIDUAL FACTORS) C7 (RISK IN FAMILY)

Fortune, Misfortune, Luck and Risk

Luck was something that the research participants suggested was crucial to one's life chances. Most of the pupils were fatalistic about luck and felt that you either got bad luck or that you had to make your own luck. Amanda suggested that, "I never had any luck in my life. That's why I'm sitting here talking with you right now. You're are not in control of anything at all." Fred noted that, "You make your own luck. Brian did not care about fortune: "Not really, just see what happens," whereas Justin felt, instead, that one "Couldn't do much to give you luck."

Money was central to many of the observations around luck and fortune with the national lottery featuring highly as a potential source of good luck. Justin believed that he could win money and move "I could win the Lotto, have a good life or live by the sea." The majority of the ex-pupils could recount examples of family members who had experienced bad luck.

> I'll give you my girlfriend's Mother, when she was younger she had two brothers, two sisters, a Mother, Father and herself and her two brothers and her two sisters died before they reached the age of thirty five, her two brothers died in one week, one of them died from TB, the other person died from a broken heart over the brother. They were so close, the two sisters died in, her whole family, her

two brothers, her two sisters and her Mother and Father were all dead within nine years of one another.

Self-Reported Career Paths of the Pupils

None of the research participants indicated that they would like to go on to study for a Diploma or Degree programme at any third level college, such as an Institute of Technology or University. All classified their preferred option as informal work where they would not have to pay tax or meet with government agencies. Fred admitted that he had no idea what he wanted to do in the future. "Oh, I don't know, probably the same thing I am doing now, sitting down doing nothing." The aspirations for career paths included becoming a child care worker, a mechanic and a shop girl. Those working at the time of the final interviews included a bar man, a security guard, three factory operatives and a sailor. In short, the self-reported expectations of the ex-pupils lacked direction.

A Positive or Negative Outlook

Some of the interviewees held a positive outlook. Shane stated, "Well, I am happy where I am, I am where I love, so hopefully I am going to stay there." Aspects of bad luck that had been experienced by the interviewees or their families featured significantly. When one of the female interviewees was asked how she could change things, Jane answered, "Forget all the past. Forget all the past." Nonetheless, Jane could also be philosophical. "Sure, no bad luck is good luck like." On the other hand, Fred felt completely fatalistic. "Nothing goes right for me though, nothing, I will tell you something though, this week now, this week now is gone alright for me, do you get me, but any other week like is all bad for me, there is nothing to do, do you get me."

CATEGORIES A11 (PERSONAL RISK/INDIVIDUAL FACTORS) B9 (RISK TO FRIENDS AND PEERS) C10 (RISK IN FAMILY)

Expressed Feelings About Social Responsibility

The area of civic responsibility is an interesting one and has been discussed in the context of promoting resiliency. This is something that the project has attempted to instil in all of the pupils and is mentioned extensively in the literature on resiliency. The majority of the ex-pupils accepted that they would be prepared to assist people in trouble, normally associated with immediate or imminent physical risk such as drowning or lying in the middle of the road. However, the will to assist was a qualified one with some interviewees commenting that they would not overly exert themselves. Reasons for this included such answers as people might not like to be offered help, to people were generally ungrateful for help given to them to the interviewees had experienced very negative reactions to offers of help in the past.

Three of the ex-pupils articulated a sense of definite civic responsibility. Justin noted that "If I thought Pat was doing something bad, I'd tell him." He extended this to a peer that might have a drug problem. "Do everything for them actually. Get them all the right help, like, if a pupil was on drugs he could get help." Joe felt that he would help most people, particularly if they were about to do something risky. "The first thing I would do is I would go over and I would give him a good nudge and I would ask him 'think before you do it,' he could go ahead and do it, but he would be warned."

Attitudes to Vulnerable Persons

All of the female interviewees stated they had been in positions where they had to mind another vulnerable person. One of the girls had to mind her mother who "was depressed" and another reported she "had to mind my nephew." One of the male interviewees had been involved minding a child who was physically and mentally handicapped for several years. "Em, about fifteen years ago, I was working with disabled kids and the family was living in Carlow, their young fella at the time was fourteen and the father was in Dublin, so he asked me for help and I said no problem, because he couldn't look after himself and told the company he couldn't walk, so every morning we used to go out there and get him out of bed and dress him, wash him, bring him to the toilet and then later on that evening we would put him to bed and I did that for four years."

However, the majority of the interviewees had not been in a position where they had to consciously mind another vulnerable person. Eamon admitted that he would not intervene in another person's problem, particularly around drug use. "I don't know. If someone was taking drugs, I wouldn't help them if it was my own family, if you know what I mean." On the other hand, Brian stated that he would intervene if he felt the situation warranted it. "You could help someone." Justin had actually intervened to save a young boy from drowning. "Yeah, I had to look after a kid or two when they got caught swimming and nearly drowned."

CATEGORIES A12 (PERSONAL RISK/INDIVIDUAL FACTORS) B10 (RISK TO FRIENDS AND PEERS) C8 (RISK IN FAMILY)

Sense of Local Identity: Belonging

All of the participants had a very strong sense of local identity both to their geographical areas of origin and to the project. This is not to say that the interviewees felt that their peers would necessarily show solidarity with them, as noted by Jane. "No. In Southill they don't want anything at all to do with it, other than to rob a fella." Fred strengthened his sense of local identity when he was on a visit to Dublin.

> When I was up in Dublin like, this homo said to me, "Limerick, stab city. What is that like, stab city, like?" I never heard that in my life, do you get me, what do you call it, what was the place you said a while ago, out to Raheen and all that, they say Limerick, they are all messers. You start rowing and all that, do you get me? You know the city has a bad name anyway, no matter what happens in here like, it is going to have the same name forever.

It was also the case that some of the interviewees expressed a desire to move out of their areas of origin. "Move out of Southill."

Being Minoritised: Belonging, Finding Opportunity

The research participants were very clear that they felt the same social and personal difficulties took place outside their areas. "My family have done enough for me. We are normal people. We are just in a situation. You're writing books, but it doesn't really benefit us. JH might get an extra teacher from you writing these books. He needs money and they have cut down on money again. In general it is different from other schools." Some of the interviewees felt that the media continually gave their areas "bad press." On the other hand, the research participants realised that children from all areas could experience adversity: "... Some families like that, their mothers and fathers are on drugs, they're 'druggies.' You've mothers and fathers who are alcoholics, then you've some children that are being starved or abused, you've got a lot of cases. So, I think no, that children from other areas have as good as chance as us." Amanda felt that the situation was grossly unfair.

> Of course, but they don't come under the same control as us in Moyross. If there is a fight in Craigavon, we get blamed. That's not fair. It has a posh name. Maybe there are a few Gardai living there. Just because there's Gardai there they think it's posh, but there are people getting stabbed there too. Look at Raheen. They come to Moyross and cause trouble. Everyone blames people from Moyross and Southill. The Gardai put more pressure on us and they don't know us from Adam.

Lack of Social Mobility: Finding Opportunity

All of the interviewees felt that they were restricted by their homes of origin and addresses. "You wouldn't be out looking for a job because there aren't any. It's mad. After a while you see that you just can't get out of it." Another interviewee mentioned his family and old job in a negative context. "I was working in this dive of a chipper and I knew I could do better, you know and I knew I wasn't going to do it at home because there were other issues at home that I couldn't concentrate on getting a proper job and getting, so I had no choice but to move and I thought that myself."

Family Identity:
Safety, Self-Acceptance, Belonging, Finding Opportunity

The interviewees had mixed feelings around their family identities. One of the female interviewees was keen to move back in with her mother in an effort to rid herself of an unwelcome male partner who was also the father of her child. "It is not completely gone, I am going to get a flat in Town, it is the only way I will get rid of him, because two of us have places up in Dublin and I owned a house, but if I throw him out he will move into my Mother's." Despite this will to move in with the mother, Jane was unsure of her sense of loyalty to the rest of her family: "Any of them getting hurt or dying. Although, I'm in two minds about it. If they don't give a fuck about me, I say fuck 'em. They are your flesh and blood. They do like but they are just animals, they care about your money and that's it."

Eamon noted that he would always look out for his family and friends. "My family, anyone standing looking out for each other, mates looking out for each other, I wouldn't wear that now, you have to look out for each other like. It is a rough ould neighbourhood now I mean, so some gangs start coming up like and we stick by each other, they stick by each other like, we look out for each other." On the other hand, Fred felt that his family were not of any particular use to him and that he could get by if he only had more money as opposed to emotional support. "Eh, I will tell you one or two people now, but na, I wouldn't say so, there are a lot of snakes in this world, do you get me. Your only friend is in your pocket, I think."

Intended Destinations After Leaving the Project: Finding Opportunity

Eamon was one of the few interviewees who expressed any particular desire to move outside Limerick City for a time and explore other places. He wanted to do "Three things. Go abroad, travel, see a bit of the world anyway for one thing, can't think of nothing else, see a bit of the world really." Fred felt that he might move away for a while but would return. "I don't know, probably won't be living here, maybe in England or something." Finally, John stated that he would like to "Move to America." None of the female interviewees wanted to move far outside Limerick. Post project, three of the girls are in receipt of social welfare with a fourth attending a part-time child-care course.

Being Equal to Others: Self-Acceptance

Despite the fact that many of the participants felt excluded, a few did state that they were no different from other teenagers, but that they lacked the same chances in life. Shane was aware how much being given a chance means to the ex-pupils of the project.

> Em, if they get a break, if people can understand where they are coming from rather than judging them from the second they meet them. Like, I know some people that would judge, would look at someone and say he is a right brazen whatever and judge that person and they know nothing about that person's circumstances or background or where that child is coming from or where and they don't know and they kind of judge. If people just kind of stand back and say hang on for a second and try find out. Like most of

the lads I know, even in here, like if you sit down, I have often sat down and had a conversation with one or two of the lads and they tell you things and then you can see why they are so aggressive and why they are so tired, because they will open up to you. Anyone will if you talk to them.

CATEGORIES A13 (PERSONAL RISK/INDIVIDUAL FACTORS) B11 (RISK TO FRIENDS AND PEERS) C9 (RISK IN FAMILY)

Perceptions of the Gardai: Belonging

The general perception of the Gardai is that some of them actively seek out children and young people from disadvantaged areas and insult them. "Sure, you have, sure you have to be, cause, you know, you can't really, they are powerful like. Guards are powerful, if you go out against a Guard like that, you are probably away for a long time, as I say like, if a Guard hit you and you can't say to a Judge, Oh, he hit me first and all that like and if he turns around, if the Guard turns around and says Oh, he hit me first like, do you want to go up against the guards, like, do you get me." This point was supported by a comment from Shane who suggested that someone from his estate was bound to have a fraught relationship with the Gardai, "Because when you are brought up where we live and when you see like, do you know, you see constantly people getting arrested and getting dragged to the ground and it is just not where I live, it is Limerick in general like. You see things like that happen and I just didn't ever wanted, I just couldn't handle anyone doing that to me, being arrested, I would probably die."

It was felt that the Gardai's role was to act in an authoritarian manner. Fred explained one particular incident he witnessed. "Ah, there are one or two cheeky guards now, like I was walking there last night and I was with my friend like, my friend and he gave him three knees into the face."

Expressed Attitudes to the Gardai: Belonging

The Gardai were a source of some displeasure for the interviewees, and none of the participants articulated many positive comments about either the work undertaken by the Gardai as a collective body or their relationship with the project as individuals. This is surprising to an extent, as the project has long established contacts with some members of the Gardai. Amanda volunteered an explanation.

Of course, but they don't come under the same control as us in Moyross. If there is a fight in Craigavon, we get blamed. That's not fair. It has a posh name. Maybe there are a few Gardai living there. Just because there's Gardai there they think its posh, but there are people getting stabbed there too. Look at Raheen. They come to Moyross and cause trouble. Everyone blames people from Moyross and Southill. The Gardai put more pressure on us and they don't know us from Adam.

CONCLUSION

This chapter has provided the reader with some of the interview transcripts to illustrate perceptions of risk and at risk as articulated by the young people themselves. I have deliberately quoted from Robert at length as he represents a youth who was always considered to be at 'high risk.' The data shows that the youth do consider risk in a variety of forms.

NOTES

1. Robert was resentful towards his family and felt that he had learnt little of any value from them.
2. Knockryan is a fictional name.

REFERENCES

Garfat, T. (2005, June). Reflective child and youth care practice. *CYC-Online, 77*, [available cyc.net].

Garfat, T., & McElwee, N. (2004). *Effective interventions with families.* Cape Town: Pretext.

Krueger, M. (1994). Framing child and youth care in moments of rhythm, presence, meaning, and atmosphere. *Child and Youth Care Forum, 23*(4), 223-229.

McElwee, N., & Monaghan, G. (2005). *Darkness on the edge of town.* Athlone: Centre for Child and Youth Care Learning.

Rutter, M. (1987). Psychosocial resilience and protective mechanisms. *American Journal of Orthopsychiatry, 57*, 316-331.

Schon, D. A. (1983). *How professionals think in action.* New York: Basic Books.

Schon, D. (1996). *Organizational learning II: Theory, method and practice.* Reading, Mass: Addison Wesley.

Stokes, D. (2004). *Submission to the youth justice agency.* Dublin: Youthreach.

doi:10.1300/J024v29n01_08

APPENDIX. Interview Transcript Codes

A Personal Risk/Individual Factors	B Risk to Friends and Peers	C Risk in Family
1 School–Safety, Self-Acceptance, Belonging, Finding Opportunity I. Primary role is diversion II. Source of peer support III. Temporarily removes children from at-risk environment IV. Sometimes acts to maintain outcast status V. Entry to the project VI. Relationship with project VII. Length of time on project VIII. Summer camp IX. Truancy	**1 School–Safety, Self-Acceptance, Belonging, Finding Opportunity** I. Primary role is diversion II. Source of peer support III. Temporarily removes children from at-risk environment IV. Sometimes acts to maintain outcast status V. Entry to the project VI. Relationship with project VII. Length of time on project VIII. Summer camp	**1 Crime–Belonging, Finding Opportunity** I. Opportunistic II. Learned familial behaviour III. Proceeds not particularly important IV. Risk acceptance V. Innocent involvement in crime
2 Childhood–Finding Opportunity I. A time to do mad things II. A time when criminal behaviour is excused	**2 Childhood–Finding Opportunity** I. A time to do mad things II. A time when criminal behaviour is excused	**2 Having a Child–Belonging, Finding Opportunity** I. Provides an individual with status II. Insignificance of a child III. Grounds an individual IV. Irresponsibility around the father role
3 Crime–Belonging, Finding Opportunity I. Opportunistic II. Learned familial behaviour III. Risk acceptance	**3 Crime–Belonging, Finding Opportunity** I. Opportunistic II. Learned familial behaviour III. Proceeds not particularly important IV. Risk acceptance V. Innocent involvement in crime	**3 Issues of Consequence–Safety, Belonging, Finding Opportunity** I. Death II. Prison III. Becoming addicted to drugs IV. Fatherhood V. Motherhood VI. Being isolated from one's peers VII. Behavioural disapproval

<table>
<tr>
<td>

4 Having a Child–Belonging, Finding Opportunity
- I. Provides an individual with status
- II. Insignificance of a child
- III. Grounds an individual
- IV. Irresponsibility around the father role

5 Issues of Consequence–Safety, Belonging, Finding Opportunity
- I. Death
- II. Prison
- III. Becoming addicted to drugs
- IV. Fatherhood
- V. Motherhood
- VI. Being isolated from one's peers
- VII. Behavioural disapproval
- VIII. Concerns regarding consequence

6 Risk Avoidance/Risk Acceptance–Safety, Self-Acceptance, Belonging, Opportunity
- I. Fighting
- II. Weapons
- III. Robbing
- IV. Using needles to inject drugs
- V. Unsafe locations
- VI. Facing fears
- VII. Avoiding conflict
- VIII. Personal safety
- IX. Gangs
- X. Knowledge
- XI. Taking drugs
- XII. Drinking
- XIII. Safe sex
- XIV. STD
- XV. Smoking
- XVI. Medical/Health issues
- XVII. Threat of violence on the roads
- XVIII. The Buzz

</td>
<td>

4 Having a Child–Belonging, Finding Opportunity
- I. Provides an individual with status
- II. Affirms male status
- III. Grounds an individual
- IV. Responsibility stops at giving money

5 Issues of Consequence–Safety, Belonging, Finding Opportunity
- I. Death
- II. Prison
- III. Becoming addicted to drugs
- IV. Fatherhood
- V. Motherhood
- VI. Being isolated from one's peers
- VII. Behavioural disapproval
- VIII. Parental punishment

6 Risk Avoidance/Risk Acceptance– Safety, Self-Acceptance, Belonging, Opportunity
- I. Fighting
- II. Weapons
- III. Robbing
- IV. Using needles to inject drugs
- V. Not including peers
- VI. Drinking
- VII. Taking drugs
- VIII. The Buzz

</td>
<td>

4 Significant Persons–Safety, Self-Acceptance, Belonging, Finding Opportunity
- I. Parents
- II. Siblings
- III. Peers
- IV. Director of Project
- V. Teachers in Project

5 Sources of Concern–Safety
- I. Death of a parent
- II. Injury to parent
- III. Death of sibling
- IV. Injury to sibling
- V. Death to oneself
- VI. Injury to oneself
- VII. Death of a grandparent
- VIII. Death of one's own child
- IX. Injury to one's own child

6 Work–Finding Opportunity
- I. Life improvement
- II. Money to buy freedom
- III. An avenue out of Limerick
- IV. Enables one to travel

</td>
</tr>
</table>

245

A Personal Risk/Individual Factors	B Risk to Friends and Peers	C Risk in Family
7 Significant Persons—Safety, Self-Acceptance, Belonging, Finding Opportunity I. Parents II. Siblings III. Peers IV. Director of Project V. Teachers in Project	**7 Significant Persons—Safety, Self-Acceptance, Belonging, Finding Opportunity** I. Parents II. Siblings III. Peers IV. Director of Project V. Teachers in Project	**7 Fatalism—Self-Acceptance, Finding Opportunity** I. Expressed attitudes to life chances II. A positive or negative outlook
8 Sources of Concern—Safety I. Death of a parent II. Injury to parent III. Death of sibling IV. Injury to sibling V. Injury and/or death to oneself	**8 Sources of Concern** I. Death of a parent II. Injury to parent III. Death of sibling IV. Injury to sibling V. Death to oneself VI. Injury to oneself VII. Injury to peers	**8 Identity—Belonging, Finding Opportunity** I. Sense of local identity II. A sense of being minoritised III. A perceived lack of social mobility IV. Family identity V. Intended destination
9 Work—Finding Opportunity I. Life improvement II. Money to buy freedom III. An avenue out of Limerick IV. Enables one to travel	**9 Civic Responsibility** I. Attitudes to society II. Attitudes to vulnerable persons	**9 Gardai—Safety** I. Perceptions of Gardai II. Expressed attitudes to Gardai
10 Fatalism—Self-Acceptance, Finding Opportunity I. Expressed attitudes to life chances II. A positive or negative outlook	**10 Identity—Belonging, Finding Opportunity** I. Sense of local identity II. A sense of being minoritised III. A perceived lack of social mobility IV. Family identity V. Intended destination	**10 Civic Responsibility** I. Attitudes to family members

11 Civic Responsibility I. Attitudes to society II. Attitudes to vulnerable persons	**11 Gardai–Safety** I. Perceptions of Gardai II. Expressed attitudes to Gardai	
12 Identity–Belonging, Finding Opportunity I. Sense of local identity II. A sense of being minoritised III. A perceived lack of social mobility IV. Family identity V. Intended destination VI. Being equal to others		
13 Gardai–Safety I. Perceptions of Gardai II. Expressed attitudes to Gardai		

Chapter 9

Framing the Future for Children and Youth in the Risk Society

SUMMARY. This chapter sets out to explore the six significant findings of this study by relating the interview content to the sociological risk literature. It examines thinking behind loss zones and gain zones and then moves on to look at individual versus collective risk and perceptions of risk. A child and youth care understanding is noted within the context of the Youth Encounter Project environments. doi:10.1300/J024 v29n01_09 *[Article copies available for a fee from The Haworth Document Delivery Service: 1-800-HAWORTH. E-mail address: <docdelivery@haworthpress. com> Website: <http://www.HaworthPress.com> © 2007 by The Haworth Press, Inc. All rights reserved.]*

KEYWORDS. Zones of loss and gain, engagement with youth, Youth Encounter Projects, risk and resiliency, at-risk youth

Zuckerman (1979) suggests that adolescents have "a need for varied, novel, and complex sensations and experiences and the willingness to take physical and social risks for the sake of such experiences" (p.10), and the Carnegie Council on Adolescent Development (1995) has identified adolescence as a particularly risky period for a range of behaviours.

[Haworth co-indexing entry note]: "Framing the Future for Children and Youth in the Risk Society." McElwee, Niall. Co-published simultaneously in *Child & Youth Services* (The Haworth Press, Inc.) Vol. 29, No. 1/2, 2007, pp. 249-268; and: *At-Risk Children & Youth: Resiliency Explored* (Niall McElwee) The Haworth Press, Inc., 2007, pp. 249-268. Single or multiple copies of this article are available for a fee from The Haworth Document Delivery Service [1-800-HAWORTH, 9:00 a.m. - 5:00 p.m. (EST). E-mail address: docdelivery@haworthpress.com].

Available online at http://cys.haworthpress.com
doi:10.1300/J024v29n01_09

Does this piece of research confirm or disconfirm the international literature? Past areas of research have tended to concentrate on eight categories of risk profiles with varying emphasis in different systems.[1] Perhaps a central difficulty now for policy makers is the conflicting research and what this means for implementing change. Arnett (1992), for example, argues that adolescence is characterised by "sensation seeking," but Lightfoot (1994) rejected Arnett's thesis. She suggested instead that adolescents tended to rationalise their risk taking. The latter was also the case in this study, where we saw the interviewees actively navigating risky behaviours such as not getting involved in potentially serious physical fights with peers that might involve the use of knives and baseball bats, not using needles to inject drugs, not walking around what interviewees felt were unsafe locations, and, generally using their "street knowledge" in avoiding situations or people that might pose a threat to them. Thus to simply state that the youth have no regard for their risk-taking behaviours is inaccurate and misleading. One also has to acknowledge that aspects of youth behaviour have changed over the years and what was deviant just a decade ago is not the case now.

A number of commentators argue that risk is not always a bad thing. Norman (1988) suggests that risk is not, as it is often taken to be, an evil in itself, and Wynne-Harley (1991) observes that an overly cautious life style can bring its own hazards. The children and young people examined in this study have been termed high-risk in government literature and may be said to invoke symbolic meanings of otherness. It has been suggested that this high-risk tag frequently denotes moral failure, weakness, and a lack of control over the self that detracts from a resiliency approach to understanding risk behaviour and client groups (Lupton, 1995). Such high-risk children are regularly depicted in both the Irish and UK media at ends of a continuum, a point noted by Hendrick (1994), who sees children occupying three distinct roles in modern social policy formulation including threat, victim, and investment.

The interviewees equated most with threat and then with victim. They did not see much investment in their future from external sources with the exception of the Youth Encounter Project,[2] and this should not be seen as unusual given their life and familial circumstances.

GIDDENS' ENGAGEMENT

Giddens' theory of engagement (1990) could be re-worked in an analysis of the interviewees' responses to risk society from the point of view of "pragmatic acceptance," "cynical pessimism," and "radical engagement." The interviewees reflect a combination of familial, geographical, peer, educative, and personal vulnerability in their lives. They are disadvantaged at every level, and psychological protective barriers, at point of contact with the project, are notably absent. The typical coping mechanisms for the interviewees in this study, at least prior to their involvement with the project, is one where rebellion and dropping out were seen as viable options to a consumerist and external system considered to be largely unattainable to them in the first instance. Indeed, this was actively supported by peers.

Pragmatic Acceptance/Participation

Giddens (1990) claims that some people repress feelings of angst and anger and concentrate, instead, on surviving in risk society by becoming numb. The focus for an individual remains on day-to-day tasks and problems (p. 135) and, in street parlance, this is commonly known as "ducking and skiving, dipping and diving." It has connotations of living in the black economy, psychologically and economically marginalised from the wider law-abiding world. Giddens claims that this may reflect "… deep, underlying anxieties, which in some individuals repeatedly surface at a conscious level" (p. 135). Paradoxically, *pragmatic acceptance* can result in either a sense of pessimism or it can nourish hope.

We see this in the interview data particularly in relation to the views expressed in sections around Personal Risk Factors/Individual Factors and Fatalism and Risk in Family and Fatalism where there is a curious sense of fatalism expressed. I have already alluded in this chapter to a culture of hope, which exists both in the project and amongst the staff and acts as a buffer to at least some of the personal characteristics identified by Giddens.

Cynical Pessimism

Giddens (1990) observes that, in some cases, *cynical pessimism* may manifest itself in "a kind of desperate hopelessness" (p. 136). He further notes a "direct involvement with the anxieties provoked by high consequence dangers" (p. 136). This may be seen in some of the activities the interviewees participated in, despite the fact that they were keenly aware that such activities were dangerous or risky. The youth may have been unconsciously dampening the emotional impact of anxieties by directly engaging with them, i.e., confronting their fears.

Radical Engagement

Giddens further claims that some people use protests and demonstrations as effective models of drawing attention to unacceptable and indefensible events or situations. The pupils of the school are well aware of their poor social status and claim that they sometimes react to this by deliberately behaving in ways that they feel "posh people expect us to behave." For example, they may protest their poverty by stealing motorcycles and cars because they know the likelihood is that they may never own such vehicles themselves. In Giddens' terms, they illuminate established constellations of power by attempting to "show them up for the community" as being "no-hopers in trying to solve anything–they say we are supposed to be no hopers." This prolonged and sustained action based critique of social power and controlling mechanisms is intended to effect social change.

MARY DOUGLAS AND RISK

I have referred to her work in an earlier chapter, and this study ultimately supports the work of the anthropologist, Mary Douglas (1992), who makes the point that what most people mean by risk in technologically advanced societies has little to do with probability calculations but much more to do with concepts of danger, avoidance, and prevention. Douglas argues that risk has emerged as a key idea for modern times because of its many uses as a forensic resource and because it "is invoked for a modern-style riposte against abuse of power" (p. 3). In short, high risk means a lot of danger. Certainly, the youth feel that they are surrounded by danger (albeit, a significant amount of this danger is self-created) as seen in their comments that simply leaving their houses could put them at risk. In fact, for some of the youth in this study, it is entirely reasonable to argue that their choices were very limited for there was danger both at home in terms of family violence and alcohol misuse by parents and danger on the streets right outside their homes.

Risk perceptions are explained functionally in terms of the contribution that those perceptions have for maintaining a particular way of life (Pratkanis, Breckler, & Greenwald, 1989). Douglas (1980) argues that the more we know about risk, the more we will come to realise that all our physical, moral, and social worlds are interdependent. We must look to all worlds to understand risk in a total context. She suggests that all of our social weapons of control emerge from the way in which we mentally construct our physical environment. She places great emphasis on the shared artefact of human life and on moral development and responsibility in the risk society. As we saw from the analysis of the interview data in this study, the participants have varying levels of social conscience. The youth stated they would not help someone in need. All cited the belief that their help would not be appreciated in the first instance and this influenced their decision not to intervene. Of course, this has much to do with their experiences of life in Limerick City where they have a strong sense of having to continually create their own opportunities due to public indifference displayed towards them.

Douglas and Calvez (1990) reassert that anthropology (rather than psychology) has the answers illuminating how the community "forces sharp and clear ideas about the self upon its members" (Douglas & Calvez, 1990, p. 445). Their explanation of risk-taking draws from a "centre and peripheral communities" thesis. The authors make an important point for this study that risk rejection or acceptance is a matter of *individual preference* even when confronted with a damning knowledge base from the "centre culture" (emphasis mine). It is worth noting that many at risk individuals choose to ignore the risks of their behavioural patterns because they cannot perceive the threat of risk or tragedy in a *personalised* context. When the centre culture fails (because it is not homogeneous itself) to alter the behaviour of the people it is directing its received attention towards, the authors liken this to "colonial misperception of native superstition" (1990, p. 455). The mood toward the centre culture is one of hostility and mistrust.

It is obvious from this study that some people from disadvantaged backgrounds will probably experience more risk in their daily lives than others, but risk is also opportunity (a point developed by Giddens). Douglas and Wildavsky (1983) cite the work of Oscar Lewis (1966), who maintained that the condition of poverty foreshortens the future. Comparison of risk perception should allow for social influences on perceptions of time (p. 85). In their concluding chapter they develop the concept of risk in different directions: If some degree of risk is inevitable, suppressing it in one place often merely moves it to another. "Shifting risks may be more dangerous than tolerating them, both because those who face new risks may be unaccustomed to them and because those who no longer face old ones may become more vulnerable when conditions change … If the selection of risk is a matter of social organisation, the management of risk is an organisational problem …" (p. 197).

Dake (1992) suggests that the work of Douglas and her colleagues can be located in plural social constructions of meanings. "Competing cultures confer different meanings on situations, events, objects, and especially relationships" (p. 27). Douglas and Wildavsky's thesis is not uniformly accepted. Dowie (1984), for example, notes the assumption that a "cultural fixes" explanation is naive in itself and actual ways of *thinking* are important. He acknowledges how little the experts know about anything and postulates that this may be the first step in radicalising the risk debate.

A Link Is Established

Two of the linking themes of interest to my own study between Giddens, Beck, and Douglas are (a) the desire for certainty in the face of uncertainty, and (b) connections between late modernity's "globalisation of doubt" (Beck, 1992, p. 21). As with Bates' (1996) study of Irish Open Centres for young offenders and the more recent Task Force Report on Discipline (2006), the poor school academic performance common to the interviewees in this study may be attributed largely to sociocultural, maladaptive patterns of family interaction and/or individual psychological factors. Such pupils, demotivated by formal academic underachievement, are unlikely to relate their formal school subjects to their later lives, if they can visualise their future lives at all, as noted by Lewis (1966). Lynch (1999) argues that "the distributive model of justice for the promotion of equality in education is necessary, but not sufficient" (p. 252). She acknowledges that the education system itself may require change so that it may accept and promote the differences between pupils.

A Preoccupation with Physical/Immediate Risk

There are three questions that need to be addressed in discussing the significance of the results of this analysis in relation to the perception of risk and how this is lived out in the context of Limerick City Corporation housing estates, the school environment, the after-school programmes and the summer programmes, and how policy might be changed. The first question is, "What factors act positively to promote the Youth Encounter Project as a source of resiliency to the pupils?" The second question is, "What are the shared factors that act to discourage participation in the Youth Encounter Project? Finally, what does the analysis inform us about risk and resiliency?

Beck (1992, p. 44) argues that the driving force in a class society is, "I am hungry," and the collective disposition of the risk society could best be summarised as "I am afraid." How afraid of external risks are the research participants in this study and what are the implications of this for policy? Do the interviewees feel part of a global collective consciousness where various ecological catastrophes await them like circling vultures, as suggested by social scientists, and what should be done to assist vulnerable young people? A key finding of my own study is that Beck's (1992) expressed social preoccupation with the failure of technology means almost nothing to the interviewees. Most end-of-century risks (as seen in Limerick City) are neither "cataclysmic" nor "democratised" as Beck suggested, nor do they appear organised around the gap in scientific expertise between theory and decision-making.[3]

A second significant finding is that the interviewees have little sense of risk *external* to their lives in Limerick. Only one of them mentioned such global risk hazards as nuclear war, toxic dumping, or environmental meltdown as a potential source of concern (Beck, 1992), and this was only after prompting. For the majority of the interviewees, life begins and ends around Limerick City and County—with the familiar.

A third significant finding is the apparent understanding participants hold of risk which is immediate, real, physical and is clearly seen in a negative, injurious, or fatalistic context. The interviewees were much more concerned with risk as it threatened their (immediate) physical activities, i.e. "falling out of trees," "falling off buildings," "getting caught by the Gardai" if they had stolen a car, "being crushed in a stolen car," "getting knocked down by lorries," or "being hurt in a street fight" as noted in the interview data.

A fourth significant finding is that participants feel that they have fewer sources of information than their peers living both inside and outside their environs. This sense of isolation tends to pervade their answers and takes away from a potential culture of hope. Although there are social services and community development projects based in and around the housing estates where the interviewees reside, many of these are not seen to work as well as they might. Policy could reorient these services to adopt a more democratic negotiating process around opening times, selection of staff, and the like.

A fifth significant finding is that the majority of the participants associated risk with *danger* and rarely equated risk with *opportunity* (Douglas, 1992). This was apparent with answers to the question, "Tell me a safe thing to do during the day and a dangerous thing to do during the day." All of the interviewees either answered with responses such as "Staying at home watching television was a safe thing to do," because they would not be out on the streets during this time, or that "Going out onto the streets could be dangerous."

This brings me to the sixth significant finding of this research, and that is the majority of the interviewees believed that they have significant responsibility for certain kinds of risk (lifestyle, intimate); but they also tend to nominate and blame others for broader risks like economic risk and even crime. This invites two questions: Who do the interviewees see as causing or having (some) responsibility over risk? Which of these risks do they perceive themselves as having personal control over and which not?

Zones of Gains versus Zones of Loss

I was particularly struck by two of the interviewees, but for very different reasons. One, Siobhan, up to age 19 had managed to stay out of trouble, stay in school, and not yet have a child on her own (which was the norm for many of her peers). Siobhan could be considered resilient. On the other hand, Robert had graduated from four residential placements, including the maximum-security unit in Ireland for young offenders, and was in an adult jail by the age of seventeen. How might one explain such diverse outcomes? It seems that Siobhan had two factors in particular that marked her out from her less fortunate peers. Her family was supportive to her staying in the project and valued education and she wanted to stay in school herself. Thus, she had two of the key resiliency factors present in her environment.

Robert is a good example of an individual attempting to make sense of living and operating in Beck's risk society (1992). One could reasonably argue that he adopts risk behaviours because he understands life in Limerick more as what is described in the risk literature as "a zone of loss rather than a zone of gain" (Strachan & Tallant, 1997). Robert claims that he takes risks, not because he necessarily feels that there will be a potentially positive outcome, but because he feels that he has little choice and has been forced into the risk situation. Robert is likely to have a range of possible outcomes when he takes a risk as identified by Lopes (1997) as "real world risks ... hardly ever have just two outcomes. More often, they range continuously over the outcome variable" (p. 690). Robert understands that taking risky decisions has a number of possible consequences but, strangely, taking serious risks can actually provide a greater sense of security for the future than not taking risks at all, as he might come away with a profit. Thus, to rob a petrol station with a shotgun is physically risky (the gun could go off accidentally, the store owner or police could shoot him in retaliation) but the experience of Robert's friends is that store owners are unlikely to confront an armed robber as both the finances and the stock are insured and the police are trained to evaluate such situations before shooting. The potential outcome is controlled to some degree based on him actively weighing up the situation to a degree.[4]

Such a conclusion is also drawn in Lewis' (1961) earlier research on poor barrios of Latin American cities. Many commentators have suggested that in areas of significant poverty, a particular subculture emerges which tends to erode personal ambition and achievement. A result of this may well be that people tend to live for the moment and deferred gratification is largely rejected.

Individual versus Collective Risk Behaviour: Peer Influence

There is a considerable difference between those who take risks and those who are victimised by risks others take (Beck, 1997). The challenge then, for the risk society and our policy makers, is to create political regimes capable of meeting and absorbing public fears and disquiet over increasingly complex risk discourses in the context of ethical, political, and economic undercurrents (Kasperson & Kasperson, 1996). As is now the norm for teens throughout the western world, the predominant point of reference for the interviewees was their peers and, as borne out in the national and international literature, they claim to have often felt pressurised to conform to the expected behaviour established by older peers.

Perhaps unsurprisingly, the majority of the research participants stated that they would prefer to engage in risk behaviours with their friends and peers than by themselves, a finding in other Irish studies such as Forkan (2001), who notes that 60% of his Irish New Ross youth study group articulated that winning trust and friendship were the most important things for them. The parents of youth in Forkan's study also noted that developing friendships with peers ranked in the top three perceived needs of youth.

Peers are considered very important amongst developmental and educational psychologists. By the mid-teens, adolescents say that their relationships with their peers are closer than those with their parents (Hunter & Youniss, 1982). What is important to this study is that peer influence is not merely a matter of what is said and done by one's friends, but rather what is *believed* to be done and who is or is not favoured.

The international experience is that if an adolescent's peers use drugs, so too might the adolescent (McElwee & Monaghan, 2005; Myers, 1999) as noted in this study. Although drug use is generally viewed as a risk-behaviour (Ennet et al., 1999), some degree of drug taking is considered normative (Gaffney, 2001; McElwee & Monaghan, 2005). Experimentation with drugs during the period of adolescence is described as widespread (Cullen, 1997) and affects adolescents from a number of diverse socio-economic backgrounds. Researchers such as Swadi (2000) argue that some youth "mature out" of substance misuse.

In a Dublin study, Mayock (2000) found that adolescents in her study group tended to reduce their drug intake between the ages of sixteen and seventeen. Nonetheless, global research indicates that early exposure to drugs can be "damaging for the emotional, social, psychological, and academic growth of the (developing) child" (McElwee & Monaghan, 2005; Wabaunsee & Williams, 1995). In an educational context, Grube and Morgan (1986) suggest that if drug use overlaps with school hours or interferes with school performance, the child or young person is at risk. My study reflects the findings of Mayock's (2000) research, where cannabis was considered to be a normal and accepted feature of youth interaction. Indeed, my experience with the project is that what might be termed soft drugs have been normalised amongst the interviewees such is their familiarity with them within their own cultures. As with Mayock's (2000) findings, peers in my study were sometimes reported as tending to encourage, endorse, and recommend drug-taking activities.

A worrying trend is the correlation between substance use disorders with other psychiatric disorders such as anxiety and affective, antisocial, and other personality disorders and the increased risks of the girls having babies with fetal alcohol syndrome as the chronic use of alcohol becomes more and more endemic.

When the interviewees stated that they would not involve a peer in risky activities, it was for two reasons: They were fearful the peers would report their activities to authorities or, in their own language, "squeal." However, there was also the desire amongst some interviewees not to involve peers in dangerous activity for fear that the peers would get into trouble or become injured.

Thus, policy makers will need to identify clear strategies that involve peers in at risk educational strategies and how these peers may effectively be reached and engaged with as advocates for change. These strategies must be measurable.

Perceptions of Risk

A number of factors have been identified in research in this area. Newman's (1972) concept of defensible space seems apt in the context of this study. Newman was concerned with the sense of safety from assault people feel when living in residential areas. The interviewees in my study noted that leaving one's own house could be seen as risky as one could get into a fight, be run down by another teenager joyriding in a car, or be stabbed.

Caring for and About Youth:
The Importance of the School Environment
in Promoting Resilience

A protective factor (resilience) in relation to the academic performance of at risk children is parents who value school and encourage a positive attitude towards learning. This has a mirrored or modelling effect on children. The Director of the project suggests that, prior to their involvement with the Project, *all* of the parents held negative attitudes to school. He estimates that this was reduced to 50% after contact with the Project (John Hanna, personnal communication).[5]

In St. Augustine's, as we have seen in an earlier chapter, the curriculum has been actively (re)developed and negotiated with the participants to transform pupils' pathologies into strengths. Drawing from an ecological perspective, the educational polices and structures have been developed with both the pupils and families of pupils in mind. The children that require additional assistance are given it by staff that consistently gives the message that they care about the pupils and will always go the extra mile for them. This reinforces the pupils' sense of self-esteem.

The importance of the teacher as a protective influence is widely noted in the literature on risk and resilience (Gilligan, 1998; Pianta & Walsh, 1996; Rutter, 1991; Werner & Smith, 1992). Teachers are particularly well placed to observe signs of abuse, changes in behaviour, or failure to thrive (Home Office et al., 1991). Students who experience one or more conditions of disadvantage can have a solid protective mechanism *if* they receive support from school personnel. Such a relationship can have a number of "positive and socio-emotional outcomes" (DuBois et al., 1994). Pianta and Walsh (1996) note that relationships between the child and young person and the school often fail because "attempts to fix it have been narrow, reflective, and reactive" (p. 2).

The culture of the school itself is dependent on the attitudes of staff and their professional ideologies (Handy & Aitkin, 1986) as culture pervades the decision-making and problem-solving strategies employed by teachers. Teachers are uniquely positioned to establish three protective factors: constructing, nurturing and fostering caring relationships; having positive expectations from their pupils that take into account each life history of each child (Delpit, 1996); and providing opportunities to participate and contribute to the community (Kohn, 1993).

Stringfield (1997) identifies six areas where change may be instigated at institutional level in schools for high challenge children including specifying the problem, seeking solutions that have been proven to work in similar situations, seeking solutions that are compatible with the current strengths of the schools, understanding the demands and limitations of the chosen programme, and understanding the requirements for full implementation. In terms of social policy, government proposals could include redesigning the curriculum to become more child centred, reviewing the role of adults in teaching at-risk children, changing the manner and focus of assessment, reviewing school organisation on a series of levels, and forging links between school and colleges.

Prevention and intervention projects that are school-based have been explored since the 1970s. Zins and Ponti (1990) acknowledge that the most successful interventions are ones that are theory-driven, and Natriello et al. (1990) suggest that the social context of the school is the major source of advantage or disadvantage with regard to educational outcomes. The climate and norm structure of the school is crucial. The Consortium on the School-Based Promotion of Social Competence (1996) notes that children should be taught a range of cognitive, affective, and behavioural skills. This would facilitate the promotion of positive social, psychological, personal, and health outcomes.

It is now well recognised that a collaborative school culture facilitates development (Fullan & Hargreaves, 1992). Pupils are enabled to concentrate on their strengths if the school promotes the need for learning, good citizenship, and consideration for others. It can do this with a negotiated curriculum. A culture of achievement is constructed when the pupils are consistently rewarded for both small and large achievements through recognition, certification, and celebration of achievement (Sattin, 1999). The fact that the ex-pupils recognise this in the interview data is telling.

A Caring for and Commitment to Youth:
The Importance of Effective Leadership

The Director of the project was singled out time and time again by the ex-pupils as a figure of major importance to them. This is consistent with international findings on risk and resiliency. Hopkins et al. (1996) suggest that there are a number of factors in effective leadership including vision building, relevant expertise added to a quality of communication, and participation. Ricks (1992) surveyed child and youth care workers in relation to caring and developed a model where she distinguishes the professional caring relationship having "... three critical factors: (1) the condition of need, (2) an attitude of concern, and (3) intentional involvement in intervention" (p. 52). It is difficult to see how the Director could have been more involved in the project as all three factors are present in his relationship with the pupils. A deep sense of care permeated all conversations I had with the Director in relation to his work with the youth in the project, their siblings, and their families. Ultimately, the Director wanted the youth "to have a better experience of themselves."

It is worth providing an example of this intentional involvement. In the early stages of the project's existence (the late 1970s and early 1980s) when there was little funding available from the Department of Education, the Director and his wife cooked dinners at home for the pupils and brought these dinners into the school. This involved considerable personal expense and time. It also involved a round journey of some twenty miles each day. In this way, the Director of the project gave a positive example to both the staff and the pupils. This was remembered over a decade later in a discussion held with some of the ex-pupils. Perhaps most importantly, the Director of the project entertains a concept of hope (Fullan, 1998). Havel (1993) described it as the certainty that something makes sense regardless of how it turns out. Thus, the Director demonstrated through action in relation to the youth that he genuinely cared for them.

Engaging with Families of At Risk Youth

The family environment that a child lives in should be as supportive as possible as the family is considered the most important sub-system in ecological literature. Child and youth care, like most helping professions, has come to realize that the young person is a member of a socially interacting system and that the development of the young person and the young person's thoughts, actions, values, beliefs, and experience of self occur within this system (Garfat, 1998). As youth at the Youth Encounter Projects overwhelmingly live with family members, we have come to realize that lasting change is only facilitated when helping professionals interested in the troubled young person are involved with the total family system (Garfat & McElwee, 2004; Gilligan, 2000). Teachers and child and youth care staff at the project daily enter the life space of pupils and attempt to engage with the pupils on their own terms.

Relationships are the essence of truly effective practice, for it is within the context of meaningful relationships that young people and their families frame their experiences and find new ways of living together successfully. In the context of genuinely caring and mutual relationships, they find new ways of (re)structuring their experience of the world and the encounters they have had and may have in it. The attention to relationship and being-in-relationship while utilizing everyday life events as they are occurring for therapeutic purposes is a key to unlocking at least some problematic behaviours. Parents are increasingly considered as individuals affected by the larger systems of which they are a part and within the family. For example, they are seen as people involved in relationships of love (e.g., as couples), as parents, and as individuals with their own needs and experiences. In essence, social policy has begun to recognize the parent as a person in his or her own right. As a result the purpose of contact with the parents has again shifted. Special educational initiatives should attempt to contact parents of pupils to offer support, guidance, and family intervention where possible.

It should be common practice for the whole family to be considered in the role of client or pupil as staff at educational projects concern themselves with the dynamics of interaction, roles, and positions of all the members of the family in the systems of which they are a part. Parents should be understood and reached as potential collaborators in the development of general intervention plans and daily and weekly educational goals. Where possible, family members should be actively involved in all aspects of a child or young person's program, and all family members should be considered for their potential role as co-helpers. In short, the family, as an interacting, dynamic system, is considered by many of the more advanced child and youth care educationalists to be the client or pupil, not just the context.

If child and youth care workers and teachers in special educational projects are to continue this movement toward engaging the whole family and become effective family interventionists, specific areas of education and training need to be targeted. These include:

- systems thinking and intervention
- family development and dynamics
- the translation of a child and youth care approach in to the area of working with families

- working independently in the home or community
- ways of engaging with families and individual family members
- the inclusion of family values into service programmes
- self-awareness in the area of family work
- shifting the perception of family
- re-defining the roles of child and youth care worker

As with parents and family members, if this shift is to continue, child and youth care workers and teachers at the special educational projects will require support in moving from the project-programme to the family environment.

CONCLUSION

A strengths-based approach to research and policy is based on the recognition that there is substantial variation in the adjustment of individuals, families, and communities experiencing adverse circumstances. Four themes have emerged in the study of risk and coping over the past decade: interrelatedness of risk and problems, individual variability in resilience and susceptibility to stress, processes and mechanisms linking multiple stressors to multiple outcomes, and interventions and prevention. All of these have been a part of this study. Resilience is a term used to describe a set of qualities that foster a process of successful adaptation and transformation despite risk and adversity (Benard, 1995; Masten & Coatsworth, 1998).

Lash and Urry (1994) acknowledge that policies of (post)modern nation-states are a product of complex processes between globalisation and localisation. This seems particularly relevant to children and youth at risk. The fate of the pupils in St. Augustine's Special School lies with the results of a centralised social policy based in the Department of Education and Sciences Offices that appears to ignore the complexities of living and working in a localised risk society, where something as basic as staying indoors is considered safe and going outside to play is risky.

Four dimensions for a comprehensive policy reform strategy have been identified in international research with regard to at risk youth. These include academic success, subject relevance, positive relationships within schools, and supportive relationships beyond schools (Legters, McDill & McPartland, 1997). Child and youth care staff have to consider three types of risk as they go about their daily interventions in special educational projects such as St. Augustine's: risk to service users from other people (including children at risk), usually their own relatives; risk to users themselves (self-neglect, self-injury), and; risks to known or unknown others from service users (substance users, people with a mental illness).

It is clear from this analysis that the research participants feel keenly that their backgrounds militate against them in a number of spheres of their lives. The interviewees realise that they are simply not in a position to avail themselves of the educational opportunities many of their middle-class peers take for granted and feel alienated from the system which favours those youth with the right address, the right accent, two parents, a history of employment, and good standing in the community. One includes here what is often taken as a natural movement from the national school system to the secondary school system and from there on to third level education.[6]

On the other hand, the interviewees had a very strong sense of loyalty to the school and realised that the teachers, support staff, and Director daily attempted to reduce risks and promote resiliency in their lives. The staff at the project accept and embrace the social and cultural backgrounds of the pupils and this is uniformly recognised by the youth. In this regard, the project may be said to be resiliency focused.

NOTES

1. These include prenatal stress and potential consequences for subsequent growth and well being in infants and children; delinquent children and adolescents (with varying emphasis on family environment as a source of stress and inadequate parenting); delinquent and criminal career paths; parental schizophrenia; affective disorders; anti-social behaviour; hyperactivity and attention deficit disorder, and socially isolative behaviour.

2. Harding (1991) notes four competing theoretical schools in relation to the treatment of children at risk of ill treatment:

    a. Laissez-faire: Leave the responsibility for children to parents, except in extreme cases when compulsory (achievement-conservative welfare state).

    b. Family support: The main role of the state should be to provide material and social support to all parents, particularly those who are struggling to care adequately for their children (institutional-social democratic welfare state).

    c. Children's rights: It is most important to give priority to the interests and especially the expressed wishes of children.

3. It is ironic that during the life of this study, several scandals broke in the public arena in child and youth care and agricultural practices and involved extensive dialogue by experts, and yet the interviewees did not see these as affecting them.

4. Of course, one could argue that this is negated somewhat by his drug use.

5. Furthermore, in matters relating to the care and education of the children, it was generally the mother figure who displayed interest.

6. A three-year study conduced by the Higher Education Authority (1995) acknowledges that students from middle-class backgrounds are more likely to transfer to higher education with a modest Leaving Certificate as opposed to working-class students who transfer only when they achieve results at the higher end of the scale.

REFERENCES

Arnett, J. (1992). Reckless behaviour in adolescence: A developmental perspective. *Developmental Review, 12*, 339-373.

Bates, B. (1996). *Aspects of childhood deviancy: A study of young offenders in open settings.* Unpublished doctoral dissertation. Dublin: University College Dublin.

Beck, U. (1992). *Risk society. Towards a new modernity.* London: Sage.

Beck, U. (1997). *The reinvention of politics: Rethinking modernity in the global social order.* Cambridge: Polity.

Benard, B. (1995). *Fostering resilience in children.* ERIC/EECE Digest, EDO-PS-95-9.

Carnegie Council on Adolescent Development. (1995). *Great Transitions: Preparing adolescents for a new century. Concluding report of the Carnegie Council on adolescent development.* New York: Carnegie Corporation.

Consortium on the School-based Promotion of Social Competence. (1996). The school-based promotion of social competence: Theory, research, practice, and policy. In R. J. Haggerty, L. R. Sherrod, N. Garmezy, & M. Rutter (Eds.), *Stress, risk, and resilience in children and adolescents: Processes, mechanisms, and interventions* (pp. 268-316). New York: Cambridge University Press.

Cullen, B. (1997). *A report for integrated services initiative on models of integrating services for young families in the community.* Dublin: Unpublished Paper for Integrated Services Initiative.

Dake, K. (1992). Myths of nature: culture and the social construction of risk. *Journal of Social Issues, 48*(4), 21-37.

Delpit, L. (1996). The politics of teaching literate discourse. In W. Ayers & P. Ford (Eds.), *City kids, city teachers. Reports from the front row.* New York: New Press.

Douglas, M. (1980). Risk and environment. In J. Dowie & P. Lefrere (Eds.), *Risk and chance. Selected readings.* The Open University.

Douglas, M. (1990). Risk as a forensic resource. *Daedalus, 119*(4), 1-16.

Douglas, M. (1992). *Risk and blame: Essays in cultural theory.* London; New York: Routledge.

Douglas, M., & Calvez, M. (1990). The self as risk taker: A cultural theory of contagion in relation to AIDS. *The Sociological Review, 38*(3), 445-464.

Douglas, M., & Wildavsky, A. (1983). *Risk and culture. An essay on the selection of technological and environmental dangers.* University of California Press.

Dowie, J. (1984). Perceived risk. A chimera? In L. Zuckerman (Ed.), *Risk in society.* John Libbey & Co. Ltd.

DuBois, D., Felner, R., Meares, H., & Krier, M. (1994). Prospective investigation of the effects of socioeconomic disadvantage, life stress and social support on early adult adjustment. *Journal of Abnormal Psychology, 103*, 511-522.

Ennet, S. T., Bailey, S. L., & Freedman, E. B. (1999). Social network characteristics associated with risky behaviours among runaway and homeless youth. *Journal of Health and Social Behaviour, 40*, 63-78.

Forkan, C. (2001). *Needs, concerns and social exclusion: The millennium and beyond.* Waterford: Centre for Social Care Research, Waterford Institute of Technology.

Fullan, M. (1998). Leadership for the 21st century: Breaking the bonds of dependency. *Educational Leadership, 55*(7), 1-6.

Fullan, M., & Hargreaves, A. (1992). *What's worth fighting for in your school?* Buckingham: OUP.

Gaffney, M. (2001). *Substance misuse: Separating adolescents and adults.* Unpublished diploma dissertation. Waterford: Centre for Social Care Research. Waterford Institute of Technology.

Garfat, T. (1998). The effective child and youth care practitioner: A phenomenological inquiry. *Journal of Child and Youth Care, 12*, 1-2.

Giddens, A. (1990). *The consequences of modernity.* Cambridge: Polity Press.

Gilligan, R. (1998). The importance of schools and teachers in child welfare. *Child and Family Social Work, 3*, 13-25.

Gilligan, R. (2000). Adversity, resilience and young people: The protective value of positive school and spare time experiences. *Children and Society, 14*, 37-47.

Grube, J. W., & Morgan, M. (1986). *Smoking, drinking and other drug use among Dublin post-primary pupils.* Dublin: ESRI Paper No. 132.

Handy, C. B., & Aitken, R. (1986). *Understanding schools as organisations.* Harmondsworth: Penguin.

Harding, L. F. (1991). *Perspectives in child care policy.* London: Longman.

Havel, V. (1993). Never against hope. *Esquire*, 65-69.

Hendrick, H. (1994). *The history of childhood and youth: A guide to the literature.* Oxford Polytechnic, Faculty of Modern Studies, Occasional Papers, 1.

Higher Educational Authority. (1995). Dublin: Author.

Home Office, Dept. of Health and Dept. of Education and Science and Welch Office. (1991). *Working together under the Children Act 1991. A guide to arrangements for interagency co-operation for the protection of children from abuse.* London: HMSO.

Hopkins, D., Ainscow, A., & West, M. (1996). *School improvement in an era of change.* London: Cassell.

Hunter, F. T., & Youniss, J. (1982). Changes in functions in three relations during adolescence. *Developmental Psychology, 18*, 806-811.

Kasperson, R. E., Renn, O., Slovic, P., Brown, H. S., Emel, J., Goble, R., Kasperson, J. E., & Ratick, S. (1988). The social amplification and attenuation of risk. *Risk Analysis, 8*(2), 177-87.

Kohn, A. (1993). Choices for children why and how to let students decide. *Phi Delta Kappan, 75*(1), 8-16.

Lash, S., & Urry, J. (1994). *Economies of signs and spaces.* London: Sage.

Letgers, N., McDill, E., & McPartland, J. (1997). Rising to the challenge: Emerging strategies for educating children at risk. In *Educational reforms and students at risk: A review of the current state of the art* (pp. 47-92). Washington, DC: Office of Educational Research and Improvement.

Lewis, O. (1961). *The children of Sanchez.* New York: Random House.

Lewis, O. (1966). The culture of poverty. *Scientific American, 215*(4), 46-47.

Lightfoot, C. C. (1994). *Playing with desire: An interpretive perspective on risk-taking.* Paper presented at the Annual Meeting of the American Educational Research Association. New Orleans: LA.

Lopes, L. L. (1997). Between hope and fear: The psychology of risk. In W. M. Goldstein & R. M. Hogarth (Eds.), *Research on judgement and decision making: Currents, connections and controversies.* Cambridge: Cambridge University Press.

Lupton, D. (1995). Risk as a sociocultural construct. *Touch. Public Health Association of Australia Newsletter Series, 12*(6), 10-13.

Lynch, K. (1999). *Equality in education.* Dublin: Gill and Macmillan.

Masten, A. S., & Coatsworth, J. D. (1998). The development of competence in favorable and unfavorable environments: Lessons from research on successful children. *American Psychologist, 53*(2), 205-220.

Mayock, P. (2000). *Choosers or losers? Influences on young people's choices about drugs in inner city Dublin.* Dublin: Montague Street.

McElwee, N., & Monaghan, G. (2005). *Darkness on the edge of town. An exploratory study of heroin misuse in Athlone and Portlaoise.* Athlone: Centre for Child & Youth Care Learning.

Myers, D. G. (1999). *Exploring psychology.* New York: Worth Publishers.

Natrillio, G., McDill, E., & Pallas, A. (1990). *Schooling disadvantaged children: Racing against time.* New York: Teachers College Press.

Newman, O. (1972). *Defensible space.* New York: MacMillan.

Norman, A. (1988). Risk. In B. Gearing. (Ed.), *Mental health problems in old age: A reader.* Chichester: Wiley.

Pianta, R., & Walsh, D. (1996). *High-risk children in schools.* Routledge.

Pratkanis, A, Breckler, S., & Greenwald, A. (Eds.). (1989). *Attitude, structure and function.* Hillsdale. NJ: Erlbaum.

Ricks, F. (1992). A feminist's view of caring. *Journal of Child and Youth Care, 7*(2), 49-58.

Rutter, M., & Casaer, P. (1991). Biological risk factors for psychological disorders. In M. Rutter & P. Casaer (Eds.), *European network on longitudinal studies on individual development* (pp. 331-374). Cambridge: Cambridge University Press.

Rutter, M. (1991). Childhood experiences and adult psychosocial functioning. In G. R. Bock, & J. Whelan (Eds.), *The childhood environment and adult disease.* Ciba Foundation Symposium No. 156. Chichester: Wiley.

Sattin, R. (1999). Effective ed schooling. A view from the inside. *Emotional and Behavioural Difficulties, 4*(3), 10-13.

Strachan, R., & Tallent, C. (1997). Improving judgement and appreciating biases within the risk assessment process. In H. Kemshall & J. Pritchard. (Eds.), *Good practice in risk assessment and risk management 2: Protection, rights and responsibilites.* London: Jessica Kingsley Publishers.

Stringfield, S. (1997). Barrriers and pathways to meaningful reforms: The need for high reliability organisational structures. In *U.S. Department of Education. Educational reforms and students at risk: A review of the current state of the art.* Office of Educational Research and Improvement. Washington, DC.

Swadi, H. (2000). Substance misuse in adolescents. *Advances in Psychiatric Treatment,* *6*, 201-210.

Task Force Report on Discipline. (2006). Dublin: Government Publications

Wabaunsee, R., & Williams, H. J. (1995). At risk students: drug prevention through latch-key programs. *Drugs: Education, Prevention and Policy, 2*(1), 65-75.

Werner, E. F., & Smith, R. (1992). *Overcoming the odds: High-risk children from birth to adulthood.* Ithaca, NY: Cornell University Press.

Wynne-Harley, D. (1991). *Living dangerously: Risk taking, safety and older people.* London: Centre for Policy on Ageing.

Zins, J. E., & Ponti, C. R. (1990). Best practices in school-based consultation. In A. Thomas & J. Grimes (Eds.), *Best practices in school psychology 11* (pp. 673-694). Washington DC: National Association of School Psychologists.

Zuckerman, M. (1979). *Sensation seeking: Beyond the optimum level of arousal.* Hillsdale, NJ: Erlbaum.

doi:10.1300/J024v29n01_09

Chapter 10

Children and Youth:
The Evolution of At Risk
to "High Promise" Youth

SUMMARY. It is impossible to make global generalisations about children and youth from a phenomenological inquiry into the experiences of such a limited number of participants in just one city, Limerick, Ireland, and one case, St. Augustine's. The goal of phenomenological research is, however, not to seek generalisations but to expose the individual case, so I have endeavoured to use a symptomatic rather than representative approach to risk biographies, in so far as we assume all biographies are composed of the partial perspectives of knowledges that are insider and situated. Truths are contingent on differences of time, space, age, gender, class, sexual preference, and other aspects of culture and context. Nonetheless, I am reminded towards the conclusion of this book of a comment made by well-known Irish economist, T. K. Whittaker (1997), who observed: "If we think about it, save for the vagaries of birth, errant biology, class and status, or simply circumstance, we are all but a half step away from the 'other' families we describe as in need of service, or 'at risk.' In the final analysis, it is not 'us' and 'them.' It is all of us. Together" (p. 138). doi:10.1300/J024v29n01_10 *[Article copies available for a fee from The Haworth Document Delivery Service: 1-800-HAWORTH. E-mail address: <docdelivery@haworthpress.com> Website: <http://www.HaworthPress.com>* © *2007 by The Haworth Press, Inc. All rights reserved.]*

[Haworth co-indexing entry note]: "Children and Youth: The Evolution of At Risk to 'High Promise' Youth." McElwee, Niall. Co-published simultaneously in *Child & Youth Services* (The Haworth Press, Inc.) Vol. 29, No. 1/2, 2007, pp. 269-290; and: *At-Risk Children & Youth: Resiliency Explored* (Niall McElwee) The Haworth Press, Inc., 2007, pp. 269-290. Single or multiple copies of this article are available for a fee from The Haworth Document Delivery Service [1-800-HAWORTH, 9:00 a.m. - 5:00 p.m. (EST). E-mail address: docdelivery@haworthpress.com].

Available online at http://cys.haworthpress.com
© 2007 by The Haworth Press, Inc. All rights reserved.
doi:10.1300/J024v29n01_10

KEYWORDS. Risk, resiliency, reclaimed youth, Youth Encounter Projects

Consider these children to have fallen among thieves, the thieves of ignorance and sin and ill-fate and loss. Their birthrights were stolen. They have no belongings.

–Karl Menninger (1982)

This study set out to examine perspectives on risk, at risk, and resiliency in children and adolescents and factors associated with greater adversity and vulnerability, or greater resiliency, in the context of a global discourse on risk theory for both children and youth and front-line practitioners. Thus, it has felt like a roller coaster at times. A sample of these children and adolescents at significant risk for a range of psychological and social difficulties was chosen in 1995 (n = 17) based on risk factors including individual factors, family factors, and support factors. The research data from this study suggests that providing for children and youth designated by authorities as being at risk or high risk with intervention programmes will enjoy only limited success unless a much more encompassing child and youth care perspective is entertained and actively supported. A variety of programmes which build on individual resiliency traits must become the norm. Nonetheless, providing physical and emotional resources matters significantly to at-risk children and young people as indicated from the four child and youth care sections uncovered in the interview data: safety, self-acceptance, belonging, and finding opportunity.

I have been truly privileged to undertake this exploratory journey from risk to at risk to resilience as one of the aims of this study has been to explore how a cohort of adolescents attempt to make sense of risk and resiliency in their lives. The interviewees refer to this in the study as "walking the roads of Limerick." What has become apparent to me (as if I needed reminding) during the life of this study is that children and adolescents can be(come) incredibly resilient even when faced with extreme personal and social adversity if there are structural supports available. This journey has reinforced for me the fact that family support must be a diverse and continuing range of interventions.

Although not often discussed in the literature until relatively recently, risk has always been central to the caring professions, and in this study I have been critical of Irish social policy which consistently failed to truly acknowledge the importance of approaching and dealing with children and youth early in their at risk cycles using a number of resiliency-led perspectives. The home life of a child, familial situation, peer group, and immediate living environment must all be targeted in any effective model of practice. The work environment of the front-line practitioner and, indeed, supervisor must also be more centred on opportunity rather than uncertainty in this "risk ledge." We should immediately begin to address the many social problems that have appeared in this study as they are seen to affect children and young people and as they have been articulated to us (adults) in studies such as this one.

The most successful *predictive* instruments concerning risk are understood to achieve an 80 percent accuracy, which leaves us with 20 percent to adopt a clinical gaze. In simple numeric terms, twenty per cent may not seem a lot, but tell that to the individual child, young person or his family. The "crux of framing's relevance to risk assessment is to move people into the zone of gains where their decision making will be less risk-seeking" (Strachan & Tallant, 1997, p. 19).[1]

EVALUATING THE YOUTH ENCOUNTER PROJECTS AS AN AT RISK INTERCEPTION

According to Catterall (1986), several general themes have emerged with respect to the ways in which schools have approached their at-risk student problems. They have tended to focus upon one or more of the following:

- importing/developing programmes for specifically targeted at-risk student populations or actual dropouts
- identifying and providing help to at-risk students as early as possible
- addressing academic deficits through remediation
- providing counselling services to address negative attitudes, to establish goals, and to develop positive self-concepts, and
- pursuing school-work linkages.

All of these are attempted in the Youth Encounter Projects. Even with this, Clancy (1995) acknowledges that despite the extensive global research on schooling, it remains difficult to identify the *essential* characteristics of the effective school (my emphasis). Many Irish commentators note the difficulties in attempting to measure the impact of interventions with at-risk children and youth. Because there remains such disagreement around defining at risk in the first instance, McKeown

(2000), for example, believes "there is often less hard scientific evidence to support the effectiveness of interventions–as opposed to either doing nothing or doing something else–than might usually be assumed ..." (p. 5).

The Director of St. Augustine's Special School confirmed that in one six month period (chosen at random from the school records), out of twenty-five pupils attending the project, *twelve* failed to complete sixth class within the formal primary school network. Nonetheless, as with the Early Start programme discussed in this study, it is clear that the pupils within the Youth Encounter Projects have a very strong sense of loyalty to their particular schools, claim that they have a genuine desire to come to school each morning, and realise that the project is, at the very least, useful. This may be attributed to the fact that the school attempts to engage the children through richness in intellectual and emotional stimulation and sustained one-to-one contact. The school has a warm, friendly environment because it occupies the daily life space of its pupils. This is the effective child and youth care intervention.

The loyalty factor is also supported by the very low rates of truancy whilst attending the Youth Encounter Projects. Perhaps surprisingly, non-attendance at the project does not differ radically from the general population in the formal primary school, which has surprised many casual observers of the system. In fact, at times, the attendance rate is better than the formal education system (Hanna, 2006). One of the strengths of the Youth Encounter Projects is their aim to improve the ability of children and youth to cope with their (total) environments and to develop their scholastic and vocational aptitudes whilst giving *both* the children and parents a more positive school experience. It seems to me that the children's sustained participation in the schools, at all, should be seen as a positive outcome, as it was admitted that some pupils were only written into the school rolls more in hope than expectation and some other children only stayed in the projects for very brief periods (Egan & Hegarty, 1984) and the parents of the pupils were distrustful of the project at the time of initial involvement. In addition, there has been a measured reduction in incidences of juvenile delinquency across the Projects. A clear lesson for policy makers in the Department of Education and Science is to be wholly inclusive of parents and caregivers in the lives of the YEP youth.

HOW DO THE PUPILS COMPARE
TO INTERNATIONAL LITERATURE?
EVERYTHING IS RELATIVE

Based on the overlap among risky behaviours in her American cohorts, Dryfoos (1990) classifies 14 year olds into different risk groups.

Very High-Risk. These youth "do it all." They have already entered the juvenile justice system, carry guns, and use illegal drugs such as cocaine. This is not the case with the majority of the St. Augustine's pupils and certainly not at such a low age. Whilst some of the youth had entered the juvenile system, only one reported that he had carried a gun and none reported taking hard drugs such as cocaine or heroin. The opposite was the case where, for example, one interviewee pointed out that he would not inject due to the potential health hazards and there was a general feeling that hard drugs were destructive to one's health.

High-Risk. These youth "do most of it." They have not entered the juvenile justice system yet but engage in heavy drinking, smoking and marijuana use, are behind in school, often truant, and have frequent unprotected sex.

This category, perhaps, fits the majority of my interviewees, particularly with regard to males (with the exception of unprotected sexual activity as there is insufficient data to comment). One might argue, of course, that many school-going youth take some drugs and consume alcohol so in this regard the YEP pupils are no different.

Moderate-Risk. These youth "do some of it." They are engaged in one or two high risk behaviors such as experimenting with marijuana and alcohol, occasionally truant, have sex (usually without contraception), and occasionally feel depressed.

Again, this fits the YEP cohort. Only a couple of the female interviewees could be described as moderate risk. We have already seen in an earlier chapter how self-reported youthful depression is no longer exceptional.

Low-Risk. These youth experiment with risky behaviours. They may have an occasional drink or cut class once in a while. A few of these youth are sexually active, but they always use contraception. They are, for the most part, protected from the dangers of risky behaviors.

Sadly, none of my interviewees could be described as low-risk. If they were, they simply would not qualify for entry into the project.

No-Risk. These youth do not engage in any risky behaviors. Except for being surrounded by many negative or risky activities, these youth are protected from the dangers of risky behaviours.

None of my interviewees could be described as no-risk.

THE VIEWS OF TEACHING REPRESENTATIVES

The Youth Encounter Projects, along with some other dedicated youth projects, received funding from the Department of Education and Science of approximately 13 million euros in 2003. The Irish National Teachers Organisation cited disappointment at the closure of the Youth Encounter Project in Dublin's inner city by the Department of Education in 1995.[2] The INTO's recommendations regarding the Youth Encounter Projects were:

1. The operation of the Youth Encounter Projects to be reviewed, with a view to establishing their place as part of a continuum of provision for pupils with special emotional, behavioural, or psychological needs. Such a review is to be carried out with the involvement of all interested parties (still has not happened although the Department of Education and Science and Finance have recently visited the Limerick Project).

2. The current Youth Encounter Projects be kept and improved while the review is being conducted. It was felt that an additional Youth Encounter Project should be re-introduced in Dublin's inner city to cater for children who no longer have access to the Rutland Street Project (the projects have been kept and, indeed, are scheduled to be expanded if one believes the recent national reportage).

3. It was agreed that all Youth Encounter Projects should be properly funded and resourced in terms of equipment, personnel, and facilities. Sub-standard buildings should be replaced immediately (certainly not the case with the Limerick YEP which has had to endure an inappropriate location since its establishment).

4. It is the belief that special classes for pupils who are socially and/or psychologically disabled be established in designated schools. Pupils in such classes should have access to play-therapy, art-therapy, drama, and support services as required.

5. Special units on the school premises should be included in designated areas as required. Pupils attending such units should be able to avail of support services and to integrate with the pupils of the mainstream school as appropriate.

PARENTS AS EQUAL PARTNERS IN THE EDUCATIVE PROCESS

The fundamental principle of supporting family life was articulated by the Irish Commission on the Family in 1996, where it was stated: "The experience of family living is the single greatest influence on an individual's life ... [because] ... it is in the family context that a person's basic emotional needs for security, belongingness, support, and intimacy are satisfied" (p. 13). Other Irish commentators, such as Keenan (1998) suggest that regardless of the apparent difficulties in families, they "contain within them resources and strengths that, if harnessed and nurtured, can produce beneficial outcomes" (p. 5). We must return and embrace parents and caregivers whenever and whereever possible because the underlying common denominator in raising socially competent children appears to be the emotional availability of parents and caregivers.

Positive, imaginative programmes (both school and community based) with realisable and mutually satisfactory outcomes (such as the handing out of certificates on completion of each part of a course or subject by teaching staff to pupils) could be more formally integrated into the school curriculum. Current practices within the project, for example, of teachers formally writing to parents could be reviewed with an emphasis toward actively including parents in disciplining but also in rewarding pupils within the formal school network. If a parent of an at-risk child only remembers negative experiences of school, we could direct some energy into creating a more tolerant and positive image of school life today. Parents, or significant adults in the child's life, must be seen to be equal partners in the education process and must be assisted in the courageous first step of turning up to support their children in what is understood to be a very formal environment.

A RECLAIMING ENVIRONMENT

'Tis the custom of schoolmasters to be eternally thundering in their pupils' ears, as though they were pouring into a funnel, while the business of pupils is only to repeat what others have said before.

–Michel De Montaigne, *On the Education of Children* (1580)

Many parents and pupils connected to the project remain largely marginalised (Hanna, 2006).[3] Having said this, the results of this study support the widely held views in resiliency literature that school can be a major protective factor for disadvantaged children. A school with a positive environment can negate very significant home-life adversity where children and adolescents can form secure attachments with adult figures that will positively influence them in the long term. For children to survive significant adversity is testimony to their resilience and, crucially, a testimony to St. Augustine's Special School, which may be called a "reclaiming" environment (Wolins & Wozner, 1982).

Nonetheless, the disproportionately high numbers of male ex-pupils going on to serve prison sentences over the years in this study indicates that "at risk" children and youth (particularly males) are being targeted too late in their lives, as many have learned to survive adversity through negative societal behaviour (Bates, 1996; Murray, 1984; West, 1974) but behaviours which are seen as positive by peers. The lack of a structured formal aftercare after pupils graduate from St. Augustine's in and around Limerick City is deplorable. If children and youth from the inner-city areas and sprawling housing estates are to be given an opportunity to develop as emotionally and morally sound individuals, there must be adequate investment in facilities for them. Many neglected children end up "walking the roads" because it appears too much effort for them to do anything else. This perception must be addressed by social services and policy analysts.

It is clear that Irish national school provision has been under-funded and under-resourced in the past, and this has been particularly the case with special educational initiatives. A major problem is not so much the well-documented pupils who fail to pass their end-of-school Leaving Certificate examinations annually (20% nationally), but it has, unfortunately, become whether or not some pupils will finish out their national school education. In 1994, for example, 2,700 children left school before completing their Junior Certificate examinations with 8,000 pupils leaving directly afterwards. Figures for 2006 suggest that 1,000 children would not make the transition from primary to secondary school.

ST. AUGUSTINE'S SPECIAL SCHOOL:
SUCCESS OR FAILURE?

Far from disheartening your pupils' youthful courage, spare nothing to lift up their soul; make them your equals in order that they may become your equals.

–Jean Jacques Rousseau

Success of failure? This is, of course, a central issue to this study. One senior official at the Irish Department of Education and Science informed me that *"The YEP's have filled an important gap in provision, but in our review we will have to recast some of the original objectives."* Interestingly, he felt that the YEP's had become more political in recent years and observed that *"The State has been able to fulfil its constitutional obligations to 'at risk' children particularly in relation to delinquency."*

It is important to note that in Farrington and Welch's (1999) study of 24 family-based prevention programmes, there were mixed results. Many of the programmes they viewed showed desirable effects with some outcomes but not with others. There have been some spectacular international failures such as the *Infant Health and Development Programme* carried out with 985 low-birth weight infants in eight sites across North America. By age eight, the experimental and control children were not significantly different in behaviour problems (McCarthon et al., 1997). The *Children at Risk* study across five American cities is another useful example. Experimental youths showed no significant improvements in self-reported delinquency, police arrests, drug use, or other problem behaviours. A key factor in the failure of this programme was low levels of parental involvement, which brings us back to the family (Harrell et al., 1997).

THE IMPORTANCE OF PREVENTION
AND INTERVENTION PROGRAMMES

So, to remind the reader, three qualities are consistently marked out in the international literature on being resilient. These include a positive sense of self, a sense of academic competence with an appropriate attribution of failure, and a sense of responsibility and determination to overcome obstacles (Werner, 1990). These have been re-articulated in the interview data in the sections about safety, self-acceptance, belonging, and finding opportunity. If children and youth can appraise a situation and seek positive pathways that lead away from problem behaviours, they stand a fair chance of being resilient in the face of adversity, because they can make more prosocial and personally healthy decisions than their peers who succumb to risk.

It is now uniformly accepted that prevention and intervention programmes are useful if they employ a multi-perspective approach. In particular, two facets of interrelatedness may be seen: "... the linkages among variables that yield a holistic understanding of context, and the interplay of risk, protective factors, and mental health over time" (Gore & Eckenrode, 1996, p. 54). Having said this, Millner et al. (1998) say that "Although demographic or case variables may statistically predict [at-] risk status, many variables (e.g., gender, severity of past incident, SES, caretaker's childhood history of abuse) are not responsive to intervention and therefore are useless to treatment planning" (p. 102). The research completed for this study indicates that individual psychological and emotional coping mechanisms reside side-by-side with environmental context in predisposing children and youth to risk or resiliency. Thus, some of the interviewees in this study resorted to crime whilst others did not, despite the fact that they all attended a special project established specifically for children at risk. Gore and Eckenrode (1996) suggest that "an early emphasis on discrete life stressors has been complemented with attention to chronic adversity and microstressors" (p. 55). Literature on risk and resiliency that assumes existing protective resources can overcome serious long-term stressors deserves more attention and empirical validation.

RISK AND RESILIENCY: OPPOSITE SIDES OF THE SPECTRUM?

So it turns out that resiliency is not necessarily at a polar extreme to risk; indeed, both may exist on a continuum, with Emery and Forehand (1996) noting that "different models of risk and resilience suggest different approaches to measurement and statistical analysis in empirical research" (p. 92). They ask the enlightened questions, "Do temperamentally difficult children require special interventions to counteract risk? Do temperamentally easy children require little or no intervention because they are protected against risk? What marks the difference between adaptive and maladaptive survival techniques?" It is worth noting that the interviewees in this study may not be so different from the general population than appears on the surface. Such a view is supported by Achenbach (1990), who comments that,

> Many behavioural/emotional problems for which professional help is sought are not qualitatively different from those most individuals display to some degree at some time in their lives. Instead, many problems for which help is sought are quantitative variations on characteristics that may normally be evident at other develop-

mental periods, in less intense degree, in fewer situations or in ways that they do not impair developmental progress. (p. 4)

CONNECTING THE THEORETICAL WITH THE EMPIRICAL

Defining risk taking in terms of comparing and balancing likely benefits with likely harms may be a useful approach. This is certainly the case with Robert, who clearly associated risk with potential profit despite the fact that he might, quite easily, be shot dead during an armed robbery by the police or shot later by one of his "competitors." At the conclusion of this study, the reader may feel that it is timely to ask, how could the Limerick Youth Encounter Project be considered a success as, historically, so few of the pupils have achieved a pass in their Leaving Certificate examinations over the near thirty years of its existence or gone on to take up places in university programmes later in life.[4] This is the wrong question, in my opinion, as I feel we need to think of the school more as a reclaiming environment for at-risk youth than in the traditional sense of it simply being a place where pupils go to study so that they can pass formal State examinations. The project is a place of safety.

DEBATING POSSIBLE EXPLANATIONS FOR THE FAILURE OF RESILIENCY PROGRAMMES

One possible explanation for the *apparent* failure of St. Augustine's Special School to adequately prepare pupils to achieve the much sought after five passes in the State Leaving Certificate examination is found in the work of Schneider (1992), who suggests that the integrity of intervention programmes that are run over a considerable period of time lend themselves to being difficult to maintain. This is because they tend to become more and more "procedurally involved." Hamovitch (1996) argues that modifying curricula systematically disadvantages children, particularly when it comes to competing with their middle-class counterparts. On the other hand, Schorr (1988) and Dryfoos (1990) are more positive and acknowledge that at-risk students will benefit from intensive, narrowly targeted programmes that are carried out over a significant period of time.

Again, let us look to a child and youth care perspective. Two child and youth care practitioners who had worked in the project during the life of this study acknowledged that the best the school could hope to do was provide a safe place for the pupils between the hours of 9:30 am and

3:30 pm (McKenna, 1995; Rehill, 1999). They argue that having other set objectives is unrealistic when one takes into account their personal and familial histories. Unrealistic but not impossible. As MacDonald and MacDonald (1999) report, "Interventions to reduce adverse risk may have the opposite or no effect" (p. 41). Perhaps the expectation of the public is too high in the first instance and requires modification.

An obvious criticism of the Youth Encounter Project structure is based directly on its implicit philosophy. Using such terms as "educational disadvantage" and "cultural deprivation" change the perception of a school's cohort (Tormey, 1999). Disadvantage is commonly thought of in terms of rough schools, i.e., schools that are poor versions of the formal schools. For example, such a cultural disadvantage perspective has been criticised as having two flaws: (1) it suggests the average low-income family is, somehow, dysfunctional, and (2) it views cultural difference as cultural deficit (see U.S. Department of Commerce, 1997, p. 39). The Youth Encounter Projects linked up with three different government departments early on and noted the crucial link between formal and informal education, which could include the wider community. There is no doubt the projects have assisted in facilitating some of the pupils to overcome disadvantaged home lives, but to what extent exactly remains unclear. The General Secretary of the Irish Vocational Educational Authority, Joe Rooney, drew attention to the monetary advantages of dropping out of school before obtaining a Junior Certificate (Irish Times, 5.3, 1996) and incentives to exit special projects by enticing them to take up Youthreach programmes has been identified. Such students are funded to sit examinations through this particular body, a European Union funded scheme run by FAS and the Vocational Education Committees, under which early school drop-outs are guaranteed further training. Schools are obliged to provide lists of their early school leavers so that Youthreach can trace them. The President of the Teachers Union of Ireland acknowledged how difficult it was for some students as they are tempted out of the school system by the State offering social welfare payments, training schemes, and training allowances (Irish Times, 5.3, 1996).

RECOMMENDATIONS

1. Perhaps the single most important finding of this study is that the positive effects of intervention programmes such as St. Augustine's Special School that are so hard won in the face of risk

lose their effectiveness when the intervention ends. This has also been found in international research where Dryfoos (1998) calls for a "Safe Passage Movement" that involves all levels of society in a concerted effort to help youth at risk become successful adults. Therefore, a structured continuum of aftercare must be made available to the youth when they leave the school. The area of after care was mooted in both the Kennedy Report (1970) and the Task Force Report (1981) but was not adequately realised in the Child Care Act (1991). This is one of the most disappointing areas of the Act. After care must be supported through legislative protection and endorsed by appropriate levels of funding.

2. The Department of Education and Science should more actively promote the Youth Encounter Projects as viable alternatives to the formal national school sector for those children and youth who have difficulty coping with the formal system of education.

3. The Department of Education and Science should cease the practice of providing what it, essentially, "negative double access." As noted in this study, many of the youth attending St. Augustine's Special School have been tempted to leave the project when they reach the age of fifteen and move to the Youthreach project in the city where they receive payment whilst attending various classes. One of the interviewees stated that she "left the school, went to Youthreach and then went back to the school even though I could have got money." This clearly illustrates the dilemma facing pupils who, on the one hand, want money, but on the other realise the security the project offers.

4. As the Consortium on School-Based Promotion of Social Competence (1996) confirms, intervention programmes must translate processes and mechanisms that promote resilience into "on-going, enduring service delivery systems" (p. 306). Programme design must incorporate needs assessments that not only evaluate risk, but also identify existing and potential protective sources such as found in a resiliency perspective. Self-esteem has been marked out as, perhaps, the single area that most leads to poor academic achievement (personal communication, John Hanna, 2006).

5. Interventions must be designed that illustrate a clear knowledge of the micro culture of the pupils attending Special Schools. Neither the project nor the pupils and their families exist in a vacuum. Structures must be further investigated.

6. Programme designs must incorporate developmental processes that accept each individual child and youth who arrives at the school with differing levels of maturity and that some pupils receive more nurturing at home that others do.

7. More imaginative employment strategies must be developed that locate employment in areas that are accessible to at risk young adults. It is clear from this study that very few of the pupils and ex-pupils have aspirations around locating formal work as dominant society understands it to be (i.e., working and paying full taxes to the government)–at least when they come into the project.

8. It is obvious from the interviews in this study that the family of origin is seen as central to the research participants' lives and is the primary source of identity. Therefore, every effort must be made to maintain the integrity of these families. One way of achieving this is by engaging in professional direct work with the families in their own environments, at times and in ways that suit them. There is a reluctance currently to change social services from the more traditional work time frames.

9. Many of the parents of the research participants in this study themselves were brought up in chaotic family environments, and it is extremely difficult to break the cycle of disadvantage. This is a point noted in the international literature. Policies that attempt to address parenting programmes must take cognisance of this and target improving positive self-esteem by including the parents and care providers of the participants in as many stages as possible. Efforts could concentrate on the provision of practical help that meets immediate physical needs and then move on to the emotional and psychological needs of parents.

10. Therapeutic strategies will need to be fundamentally re-evaluated. The interview data suggests that the research participants were unaware of where and how to go about obtaining therapeutic help in the first instance. The current focus of providing therapeutic assistance to children when they are in trouble with various authorities, as opposed to when they are at risk, is not seen to be cost effective in the Irish context, nor does it work in the long run. The provision of preventative therapy to at-risk children and youth must be prioritised. This therapeutic engagement should explore aspects of risk and resiliency from a number of perspectives and concentrate on enabling the child to identify protective factors and then be self-aware enough to use these.

11. The public health approach to children at risk remains under-developed. This is obvious in that statutory and voluntary services have yet to coordinate their efforts. Bates (1996) advocates the use of multi-systemic therapy which identifies and counter-acts risk factors whilst reinforcing the protective factors. This is, in effect, the resiliency approach.

12. The majority of the interviewees in this study have encountered alcohol and drug abuse both in the context of their families and peers and through personal experience. Indeed, "drugs" was the single most common response when the pupils were asked to talk about risky behaviour (although not always in relation to themselves). An environment where children do not feel threat-ened by their peers to ask questions about such matters is to be welcomed. It may be *"the way of an area"* (Siobhan), but this does not mean that individuals are predestined to become individual casualties. We could provide both day and residential facilities that are genuinely client-centred by embracing therapeutic approaches that take each psychological and social profile into account. In terms of legislative initiatives, it is clear when re-searching child protection and welfare issues that any form of consensus breaks down when *specific* strategies for children and adolescents at risk are placed into the public realm for discus-sion. Children's rights, parent's rights, the law courts rights, practitioner's rights, the State's rights and society's rights all compete for attention.

13. Although, the 1990s saw policy priority increasingly directed at children at risk, services for children and adolescents in Ireland exist in a state of ambiguity operating within a context of resource constraints and increasing demand. Services for youth at risk are consistently described as reactionary rather than proactive. There is an obvious need to initiate the collection of data in relation to child and adolescent mental health issues as there is little at the na-tional level and wide variance in the degree and depth of informa-tion available from the various health boards at present.

14. The experience in the UK over the past number of years has been an increased willingness of aggrieved young people to sue social services, health boards, and health districts for failure to provide adequate prevention and intervention services. A fear has been ex-pressed by a leading UK based academic that this may quickly be-come the situation in Ireland (Barrett, 1998). Children considered

to be potentially at risk must be actively sought out by child welfare services.

15. An emphasis on youth in residential care who are habitual runaways could be explored in greater depth as this category can easily disappear out of sight of social services. The infamous Fred and Rosemary West case in the UK illustrated this point clearly, as a number of the murdered victims had no one rigorously looking for them and so were not missed. Therefore, social policy needs to address who might go missing and who follows missing children up until the children are located.

16. Policy analysts could usefully address risk and intervention and prevention factors at multiple levels of the child's ecology. The personal and social characteristics of the students *and* teachers, the social and academic structure and status of the school environment, the community contexts within which these students live and socialise, and the inter-relationships between and among these variables all combine to predict an outcome or risk *and* resiliency probability indices for the children of this study.

17. A more comprehensive and integrated schools' psychological service must be developed. Limerick is particularly badly provided for in this context. Defining, targeting, and working with children at risk necessitates a more wide-ranging evaluative, imaginative, and clinical approach from educationalists than has been the case thus far. The Departments of Health and Children, Education and Science, Justice, Equality and Law Reform and Social Welfare should liaise better in this regard. Costs–both human and financial–could be alleviated by prevention-orientated psychological services (that embraces resiliency as a concept) drawing on their related professional disciplines.

18. The establishment of a dedicated research unit attached to the Department of Justice, Equality and Law Reform or the Department of Health and Children would be welcome.

19. More appropriate questions around risk management (as opposed to a concentration on danger) issues must be asked by the entire range of professionals dealing with marginalised and at risk children.

20. The potential success of the Youth Encounter Projects, however we measure this, depends on ensuring a continued sense of ownership and emotional involvement n decisions relating to intervention design and implementation.

SOME FINAL IMPLICATIONS FOR THEORISING RISK

What an age in which we live. A single fibre optic strand can transmit the entire Encyclopaedia Britannica in just three seconds, computer memory is doubling every eighteen months and Americans have more shopping malls than high schools. Agricultural processes in the USA use 2.3 billion pounds of pesticides and 20 million tons of anhydrous ammonia each year, and about 80% of the 70,000 chemicals currently in use have yet to be studied for their toxic effects to humans. (Coates, 2003, pp. 161-163)

Beck argues that modern society is one where the creation of wealth has been superseded by the production of risks and where the laboratory of society has no one in charge. Almost inevitably, the already poor and people of color continue to experience poverty. Beck wants us to consider how we might try to attempt to calculate risks when we do not even know what these risks are, from where they might come, and when they might come. Ironically, this invites potential new directions for both policy and action (Coates, 2003). Giddens, however, suggests that the risk society is really one preoccupied with the future. Science needs to no longer claim to be entirely neutral but, instead, admit its political nature. In the midst of all this, many child and youth care intervention focus on the "here and now."

What marks out the many narratives of risk experiences while living in Limerick, at least, is there sheer quantity over time. The interview data clearly illustrates the perception that risks are still not democratised but are unevenly spread according to various factors of social class, gender, age, address, and educational opportunity. None of the interviewees have attempted to locate solutions to their problems in Beck's (1992) "community among 'Earth, plant, animal and human being' in a solidarity of living things" (p. 74). Beck's contention that societal cleavages are increasingly coming to be defined by the distribution of technological risks is not the experience of those youth attending the Youth Encounter Projects.

Despite the significant developments in risk discourse and risk management, what is clear from this study is that no one model can accurately and succinctly capture the nature of risk in human decision making. The way children and young people perceive risk is conditioned by many internal and external factors and is highly individualised. Ambiguous probabilities, context and framing effects, and regret play important roles in decision-making (Neumann & Politser, 1992). A number of theories such as trait theory, which recognises the joint situation and personality characteristics in generally determining behaviour, hold currency with social and behavioural scientists, and yet few theories present coherent explanatory data for individual differences (Zuckerman, 1979, 1983). Each individual behaviour has its own inherent set of dynamics that either encourages or disencourages risk-taking behaviour.

CONCLUDING COMMENTARY

> To be reclaimed is to be restored to value, to experience attachment, achievement, autonomy and altruism–the four well-springs of courage.

> –Anonymous

Lupton and Tulloch (2001) critique Beck's risk society account stating that it is reductionist in ignoring the risk histories carried in personal memory. In their Australian study of risk narratives they found that people's response to risk is multi-layered and thus concurred with Lash and Wynne on this point. At least it is now accepted that schools have much to offer. The lack of involvement, then, by the pupils of projects such as St. Augustine's should not be surprising as this "is consistent with modernity's emphasis on dualism, dominance, and hierarchy" (Coates, 2003, p. 138).

Social competence promotion interventions assist in the development of pro-social skills. The focus of St. Augustine's on psychosocial and emotional development of the youth is validated in this study. As intervention programmes can either seek a reduction or an increase in behaviours, it can be difficult to examine their outcomes. The idea that "people are in control of their own destiny" regularly comes up in conversation, but this study has illustrated that it is not quite that simple. Risk assessment in social policy acknowledges that risk behaviours can be deterred, reformed, or even changed fundamentally or, put somewhat differently, they can be managed and/or changed. A comment from one of the pupils of the school sums up neatly the predicament of attempting to survive in a society where *"life just gets in the way."*

On completion of this book, it seems fair to suggest that my research participants understand risk as a multidimensional concept but one that *excludes* what might be termed global risk (Beck, 1992). As a whole, their understanding links risk more to the concept of loss than opportunity

(Douglas, 1992; Yates, 1990). This is clear from both their risk behaviours and expressed worldviews around fatalism. Although the teachers and staff in the school perceive much of the pupils' behaviour as risky in terms of their general discourse, this is not necessarily the way the interviewees understand their behaviour(s). In other words, a percentage of their risk behaviour(s) could be labelled as *nondeliberative* as opposed to *deliberative* (Yates, 1992) and, often, the interviewees actively engage in risk avoidance behaviours such as staying away from a particular public house or nightclub in the city, avoiding fights involving weapons, and not taking drugs. In making such choices, the interviewees exhibit strong resiliency traits. The Director of the project has been visionary and informal in his approach, and I have been fortunate to witness how such an approach can promote and foster resilience.

Although it could be argued that the research participants do not think out their risk behaviour in the manner traditionally ascribed to them by social scientists, the majority do attempt to make sense of risk in their own ways. Simply stated, risk is not something that is ignored completely. At risk children and youth may reject the traditional choice between two polarised risk choices–opportunity and danger–and elect, instead, to choose a third option. This option could be termed a *risk compromise*.

We must now move away from models of at risk to ones which embrace "high promise" children and youth. We must focus on strengths instead of weaknesses and abilities instead of limitations. I have deliberately utilised the term "at risk" throughout this book, but I want to conclude by focussing on the term "high promise" as this more accurately describes the individual journey each child and young person embarks on. My overwhelming experience in this piece of research has been that it is structures and institutions rather than the individual pathologies of children and youth that create and sustain the average "at-risk" profile.

I have learned that some children and young people can successfully navigate through life's increasingly tough obstacle course, whilst others find it much more difficult. As with any obstacle course, the amount of hints along the way, markers set down by instructors, and amount and complexity of obstacles will largely determine if it can be completed. At the end of the day, the youth in this study end up "walking the roads of Limerick" because they feel there is little else to do. We should be ashamed about that.

POSTSCRIPT

April, 2005, saw Susan, my wife, invited to the retirement party of John Hanna, the Director of the Limerick Youth Encounter Project since 1977. The party took place in a new hotel in Limerick City, which is fitting as it acknowledges the direction the project will take with the incoming Director. The room was full of people connected to the project, people from education, from government departments, from social services. There were family members of ex-pupils and, at one table, a group of ex-pupils themselves. They had come to honour John and the project.

Susan and I ended up sitting with them animatedly talking about the old days when we were all much younger and life was not about mortgages and babies! One of my former interviewees is now a young man of twenty-seven and works in the project. How wonderful is that! He can act as a positive peer and give so much in terms of his life experiences. Another one of my interviewees now has his own courier business. A third remains unemployed but is hopeful of the future. This futurist approach is crucial because it clearly illustrates the move from loss to potential gain. And, a fourth still enjoys Mario Lanza music but he has moved from vinyl to mp3 status.

We all share a few drinks and jokes and it feels good. On this evening, we all felt reclaimed.

NOTES

1. In terms of social policy, the family, the community, and the individual child must be accessed and resourced for any long-term benefits to accrue.

2. The pupils who would have been in this school were being catered for at a new project, which has been established in Henrietta Street and in some mainstream schools.

3. Of course, associated with poverty and scarce social resources is risk and the more exclusion, the more difficult it is to be resilient. The strength is sapped under sustained or acute adversity.

4. What is termed a pass Leaving Certificate is considered to be five passes out of the subjects taken but, more recently, this distinction is no longer made. In practice, a student must achieve at least five passes for entry into third level and for many jobs.

REFERENCES

Achenbach, T. (1990). Conceptualisation of developmental psycho-pathology. In M. Lewis & S. Miller (Eds.), *Handbook of developmental psycho-pathology* (pp. 3-14). New York: Plenum.

Bates, B. (1996). *Aspects of childhood deviancy: A study of young offenders in open settings.* Unpublished doctoral dissertation. Dublin: University College Dublin.

Beck, U. (1992). *Risk society. Towards a new modernity.* London: Sage.

Catterall, J. (1986). *School dropouts: Policy prospects.* Charleston: WV. Appalachia Educational Laboratory, Policy and Planning Center.

Clancy, P. (1995). *Access to higher education: A third national survey.* Dublin: Higher Education Authority.

Coates, J. (2003). *Ecology and social work: Towards a new paradigm.* Halifax: Fernwood Press.

Douglas, M. (1992). *Risk and blame: Essays in cultural theory.* London: Routledge.

Dryfoos, J. G. (1998). *Safe passage: Making it through adolescence in a risky society.* New York: Oxford University Press.

Dryfoos, J. (1990). Adolescents at risk: Prevalence and prevention. New York: Oxford University Press.

Egan, O., & Hegarty, M. (1984). *An evaluation of the Youth Encounter Project.* Dublin: Educational Research Centre. St. Patrick's College.

Emery, R., & Forehand, R. (1996). Parental divorce and children's well-being: A focus on resilience. In R. Haggerty, L. Sherrod, N. Garmezy, & M. Rutter (Eds.), *Stress, risk and resilience in children and adolescents: Process, mechanisms and interventions* (pp. 64-69). Cambridge University Press.

Farrington, D., & Welsh, B. (1999). Delinquency prevention using family-based interventions. *Children & Society, 13,* 287-303.

Gore, S., & Eckenrode, J. (1994). Context and process in research on risk and resilience. In R. Haggerty, L. Sherrod, N. Garmezy, & M. Rutter (Eds.), *Stress, risk and resilience in children and adolescents: Process, mechanisms and interventions* (pp. 19-63). Cambridge University Press.

Hamovitch, B. A. (1996). Socialisation without voice: An ideology of hope for at-risk students. *Teachers College Record, 98*(2), 286-306.

Harrel, A. V. et al. (1997). *Impact of the children at risk programme: Comprehensive final report* (Vol. 1). Washington, DC: The Urban Institute.

Keenan, O. (1998). Foreword. In S. Jones (Ed.), *Supporting Ireland's children: An independent evaluation of Barnardo's family support project, Moyross, Limerick.* Dublin: Barnardos.

Lupton, D., & Tulloch, J. (2001). Border crossings: narratives of movement, "home" & risk. *Sociology On Line, 5*(4). socresonline.org.uk/5/4/lupton.html

McCarton, C. M. et al. (1997). Results at age 8 years of early intervention for low-birth weight premature infants: The infant health and development programme. *Journal of the American Medical Association, 277,* 126-132.

MacDonald, K. I., & MacDonald, G. M. (1999). Perceptions of risk. In P. Parsloe (Ed.), *Risk assessment in social care and social work.* London: Jessica Kingsley Publishers.

McKenna, S. (1995). *Walking the roads: The children of St. Augustine's.* Unpublished Thesis: Waterford: Waterford Institute of Technology.

McKeown, K. (2000). *A guide to what works in family support services for vulnerable families.* Dublin: Government Publications Office.

Millner, J. S., Murphy, W. D., Valle, L.A., & Tolliver, R. M. (1998). Assessment issues in child abuse evaluations. In J. R. Lutzker (Ed.), *Handbook of child abuse research and treatment.* New York: Plenum Press.

Murray, C. (1984). *Losing ground: American social policy 1950-1980*. New York: Basic Books.

Rehill, K. (1999). *Young people and crime*. Unpublished Thesis. Waterford: Waterford Institute of Technology.

Report on Reformatory Schools: Kennedy Report. (1970). Dublin: Government Publications.

Schneider, B. (1992). Didactic methods for enhancing children's peer relations: A quantitative review. *Clinical Psychology Review, 12*, 363-382.

Schorr, L., & Schorr, D. (1988). *Within our reach: Breaking the cycle of disadvantage*. New York: Anchor Press, Doubleday.

Strachan, R., & Tallent, C. (1997). Improving judgement and appreciating biases within the risk assessment process. In H. Kemshall & J. Pritchard (Eds.), *Good practice in risk assessment and risk management 2: Protection, rights and responsibilities*. London: Jessica Kingsley Publishers.

Task Force Report on Child Care Services. (1981). Dublin: Government Publications.

Tormey, R. (1999). Disadvantage or disadvantaging. Conceptualising class differences in education as a disease or as a process. *Irish Journal of Applied Social Studies, 2*(1), 27-50.

Tormey, R., & Prendeville, T. (2000). *Making sense of the cacophony: Understanding the different voices on rural educational disadvantage*. Limerick: Centre for Educational Disadvantage Research.

U.S. Department of Commerce. (1997). *America's children at risk report*. CENBR/97-2. Washington: DC.

Werner, E. E. (1990). Protective factors and individual resilience. In M. Kessler & S. E. Goldston (Eds.), *A decade of progress in primary prevention* (pp. 205-234). Hanover: University Press of New England.

West, D. (1974). *The young offender*. London: Penguin.

Whittaker, J. (1997). Intensive family preservation work with high risk families: Critical challenges for research, clinical intervention, and policy. In W. Hellinckz, M. J. Colton, & M. Williams (Eds.), *International perspectives on family support* (pp. 124-139). Areana: Aldershot.

Wolins, M., & Wozner, Y. (1982). *Revitalizing residential settings*. San Francisco, CA: Jossey Bass.

Yates, J. F. (1990). *Judgement and decision-making*. Englewood Cliffs, NJ: Prentice Hall.

Yates, J. F. (1990). *Judgement and decision-making*. Englewood Cliffs, NJ: Prentice Hall.

Yates, J. E. (1992). Epilogue. In J. F. Yates (Ed.), *Risk taking behaviour* (pp. 331-330). New York. Wiley.

Zuckerman, M. (Ed.) (1983). *Biological bases of sensation seeking, impulsivity and anxiety*. Hillsdale, NJ: Erlbaum.

doi:10.1300/J024v29n01_10

Index